BIOETHICAL ISSUES, SOCIOLOGICAL PERSPECTIVES

ADVANCES IN MEDICAL SOCIOLOGY

Series Editor: Barbara Katz Rothman

Recent Volumes:

ADVANCES IN MEDICAL SOCIOLOGY   VOLUME 9

BIOETHICAL ISSUES, SOCIOLOGICAL PERSPECTIVES

EDITED BY

BARBARA KATZ ROTHMAN
City University of New York

ELIZABETH MITCHELL ARMSTRONG
Princeton University

REBECCA TIGER
City University of New York

ELSEVIER
JAI

Amsterdam – Boston – Heidelberg – London – New York – Oxford
Paris – San Diego – San Francisco – Singapore – Sydney – Tokyo

JAI Press is an imprint of Elsevier

JAI Press is an imprint of Elsevier
Linacre House, Jordan Hill, Oxford OX2 8DP, UK
Radarweg 29, PO Box 211, 1000 AE Amsterdam, The Netherlands
525 B Street, Suite 1900, San Diego, CA 92101-4495, USA

First edition 2008

Notice
No responsibility is assumed by the publisher for any injury and/or damage to persons
or property as a matter of products liability, negligence or otherwise, or from any use
or operation of any methods, products, instructions or ideas contained in the material
herein. Because of rapid advances in the medical sciences, in particular, independent
verification of diagnoses and drug dosages should be made

British Library Cataloguing in Publication Data
A catalogue record for this book is available from the British Library

ISBN: 978-0-7623-1438-6
ISSN: 1057-6290 (Series)

For information on all JAI Press publications
visit our website at books.elsevier.com

Printed and bound in the United Kingdom

08 09 10 11 12 10 9 8 7 6 5 4 3 2 1

CONTENTS

LIST OF CONTRIBUTORS

Renee R. Anspach	University of Michigan, Department of Sociology, USA
Rosalyn Benjamin Darling	Department of Sociology, Indiana University of Pennsylvania, USA
Claudia Chaufan	Social Sciences Division, University of California-Santa Cruz, USA
Elizabeth Ettorre	University of Liverpool, School of Sociology and Social Policy, UK
Lynn Gillam	Centre for Health and Society, School of Population Health, University of Melbourne, Australia
Marilys Guillemin	Centre for Health and Society, School of Population Health, University of Melbourne, Australia
Sydney A. Halpern	University of Illinois at Chicago, USA
Svea Luise Herrmann	Department of Political Sciences, University of Hannover, Germany
Barbara Katz Rothman	Department of Sociology, City University of New York, USA
Helen Kohlen	Department of Political Sciences, University of Hannover, Germany
Sabine Könninger	Department of Political Sciences, University of Hannover, Germany
Katharina Mayr	University of Munich, Institut für Soziologie, Germany

Elizabeth Mitchell
Armstrong

Department of Sociology and Woodrow
Wilson School of Public and International
Affairs, Princeton University, USA

Daniel R. Morrison

Department of Sociology,
Vanderbilt University, USA

Ananya Mukherjea

College of Staten Island, CUNY, USA

Armin Nassehi

University of Munich,
Institut für Soziologie, Germany

Erin Rehel

Department of Sociology,
Brandeis University, USA

Irmhild Saake

University of Munich,
Institut für Soziologie, Germany

Sara Shostak

Department of Sociology,
Brandeis University, USA

Janardan Subedi

Department of Sociology,
Miami University, USA

Sree Subedi

Department of Sociology,
Miami University, USA

Mark Tausig

Department of Sociology,
University of Akron, USA

Rebecca Tiger

Department of Sociology,
City University of New York, USA

Duncan Wilson

Centre for the History of Science,
Technology and Medicine,
The University of Manchester, UK

INTRODUCTORY PREFACE

I am a sociologist. It is the way I think, the way I work, and the methods and the theory and the imagination I bring to the world.

But when journalists call to get a 'quotable quote' on some reproductive issue, a surrogacy case or sextuplets, a divorce 'custody' battle over frozen embryos or a celebrity adoption, they want to identify me as a 'bioethicist'.

Now why is that? Partly it is because as sociologists we have not made ourselves darlings of the media. I organized a panel on working with the media at the American Sociological Association one year, and a journalist pointed out that her job was to make things as simple as possible. And then Behrooz Ghamari, a sociologist, said "And our job is to make things complicated." It is true: What sociologists do is complicate the obvious, cast a critical eye on taken-for-granted truths, question assumptions and leave no 'obvious' fact unturned. No wonder the media does not like us.

And perhaps that is why the medical folks are often none too fond of us either. In a culture that wants to deny power, we focus our eyes on power. In America, a country that actively denies class, claiming middle class identity for all, we do a class-based analysis. We look at an occupation that values, first and foremost, doing no harm and measuring the many harms that are done. We look at people who see themselves – and strive to be – helpers of ailing humanity, and often show a very different picture.

And now we are turning our eyes to the field of bioethics itself. It is particularly complicated: The bioethicists, like the medical sociologists, are standing outside of medical practice and research, and offering a critique and an analysis. The topics that were long the province of medical sociology as a subdiscipline have been increasingly taken over by bioethics: the doctor–patient relationship, the concept of the self in illness and the institutional constraints on clinical practice. Whether at that level, or at the more grounded level of 'issues', from care of the dying to creating embryos, the person at the bedside taking notes, *not* in a white coat, is increasingly more likely to be a bioethicist than a medical sociologist. And so, small wonder, we medical sociologists started looking at the bioethicists themselves, taking that occupation as a subject of study, and that discipline as a body of knowledge to be analyzed.

In this volume, the first under my editorship of the *Advances in Medical Sociology* series, Elizabeth Mitchell Armstrong, Rebecca Tiger and I are going beyond this new "Sociology of Bioethics," to refocus the sociological lens on the framing and management of bioethical issues at the micro- and the macro level. We think that looking at bioethics with a sociological imagination is a key way to advance the field of medical sociology. *Bioethical Issues, Sociological Perspectives* looks at what gets counted as 'bioethics' and – equally or maybe even more important – what gets left out of a traditional bioethical analysis that a medical sociological perspective can highlight.

We have organized this volume into four broad areas, and offer detailed introductions and overviews to the articles themselves for each section. But in brief, we begin by "Placing Bioethics Historically." This is a new discipline, which has achieved national and international prominence with startling speed. A particularly American version of bioethics is being distributed around the world, and echoes of that show up throughout this volume.

The second section is perhaps the most traditionally 'sociological', as we offer a series of articles that look at "The Sociology of Working Bioethics: Private Narratives." Just how does bioethics as a discipline and as a practice *work*?

In hospital committees, in the thinking of bedside practitioners, and in clinical settings, bioethics is 'done'. The articles in this section go a long way towards showing just how, and what that has come to mean.

The third section discusses "Macrosociological Perspectives: Bioethics in the Policy Arena." The new bioethics does not show up only at the bedside. Bioethicists and their way of thinking have entered into public policy. As Rebecca Tiger points out in her introduction to this section, issues picked up as 'ethical' have most often focused on individuals and individual decision making. But increasingly, discussions of bioethics inform public policy, and shape public discourse. Bioethics does so by framing issues, by highlighting some things and, as all disciplines do, by turning our eyes and our talk away from others.

The final section of the book makes a start at "Re-imagining Bioethics: Expanding the Borders of Bioethical Inquiry and Action." Most especially, a sociological imagination looks at bioethics and asks questions beyond the level of the individual. It is true that anything can happen to anyone, as I point out when I teach introductory sociology to undergraduates. But there are patterns here; there are larger forces than individuals. Right and wrong, 'ethical questions', are not just individual choices and decisions. The choices available to us, the questions that we ask, are embedded in a political economy. When we sociologists do bioethics, we do not start with the standard bioethical opening, hypothetical cases in which Patient Problem walks into Dr. Goodguy's office and presents an 'ethical dilemma'. For sociologists, there is a context, and that is how we complicate the question.

Running all through these sections are a variety of themes. Clearly, the relationship between the social and the individual is everywhere, in every article in which a sociologist looks at bioethics. Many of these also engage the issue of 'risk', a defining concept of our time. Risk society frames questions of medical practice in particular ways, as many of these articles show, from genetic counseling sessions to the use of circumcision to reduce HIV rates. Interrelated with questions of risk are questions of knowledge: These papers raise fundamental questions about knowledge itself: What constitutes medical knowledge and who is authorized to (re)produce and use it? And that, of course, segues into issues of imperialism more generally: not just occupational imperialism, but that of the nation-state. Several of these articles specifically address the uses of bioethical inquiry and framing on the export of American and European practices to under-resourced countries, and to under-resourced areas within America. Issues of justice inform a sociological perspective, asking us to see the environment(s) in which illness and medicine practices arise.

We also offer these articles as a testimony to sociological method. As sociologists, we bring to bioethics and its areas of study not only our critical voice, but also a methodological stance. Bioethicists themselves have been drawing on ethnography, and sociologists have been producing more and more ethnography of bioethical settings and practice.

This is what sociology brings to bioethics. But bioethics brings much to sociology as well. The use of narrative is an under-used technique of much value in sociology. It is no accident that much of 'autoethnography' focuses on patient narratives. Narrative has been of special interest in medical ethics and medical sociology because the illness experience is inevitably multi-layered, rich and complex. There are much data there to be constructed into a narrative. It is possible too that the inevitable helplessness one feels – as patient or as practitioner – in so much of medical work makes narrative particularly appealing and useful. To narrate is to make sense of, to order, by controlling the telling of events and experiences. By encouraging us to focus on narrative, bioethics advances our work as sociologists.

Beyond this methodological contribution, bioethics as a discipline has brought us back to some of the early work that was central in the development of medical sociology as a field. We can learn from reading the work that bioethicists are doing, as well as from observing them in practice, the value of the rich ethnographies of hospitals and medical settings that were once so central to medical sociology. Health-care institutions are important sites for sociological inquiry, teaching us lessons that go beyond 'medical' sociology.

Amazing things are happening in the world of medical practice: Every day brings more news on 'breakthroughs' and treatment options, new technologies, drugs, practices and therapies. And many of them come with questions – journalists and the rest of society call on sociologists as well as bioethicists to raise those questions for the rest of us. Bioethics provides us an impetus to rediscover and to refresh our vision as sociologists, to exercise our sociological imagination on the issues that have captured the imagination of the world.

Barbara Katz Rothman
Editor

PART I: PLACING BIOETHICS HISTORICALLY

Like all tribes, bioethics has its own origin myths. According to these myths, bioethics emerged in the latter half of the twentieth century when new technologies and scientific developments challenged the norms that had traditionally governed clinical practice. Theologians, philosophers, clergy, judges, lawyers, journalists and ordinary people – the "strangers at the bedside" in David J. Rothman's memorable phrasing – began to take an interest in moral matters that previously had been the realm of physicians alone. Codes of research ethics were formulated in response to the Nazi atrocities; hospital ethics committees were established in sensitivity to the emerging notion of "patients' rights." Bioethics was born.

The three papers by Renée Anspach and Sydney Halpern, Duncan Wilson, and Rosalyn Benjamin Darling in this first section show us in fine-grained detail who these strangers at the bedside were and how they have and have not changed the practice of medicine and biomedical research; they show us the multiple and sometimes contradictory origin points of the enterprise that today we recognize under the rubric "bioethics." Each paper takes the long view of a particular enduring issue in bioethics: the right to die, human tissue research, and decision making in the neonatal intensive care unit (NICU). Precisely because these papers focus on matters that have preoccupied and vexed bioethicists from the very beginning, they constitute an important corrective both to a linear view of the progress of the field and to universalist notions of bioethics. Each paper shows us how time, place and context matter deeply, as well as how things have changed and how they have stayed the same. Moreover, they offer a revisionist perspective on certain key moments in the official history of bioethics. Together they show us "how history can help empirically ground moral concepts as historically and culturally contingent," in the words of Duncan Wilson.

In the second paper, "From *Cruzan* to *Schiavo*: How bioethics entered the 'culture wars'," Renée Anspach and Sydney Halpern use the cases of Nancy

1

Cruzan and Terri Schiavo as a kind of "natural experiment," as they put it. The year that Cruzan's saga ended with the court-sanctioned removal of her feeding tube – 1990 – was the beginning point of the Schiavo story, with her unexplained collapse at home and subsequent lapse into a mental state that was variously diagnosed as a persistent vegetative state, "a minimally conscious state," and, most famously, "not somebody in a persistent vegetative state" by Senate majority leader Bill Frist on the Senate floor in March 2005. While both women became the focal point of national attention and crystallized widespread discussion of end-of-life issues among the general public, the Cruzan and Schiavo cases were in fact framed very differently both by the mass media and by the experts who claimed to speak as bioethicists in each case.

By examining the coverage of the two cases in a single newspaper, Anspach and Halpern are able to show that despite the parallel facts in each case, the two stories were depicted very differently in the mass media. The Cruzan case was at the time and is still today seen as a "right to die" case; indeed, the United States Supreme Court ruling is often regarded as a definitive legal moment in the history of the right-to-die movement in the United States. The Schiavo case, however, was portrayed as a "right to life" case, with Terri Schiavo's parents fighting to keep their daughter alive while her husband Michael Schiavo sought to have her feeding tube removed. Anspach and Halpern, in fact, use these disparate core frames to argue that "the discursive ground had shifted." Most notably, religious conservatives had begun to organize and present themselves as Christian bioethicists, thus implying that bioethics as a field had begun to crystallize into distinct subgroups. Right-to-life advocates – mainly abortion opponents – had been involved in the Cruzan case, mounting a series of small-scale and last-minute protests and vigils outside the Missouri Rehabilitation Center, as well as filing a series of court challenges, all of which were turned down. In contrast, right-to-life advocates acted as an organized, coordinated and influential mass movement in the Schiavo case, ultimately bringing their battle to the Florida governor's office (occupied at the time by Jeb Bush, brother of the President), the Florida legislature, the U.S. Congress, the White House, and the Vatican, all of which denounced the removal of Schiavo's feeding tube as an act akin to murder. These are some very prominent and politically powerful strangers indeed.

Anspach and Halpern note that while the medical facts in the Cruzan and Schiavo cases were virtually identical – both women were in a persistent vegetative state, without higher brain function, able to breathe unaided, but unable to swallow or eat and thus dependent on a feeding tube, with no possibility of recovery – the media depictions in the Cruzan case were "bleak and unequivocal," whereas in the Schiavo case, the media were more apt to present the controversy around her diagnosis, depicting her as "brain damaged," or "incapacitated," or even "clinging to life." Moreover, medical opinion in the Cruzan case was not only uniformly dire, but also the only accepted opinion, whereas in the Schiavo case the media privileged a wide range of opinions and assessments from professionals and laypeople alike. The contrasting frames in the two cases are in large part a consequence of broad social shifts, including the political ascendancy of social conservatives and their alliance with elected leaders, the emergence of a "culture of life" social movement (in opposition to the so-called culture of death manifest in liberal policies around abortion and physician-assisted suicide), and the growing strength and voice of disability rights advocates like "Not Dead Yet." It is no small irony that the social forces that played such a large role in the case of Terri Schiavo had roots in the much less contentious resolution of Nancy Beth Cruzan's destiny. The right-to-life movement that proved so consequential in the Schiavo controversy was itself both invigorated and propelled by what mainstream bioethicists had long regarded as the definitive establishment of the right to die encapsulated in the Cruzan case. Whether setback, backlash, or countervailing force, the Schiavo case, which at first glance may seem utterly uninformed by the Cruzan case, is in fact a direct consequence of the history made by Cruzan.

Like Anspach and Halpern, Duncan Wilson investigates the historical trajectory of a defining issue in bioethics in his chapter, "Whose body (of opinion) is it anyway? Historicizing tissue ownership and examining 'public opinion' in bioethics." Wilson's analysis of public discussions spanning the 1970s and 1980s in the United States and the United Kingdom concerning the use of human tissues in biomedical research will undoubtedly come as a surprise to most American readers, who typically date the beginning of bioethical debates about property rights in human tissues from the famous John Moore vs. the Regents of the University of California case which played out from 1984 to 1990. Wilson asserts that most researchers and commentators have used the Moore case as a starting point for ownership debates and as "evidence of a broad public pre-occupation with ownership in tissue." He goes on to show that neither is correct. Ownership disputes first arose in the decade preceding Moore, during debates about abortion and fetal tissue research. And public opinion polls from this period demonstrate considerable ambiguity – rather than universal repugnance – over the commodification of the human body. Contrary to the prevailing storyline in bioethics, which uses the Moore case to anchor both scientific engagement in tissue debates and a groundswell of public disgust with this scientific appropriation, Wilson argues that Moore is but "one, much-reported, instance in a gradual development of a multifaceted, malleable concept – that garnered no consensus in either scientific or public social worlds." He anchors his analysis in how bioethicists and scientists themselves construct that amorphous social phenomenon, "public opinion." Here the strangers at the bedside – or the lab bench – are the public writ large. But who or what counts as "the public"? Is there a single unitary public, or multiple conflicting publics? And how is the notion of the public deployed by scientists, politicians, bioethicists and other social actors to advance a cause? These questions are at the center of Wilson's analysis.

While the use of human tissue in research accelerated rapidly in the 1970s and 1980s, it certainly did not originate in this period. Wilson argues that for much of the twentieth century, the biomedical acquisition and use of human tissues was "never intentionally hidden from public view." Scientific practice "reflected cultural norms, and the broad conception here was of extant tissue as waste material." He points to the drive to develop the polio vaccine and the quest to find a cure for cancer as examples of public awareness and sanctioning of scientific use of human tissue. Indeed, Wilson notes that the nascent animal rights movement actually lauded the increasing reliance on human tissue as a welcome development. Yet by the late 1960s, "certain human tissues were gradually now being transformed from non-contested waste to the subject of political and press attention, with their use controversial in certain quarters."

In fact, Wilson argues that to the extent that public opinion about scientific uses of human tissues and ownership rights shifted in this period, the shift was driven by the abortion controversy and a growing critique of the scientific research enterprise more broadly. Ownership questions arose not from bioethical engagement, but from a "cultural milieu specific to America in the mid-1970s, from linked debates surrounding regulation of research, abortion and informed consent." In the United States and in Great Britain alike, abortion opponents began to raise red flags about the use of fetal tissue in research, contending that the use of such tissue was "intimately bound with abortion." Yet their concerns found very different audiences in each country. In the United Kingdom, most commentators were themselves scientists and the press portrayed fetal research in a positive, humanitarian light, in distinct contrast to the United States, where outsiders to the biomedical enterprise – theologians like Paul Ramsey – were most vocal and where the pro-life social movement led public protests and pickets, dramatically raising the visibility of the controversy in the public arena. Moreover, in the United States, debates about fetal tissue became tied to a broader set of emerging concerns about the matter of informed consent for human subjects, raised most viscerally in the exposé of the Tuskegee syphilis study. Once the argument shifted to the matter of "who could legitimately consent to experimentation on behalf of the fetus," surgically excised tissue could no longer be regarded as mere waste, a development that not only disturbed many scientists but also betokened "a state of legal and moral confusion," in the words of one. Questions of consent led inexorably to questions of ownership, which in turn led to the questions of compensation that so vividly drove John Moore's claim against the University of California.

As Wilson convincingly shows, the matter of tissue ownership is local, contingent and historical. "Ownership issues were a symptom of questions regarding patient autonomy, abortion, research practice and, later, commerce," he says. "Ownership was a multivalent concept; it always embodied some wider cause or context, such as anti-abortion politics, scientific self-interest, financial inequity, or a means of ensuring public trust." Neither scientists, nor bioethicists, nor the public at large were ever of one mind on this matter. Despite bioethicists' highest aspirations, there is no universal ethical standard for judging how to think about human tissue – whether as waste, or research material, or commodity, or personal property – nor could there be.

In the final paper in this section on placing bioethics historically, Rosalyn Benjamin Darling takes up a matter of perennial interest in bioethics: *Who decides?* Her paper, "The changing context of neonatal decision making: Are the consumerist and disability rights movements having an effect?" examines the intersection of bioethics with two other contemporary social movements and asks what impact these two movements have made on the context and content of decision making in the NICU. As in Anspach and Halpern's and Wilson's accounts, Darling aims to show how the broader social context – the wide world outside the NICU's confining walls – shapes and colors what happens in that rarefied and seemingly isolated social environment. Here "the strangers at the bedside" are not literally present as the protesters were outside the Florida hospice where Terri Schiavo lay dying; rather, they take the form of social catalysts precipitating subtle, but significant, shifts in the consciousness – what Darling calls the predispositions – of the actors in the NICU.

Norms around the medical treatment of infants born prematurely or with birth defects and around parental involvement in the decision-making process have shifted several times over the last 30 years. Numerous sociological accounts have documented many features of this particular social arena that persist regardless of treatment norms: The role of professional dominance and medical control over the situation, the parents' experience of anomie, grief and powerlessness and their subsequent tendency to seek expert advice for relief, contests over what counts as expertise and who might rightly be regarded as a stakeholder in the decision, the tension between technical knowledge and emotional involvement, the diffusion of responsibility that can accompany group decisions, and the stigma attached to disability in American culture. At the core of these accounts have been conflicts over not only who decides, but by what criteria – cost of treatment, quality of life for the child, impact on the family, meaning for society writ large – decisions ought to be made. Since the Baby Doe cases of the early 1980s and subsequent federal legislation, a pro-treatment bias has existed in American NICUs.

Darling points us in the direction of *how* decisions are made, rather than who makes them, arguing that we must understand the interactional process that shapes, constrains and channels the ethics of the decision making. The relevant sociological facts here are, first, the prior socialization of decision makers in a particular sociocultural environment and, second, the nature of the process itself – such as status inequality and information asymmetry between doctors and parents, or structural features of the NICU, for example, the lack of privacy, that may influence attitudes and behaviors. Furthermore, the nature of the interaction itself may dismantle or reinforce existing predisposition attitudes and beliefs on the part of the actors involved. While these sociological parameters may be constant, Darling notes several changes in the social context that inevitably impinge on this interactional process. The first, a compositional change in the newborns who populate the NICU, is a direct consequence of developments in medical technology and knowledge. Due to improvements in prenatal diagnostic imaging and testing, most infants born today with Downs syndrome, spina bifida, or duodenal atresia – the kinds of defects that characterized the Baby Doe case and that are the stuff of classic bioethical reasoning – are diagnosed *before* birth. In other words, parents who in the past might have opted to withhold treatment after birth, now have the opportunity to end the affected pregnancy, eliminating the decisional conflict that might have ensued in the NICU. In consequence, most NICU decisions today are being made in the context of extreme prematurity or unanticipated birth complications. Second, the consumerist movement has shifted the terrain that physicians and parents alike occupy. Third, although we cannot yet document the full extent of this effect, the disability rights movement, with its emphasis on a social model of disability rather than on a medical model, has begun to change how we think about quality-of-life issues in the NICU.

Yet as Darling notes, most of the classic sociological accounts of NICU decision making were written well before the disability rights movement or the consumerist movement had begun to make real inroads into medicine. After laying out some of the ways we might expect these two broad social forces to affect neonatal medicine (noting that, in fact, they may pull in opposite directions), Darling examines a set of recent parental accounts of the NICU in print and on the web. She finds evidence both of consumerism, in the form of greater parental willingness to challenge and defy medical recommendations, and of some evolution in beliefs about disability, such as a greater acceptance of a life with severe limitations as a life worth living. Yet she also notes that consumerism tends in the direction of seeing children as consumer goods, "perfectible commodities," which may be rejected if not up to standards. Moreover, she finds some evidence that class may affect both consumerist orientations and acceptance of disability, with high-SES parents more likely to challenge professional dominance and less likely to embrace a child with disabilities. "As in the past," she concludes, "whether future babies with disabilities will be treated or not will be contingent on the predispositions of the various stakeholders, as well as on the interactions that take place between stakeholders and others, both within and outside of the nursery setting." Although Darling characterizes her own analysis as "exploratory" and ends her chapter with a call for more research, her deeply sociological attention to the social context of decision making in the NICU offers yet another opportunity to examine the historical specificity and contingency of bioethics. The three papers in this section all highlight the shadowy presence of "the public" in bioethics.

All three underscore the importance of both the societal and the interactional contexts in which bioethical issues play out. In sum, Anspach and Halpern, Wilson, and Darling demonstrate the historical specificity of what counts as bioethics at any given moment – more evidence that these issues are not necessarily universal, but historically contingent and culturally bounded.

Elizabeth Mitchell Armstrong
Editor

WHOSE BODY (OF OPINION) IS IT ANYWAY? HISTORICIZING TISSUE OWNERSHIP AND EXAMINING 'PUBLIC OPINION' IN BIOETHICS

Duncan Wilson

ABSTRACT

Debates regarding patient claims to extant tissue samples are often cited as beginning with the infamous US case of John Moore vs. the Regents of the University of California *(1984–1990) – where the plaintiff unsuccessfully tried to claim title in a cell line derived from his excised spleen. Following the 1990 Supreme Court verdict, the issue of patient property in excised tissue was held by certain bioethicists as* the ethical problem inhering in biomedical research from the 1980s onward: *encompassing debates about a newly-avaricious biotechnology, consent, autonomy and identity. I show here that the concept of patient property was first mooted during the 1970s, some 10 years before* Moore, *as a response to US-based criticism of the use of foetal and human tissues in research. Rather than representing a struggle between an avaricious science and misled patients, it evolved as a result of debates between philosophers, lawyers, scientists and members of the public, amidst*

Bioethical Issues, Sociological Perspectives
Advances in Medical Sociology, Volume 9, 9–32
Copyright © 2008 by Elsevier Ltd.
ISSN: 1057-6290/doi:10.1016/S1057-6290(07)09001-8

*broader debates regarding human experimentation and abortion. More-
over, the first person to assert a patient's right to their own, or their
family's tissue, in a legal arena was a scientist. This article attempts to
investigate, through the evolution of ownership debates, how bioethicists
and scientists themselves construct what counts as 'public opinion'.*

INTRODUCTION

Most, if not all, literature on biomedicine's increasing reliance on human
tissue details at length the now infamous US case of *John Moore vs. the
Regents of the University of California.*[1] This dispute, which ran from 1984
to 1990, and was heard in three different levels of the US judicial system,
centred on property rights in a spleen cell line. Plaintiff, John Moore,
sued the research physician who removed his spleen during treatment for
leukemia and turned it into a commercially valuable cell line without
consent, signing lucrative contracts with biotechnology companies. Moore's
case was eventually dismissed in 1990, with the California Supreme Court
ruling that he had no property right in the extant cell line; it rested with
those researchers who could recognize biomedical or commercial value in
diseased tissue and then convert it into a viable tool. The case has been
approached from a number of angles by social scientists. Anthropologists
such as Landecker and Rabinow, for example, analyse it as influenced by,
and an influence to, the shifting value placed on biological objects amidst
contemporary changes in patent laws governing naturally-derived tools
(Landecker, 1999; Rabinow, 1996a). This article rather looks at how *Moore*
was, and continues to be, represented by bioethicists: as both (i) the start of
ownership disputes and (ii) as evidence of a broad public pre-occupation
with ownership in tissue.

A number of examples illustrate this. Andrews and Nelkin's *Body Bazaar*
begins by framing *Moore* as embodiment of the interlinked ethical, legal and
cultural problems that converge under the banner of 'ownership'. Crucially,
these problems are represented as arising from changing patent laws,
technological advancement and the concurrent biotechnology boom that
have together 'enhanced the value of human tissue'. This new commercial
bent to biomedicine has, to these authors, heightened professional
perceptions of human tissue as valuable commodity and its corporeal
sources as 'valuable treasure troves'. Kimbrell similarly argues that in
running up against the 'cultural symbolism' bodies are loaded with – without

fully explaining this cultural value – scientific use of tissue is pushing society toward 'ethical precipices' (Kimbrell, 1997). In such accounts, written for various audiences, Moore's admission that he felt exploited is situated amidst a seeming 'popular repugnance about the commodification of the body' (Gold, 1997; Kimbrell, 1997).[2] Such repugnance is, sometimes, refigured as part of a long-historical public resistance to the use of body parts in science and medicine (Nelkin & Andrews, 1998; Kimbrell, 1997).

I must stress that views on the *ruling* in *Moore* differ; one also finds arguments that deny patient claims to property in excised tissue (Erin, 1994; Harris, 1998). I do not wish to engage in a discussion of the relative right and wrong of the *Moore* decision here; it is my contention that the common representation of the case in ethical analyses is misleading on two grounds. In the first half of this article I show how ownership disputes first arose in US during the 1970s, amidst broader scientific, ethical, political and public debates about abortion and human experimentation – not in the 1980s, 'outside' science in patients and ethics. Indeed, I show that the first person to legally assert patient or familial ownership was a *scientist*. In the second half, I challenge the bioethical construction of broad popular support for ownership and repugnance at tissue research, using public polls conducted after *Moore* that point to a distinct popular ambiguity.

Axiomatic to much of history of science and its relation to a broader 'public' is that both are interdependent, mutually constitutive components of a particular culture, consistently interacting and exchanging rhetoric and imagery relating to research and research materials (Sturdy, 2000; Durbach, 2005). Histories of tissue research embody this, showing how practical usage of human tissue is historically and culturally contingent – and how biomedical practice is hence reflective of, not opposed to, cultural values (Lawrence, 1998; Landecker, 2000). Such work offers a challenge to representations of *Moore* that portray scientific and public views of tissue as dichotomous. By showing how ownership debates were a collaborative product of the 1970s, we can refigure *Moore* not as the beginning of a divisive issue, but as one, much-reported, instance in a gradual development of a multifaceted, malleable concept – that garnered no consensus in either scientific or public social worlds. I conclude by engaging with other literature that argues for a better appreciation of how history can help empirically ground moral concepts as historically and culturally contingent, within the lived experience and moral economy of the complex 'public' bioethics purports to represent (Belkin, 2004; Hedgecoe, 2004; Rosenberg, 1999).

FROM WASTE TO CONTESTED OBJECT: THE SHIFTING STATUS OF HUMAN MATERIAL IN THE TWENTIETH CENTURY

Analysts of biomedicine during the 1980s were in no doubt that development of new technologies and commercial incentives had directly increased research use of human tissue.[3] History, though, shows this to be an upturn in a long-standing trend; the late-nineteenth and early-twentieth century success of experimental, biological techniques had long fostered a demand for bodily materials that existed as work-objects (Clark, 1987). Aside from live experimental animals, this included human tissue, in various guises. Most coverage has thus far been devoted to embryologists, who set up networks to ensure a ready supply of foetal material – but a subset of work also examines how human tissue was now also used for new pathology techniques, how human glands were extracted for endocrinology and how various tissues were implanted and grown in vitro as tissue cultures, which functioned across a spectrum of work.[4]

Important here is the fact that such acquisition and research was never intentionally hidden from public view: then, as now, scientists in emergent fields depended on popular, as well as professional, support (Wilson, 2005). Secondary literature on these uses of human tissue, and analysis of contemporary press coverage, highlights a lack of evident distaste at this rising use of human tissues – which rather undermines the arguments for a long-standing popular repugnance. Human tissue, as Lawrence argues, could be readily obtained, exchanged and researched upon without any formal regulation because the public did not see this as problematic (Lawrence, 1998, p. 127). Scientific practice here reflected cultural norms, and the broad conception here was of extant tissue as waste material (Morgan, 2002). Only when worked upon by scientists, transformed into a tool or therapy, did the professional or public sphere conceive of potential in tissue. This was embodied in post-Second World War developments, dependent on raw human material. Endeavours such as the new polio vaccine and the widely-reported drive to 'conquer cancer' attracted popular support; practitioners in both fields counted on this enthusiasm and never made any effort to hide their reliance on human tissue (Gregory & Miller, 1998).[5]

This much is evident when we survey public representations of human tissue research in Britain during the 1970s, where scientists continued to court public attention. For instance, Robert Edwards and Patrick Steptoe, pioneers of in vitro fertilization, often pointed to the human origins of the embryos in culture, to play up the clinical potential of work that was criticized by the media for its seeming irrelevance and menace (Turney, 1998). The clinical relevance of human tissue was similarly stressed by emergent animal rights charities, which pointed to its use in vaccine development and research on the harmful effects of smoking in order to further their calls for the abolition of vivisection (Hegarty, 1995).[6] Like the claims of Edwards and Steptoe, these arguments were made in popular media and continued to find a large audience. Yet, by this point, the cultural milieu in which these representations were made, and the scientific motives behind them, had changed considerably. Certain human tissues were gradually now being transformed from non-contested waste to the subject of political and press attention, with their use controversial in certain quarters. This transformation betokened two, interlinked cultural factors from the 1960s that would influence questions of ownership: controversy over abortion reforms, and a growing criticism of scientific research.

Concurrent with growing scepticism toward traditional seats of authority, science by the late-1960s had become heavily criticized in popular coverage; due to evident strides made in areas such as genetics and in vitro fertilization, and its seemingly revolutionary potential, biology was often represented as possessing particular menace (Sandbrook, 2006).[7] Criticism of research in the press, on television or in popular works such as Roszak's *The Making of a Counter-Culture* and Rattray Taylor's *Biological Time-Bomb*, was seized upon to advance certain political agendas – not least by opponents of recent British and mooted American abortion reforms, who alleged that research on foetal tissue was dependent on, and encouraged acceptance of, abortion. Such rhetoric was also dependent on well-documented new ways of representing the foetus within biomedicine, contingent in the incorporation of ultrasound technologies and development of in utero surgical techniques (Casper, 1998; Petchesky, 1987). Though the vested goals behind respective representations clearly differed, the construction of foetuses as subjects, rather than mere objects, arose in concert from science, pro-life camps and the media.

In May 1970, in Britain, Conservative MP Norman St John Stevas alleged that the 1967 Abortion Act, which had greatly increased the number of abortions and, hence, the amount of foetal tissue for researchers, was underpinning an illegal black-market in live foetuses and foetal tissues (Stanhope, 1970; Anon, 1970a). Stevas's allegations were essentially criticisms of what he saw as the morally reprehensible consequences of abortion reforms, though the immediate press focus was on foetal-dependent research. Within a day of the initial claim, the government had ordered an enquiry into such work, headed by obstetrician John Peel.

While Stevas's allegations were certainly afforded ample media attention, it is notable that the press portrayed foetal research in an overtly positive light. Within days of the initial claim, newspapers reported the beneficial aspects of even the most extreme practice of keeping foetuses alive outside the womb, which it was reported would aid future treatment of premature babies (Anon, 1970b). Highlighting the humanitarian aspects of research on extant foetal tissues was even easier. Tabloid paper the *Daily Express* noted how 'alleged use of living foetuses' might well make some uneasy, but added that 'the use of foetal *tissue* for research purposes is, however, essential and causes no concern'.[8] The report was quick to point to foetal tissue's role in development of vaccines against polio, rubella and, possibly, rabies. Similarly, the eventual report of the governmental Peel enquiry, issued in 1972, listed benefits derived from foetal tissue research, and noted that use of foetal parts was often unavoidable; viruses for vaccines would often not grow in animal hosts, which was a far more publicly controversial practice than the use of foetal tissue anyway.[9] Like the press, the report concluded that the use of foetal tissue should continue as before. Noting that the best source of tissue for research was from abortions – miscarried or spontaneously aborted foetuses having decayed in utero – it also refuted the question of whether kin should consent to use of parts in biomedicine. Initial consent to the abortion, the report claimed, constituted abandonment of the foetus and there was hence 'no statutory requirement to obtain consent for research'.[10] As before, such tissue was waste and could be used in research. All this betokens the rather marginal status of the British anti-abortion lobby in the early-1970s; poorly organized before the 1967 Abortion Act, they did not yet possess enough influence in governmental circles and public life to significantly influence scientific practice (Yoxen, 1990, p. 37; Pfeffer, 2000).

Things in US were markedly different though. Inescapable, for one, was the fact that US pro-life lobbies were well-funded, mobilized and politically supported, even before the abortion reform that followed *Roe vs. Wade* in 1973 (Risen & Thomas, 1998). Crucially, abortion was further problematized in the public sphere by those individuals, external to biomedicine, who were now commenting on 'ethical' issues in research and clinical care. In UK, by contrast, public spokesmen on research practice still tended to be scientists themselves – often defining themselves as 'socially responsible', but acting in the best interests of their profession. American commentators, not yet collectively known as 'bioethicists', were not encumbered by issues of self-interest, and brought their own professional backgrounds to bear on the issues of abortion, and foetal experimentation, that were a collective early focus.[11]

One avid critic of foetal experimentation was Princeton theologian Paul Ramsey, who deliberately included foetal experimentation amongst the emergent discourse surrounding patient rights. This standpoint consistently granted the foetus the same rights as dying or comatose individuals; a logical extension, since, to Ramsey, the foetus was a person (Ramsey, 1975).[12] His portrayal of foetal research as 'unethical medical experimentation on possible human beings' was often replicated in the public domain, and co-opted by anti-abortionists. Unsurprisingly, then, research on tissues became far more contested in US than it did in Britain. Writing shortly after *Roe*, in 1974, Ramsey himself detailed how an increasingly acrimonious public, political, medical and legal debate was marked by claims that 'research on foetal tissue is as outrageous as research on the whole foetal being' (Ramsey, 1975, p. 67).

Ramsey noted that such claims arose from the pro-life camp – a number of whom were now, as scientists noted with horror, turning the issue of foetal *tissue* research into a 'powerful emotional weapon' in the anti-abortion cause (Chedd, 1974; Hart, 1975). Use of foetal material was explicitly targeted after *Roe* because certain campaigners claimed, as had Stevas, that research on aborted tissue was intimately bound with abortion. In US, such claims found a receptive audience. An increasingly active post-*Roe* campaign subsequently saw pickets against the NIH headquarters in Bethesda, Maryland and Philadelphia's Wistar Institute, for their collective use of foetal tissue (Hart, 1975, p. 76; Nardone, 2005).

The Wistar protests centred on a long-established foetal culture – also to be the subject of the first legal ownership dispute, illustrating how scientific objects and their trajectories are intractably tied to, and affected by, wider cultural contexts. This culture, strain WI-38, was derived in 1962, using tissue imported from Sweden to circumvent stringent US abortion laws that obstructed the supply of foetal materials. The individual who cultured the sample, Leonard Hayflick, and his Wistar patron, Hillary Koprowski, were at the time publicly endorsing the use of foetal tissue in polio vaccine production, selling foetal tissues as safe alternatives to monkey tissue, which some believed harboured viruses that could cross species barriers through vaccines (Koprowski, 1961).[13] Given this prior profile, and that use of WI-38 was often reported in the professional journals now scoured by pro-life campaigners, it is little wonder that the culture became embroiled in abortion politics. This was evinced in a pro-life protest at the launch site of the widely-hyped Skylab III satellite mission in November 1973, centring on the fact the capsule carried a specially-made closed laboratory for WI-38, for an experiment to see how space orbit affected cellular growth (Montgomery et al., 1978). Though this experiment was not reported in the national press, it is likely protestors heard of it from local newspapers that proudly reported the development of this special 'Woodlawn Wanderer' laboratory at the University of Texas, Dallas (Hayflick, 2005). Concerned NASA officials telephoned Hayflick, now at Stanford, seeking reassurance that the tissue in question had not come from a recent US abortion (Hayflick, 2004).

This unease mirrored that of the scientific community in general, which also faced public censure from the recent exposées of the Tuskegee Syphilis Study and injection of cultured tumours into terminally ill patients, as well as sizeable cuts in federal funding.[14] Its counter to existing pro-life protest, namely that research on foetal tissue was a humanitarian endeavour, was dealt repeated blows through 1974. Firstly, pro-lifers successfully indicted researchers in Boston, charging them under an 1814 grave-robbing statute for taking tissues from aborted foetuses without parental consent; secondly, congress now included foetal research in ongoing investigation of human experimentation ethics. Though certain pro-life senators urged a ban on *all* research that 'profited' from abortion, a temporary moratorium was issued on all experimentation on 'living' foetuses.[15] Prior to the moratorium, *Science* noted that pro-life campaigns had already forced many to abandon foetal-based research; after federal intervention even more refused to use foetal tissue, fearful of penalties for using in vitro material that exhibited some form of 'life' (Hart, 1975, p. 80).

THE DEVELOPMENT OF OWNERSHIP QUESTIONS

The level of biomedical unease spurred by criticism of foetal research can be evinced not only from fraught exchanges in the pages of journals, but also in practitioners' eagerness to collectively meet and discuss solutions to recent controversy. These symposia brought together scientists, lawyers, philosophers and, sometimes, non-academic members of the public, reflecting growing claims that regulation of biomedicine should no longer be left to its practitioners. While these meetings had a broad remit, often discussing human experiments, or recent advances in genetic engineering, the sensitive nature of foetal research ensured that it was a common topic. This is not to say, of course, that concerns were rigid: by now, issues in foetal research were intractable from those of research practice, and both dovetailed with newer concerns surrounding genetic engineering and eugenics.

Though not as prevalent as it would be in the 1980s, the issue of commerce and trade in foetal tissues did occasionally arise – as it had in UK during 1970. In a National Academy of Science meeting on 'Experiments and Research with Humans' one lay contributor argued that a women who had an abortion should be given the property rights in the foetus, allowing her to sell it to the commercial companies he rather erroneously believed were exploiting foetal tissue. This claim confronted 'the very important ingredient of our society – private property', presented by this individual as an important issue with regard to biomedical research that 'physicians and theologians are not prepared to grasp'.[16]

But a number of lawyers, philosophers and scientists were grappling with ownership. Questions arose from wider discussions about patient or research subject autonomy, in line with the increasing bioethical emphasis on patient *choice*, and did not generally concern marginal issues of profit from research. The fact that consent was encroaching into discussion of tissue research is a mark of how ubiquitous it was becoming in analyses of research practice. This first arose from the volatile arena of foetal research; questions concerning who could legitimately consent to experimentation on behalf of the foetus mirrored similar questions regarding the comatose, children, the mentally ill, and the ill-informed (Morrison & Twiss, 1973; Ramsey, 1975, pp. 95–96). When the moratorium was lifted in August 1975, NIH recommendations stipulated that parental consent should be sought before research on aborted material could begin; this was soon extended to use of *any* surgically-derived body tissue (Holder & Levine, 1976). Here, as elsewhere, consent functioned within and without biomedicine – tightening research practice, but also recognizing the importance of safeguarding public trust. 'Requiring informed consent for the use of tissue', one lawyer told a gathering of tissue culture researchers in 1976, 'not only removes the taint of impropriety stemming from non-disclosure, but also gives a person an opportunity to express his/her desires and provides for the values, privacy and self-determination' (Winslade, 1977).[17]

Granting a patient the opportunity to express self-determination when it came to the fate of their excised tissue was not wholly endorsed by the scientific community. Certainly, tissue in US could no longer be perceived as waste, and this perturbed many scientists. One noted, in a 1975 conference, how surgeons now refused to pass excised foreskins on to him for fear of having to ask for consent and describe any ensuing research project, while *Clinical Research* derided consent for tissue as a prime example of the increasing 'trivialization of medical ethics' (Holder & Levine, 1976).[18] Later exposure of non-consented research on tissue, not least in *Moore*, certainly raises questions of how well the NIH directives were enforced and why they were ignored. Certainly, some researchers saw consent for tissue as an unnecessary administrative burden (Holder & Levine, 1976). Important here is that it was also viewed by some as tacit endorsement of property rights. Scientists in symposia exhibited unease at the prospect of patients, or the parents of an abortus, claiming title to tissue – envisaging a falling supply when many withheld consent, or the establishment of a costly payment system to placate them. One Tissue Culture Association member stated that 'it is quite unclear who has rights in cut hair, nail clippings and cells taken from the body', adding that he believed such questions represented a general, '*state of legal and moral confusion*'.[19]

In this case, we see evidence of ownership questions arising from a cultural milieu specific to mid-1970s America, from linked debates surrounding regulation of research, abortion and informed consent. Notably, however, by no means all scientists rejected the notions of consent and ownership in tissue; the quote above is less a rejection of patient property and more a plea for clarification. Generally, though, lawyers and philosophers did little to calm scientific anxiety. Many claimed a shift to patient ownership was inevitable, due to the bioethical and regulatory emphasis now placed on individual autonomy, and also the fact that sources were already remunerated for blood and sperm, which too hinted at ownership rights (Winslade, 1977, pp. 716–717). Others argued that further developments in research would only heighten existing questions. 'Perhaps the strongest justification for considering legal control of body materials', a legal piece stated, 'is the need to take account of new developments in biomedical and medical technology' (Dickens, 1977).

Indeed, by the late-1970s, the relative merits of scientific, federal and patient ownership were receiving legal hearing – but this centred on a long-established, rather than an emergent, biomedical tool.

OWNERSHIP IN COURT AND IN THE PRESS: WI-38

Given the origins of ownership debates in abortion politics, it is apposite that the first legal wrangle over tissue should involve WI-38. The case in question centred on the actions of Leonard Hayflick who, on leaving Wistar for a position at Stanford in 1973, took the majority of WI-38 stocks with him, and established a personal company, Cell Associates Inc., to distribute them. Before applying for a job at a NIH institute for aging research in 1975, Hayflick asked the NIH for clarification on the ownership status of WI-38. After auditing Cell Associates, the NIH leaked a damning report to the press, claiming Hayflick had made over $67,000 by selling *federal property*. NIH officials immediately confiscated all stocks of WI-38, and Hayflick resigned from the university. A front-page report in the *New York Times*, clearly influenced by the NIH audit, described WI-38 as 'property of the federal government' – leaving readers in no doubt as to whom it supposedly belonged (Schmeck, 1976).

The NIH claimed that *it* owned WI-38 because the culture was established and maintained with federal money. Hayflick, on the other hand, echoed long-standing scientific conceptions of tissue, and argued that since he transformed raw foetal material into a viable tool, *he* owned it – stating in 1976 that 'I felt, and I am justified in feeling, that these cells are like my children' (Wade, 1976). The dispute went to the courts when the NIH initiated criminal proceedings, only for Hayflick to counter, alleging that they deliberately leaked his name to the press.

This novel custody battle lasted five years, eventually being settled out of court in 1981, with Hayflick being granted his title to WI-38. Hayflick has stated that the NIH's position became untenable after the 1980 *Chakrabarty* case, which allowed researchers to claim ownership and issue patents on biological material (Hayflick, 1998). While this may be so, he and his legal team certainly complicated proceedings by drawing on contemporary notions of patient ownership, arguing that the Swedish parents of the foetus also had a claim. As Hayflick attested:

> We argued, I believe for the first time, that not only did my former institution and I have a legitimate claim to these cells, but a good case could be made for title to be vested in the parents or estate of the embryo from which WI-38 was derived. (Hayflick, 1998, p. 196)

Whatever the personal motive, Hayflick's use of an emergent patient ownership concept here demonstrates that it had currency in, and linked, science and bioethics as much as it divided them.

INTO THE 1980s: REPRESENTING PUBLIC CONCERN

The next assertion of property rights on behalf of family members was again made by a scientist. This instance now evokes the shifting economic contexts that may have proved fortuitous for Hayflick. As Dorothy Nelkin noted in 1984, the new commercial potential in biomedicine was likely to foster disputes regarding tools and products of research (Nelkin, 1984). A number of controversies surrounding human tissue buttressed Nelkin's claim, shifting questions away from the propriety of foetal research, to those of commerce in biomedicine. Scientists had already disputed who should patent a cell line derived from a terminally ill leukemia patient – not, it should be said, considering the patient – when in 1983 Hideaki Hagiwara, a post-doc at University California, San Diego (UCSD), claimed ownership of a monoclonal culture, derived in part from the cells of his mother.[20]

Hagiwara's claim principally arose from the fact that his father ran a research institute in Japan, recognized a commercial potential in the culture, and was keen to wrest it from UCSD. The case was settled fairly promptly, with the university retaining original patent rights and the Hagiwaras awarded rights in Asia. Whatever the outcome, Hagiwara's assertion of *familial* property certainly troubled researchers. His UCSD supervisor made a renewed plea for legal and philosophical clarification of tissue's ownership status, claiming in *Science* that inactivity rendered further claims inevitable. Notably, he held that granting patients or their kin ownership may be a method of maintaining public confidence in biomedicine and should not be dismissed.[21]

The lack of clarification became all too prescient the following year, when John Moore filed suit against UCLA. *Science* presented Moore's claim as an extension of questions that had been circulating since the 1970s, but noted that they were become ever pressing in changing financial contexts. 'The question of person's right to bodily tissues', it noted, 'is one whose time has come in this new era of commercialization' (Culliton, 1984). Again though, when it surveyed professionals for opinions, there was no consensus. Negative representations of ownership claims were certainly prominent: a *Nature* article contained an illustration of an avaricious lawyer interrupting an operation on a 'Mr Doe' in order to secure ownership rights of the patient's tumour – embodying the arguments that such claims were a stifling threat to the humanitarian work of biomedicine (Blake, 1984). On the other hand, one does not have to look far to find counter arguments. The *Science* article cited above, for instance, contained a number of quotes in support of patient ownership, as a way of securing public good-will in the future (Culliton, 1984).

In conferences, as in print, certain scientists argued that *Moore* was nothing more than one patient trying to make a fast buck (Rosenberg, 1985).[22] Others continued to call for clarification, and noted that surgical

consent forms should ask the patient to waive right to future commercial
gain – a move that implicitly acknowledged ownership (Royston, 1985).
There was also no consensus among bioethicists. Though all agreed that
patients should have the right to consent or refuse to use of tissue, the issue
of payment for these samples was contentious. Arthur Caplan, for one,
believed consent was mandatory, stating that 'those whose materials are
to be used have a right to know and consent to such use' (Caplan, 1985,
p. 451). In this respect, the questions raised were homologous to those of
the 1970s. Questions of finance and remuneration were not novel either,
but were encountered now at a greater frequency. Caplan shied away from
remuneration – the most explicit acknowledgment of ownership – though.
He argued that a payment system would simply erode the trust between a
patient and doctor, and would render the poor vulnerable to exploitation
(Caplan, 1985, p. 451).

Lori Andrews disagreed. Arguing that 'people's body parts are their
personal property', she advocated a market in tissue (Andrews, 1986).
A prime factor in Andrews' argument was that 'people have an interest in
what happens to their extracorporeal body parts'. *Moore* served here as
evidence that the public perception of body parts had been transformed by
awareness of their new commercial value, coupled with a sense of injustice
that sources of such material could not share in profits. Yet representing
this public perception was problematic: aside from *Moore* and three
1970s cases relating to hospital disposal of body parts, Andrews relied on
a poll where only 20 per cent of respondents said they would give not body
parts to biomedicine. Could such a proportion really be refigured as
evidence of public concern? Nevertheless, that same year, Thomas Murray
told the *Wall Street Journal* that the greatest threat to such research was
'public confidence in science, and the public's willingness to support science
with ... their tissues and organs'.[23]

There were clearly problems in assessing exactly *what* the public thought.
Were they overwhelmingly opposed, as Andrews alleged? Or was John
Moore simply expressing a minority standpoint, as the poll Andrews cited
seemed to suggest? Immediately after the 1990 refusal of Moore's property
right, a number of articles criticized the Supreme Court decision, on the
basis that it ran counter to predominant popular sentiment. 'Contrary to
assertions that, one removed from the body human tissue becomes waste',
one argued, 'individuals often have genuine concerns regarding how their
tissues will be used' (Perley, 1992, p. 346; Tallerico, 1990). Commerce was
not presented as the sole cause of this concern. It was rather, now, the
perception that tissues bore 'the genetic stamp of the unique individual'

(Perley, 1992, p. 348, ft 72). Public representation of the DNA resident in *all* tissues as central to identity did occur in the 1970s, and had underpinned some unease at cloning, but increases in this portrayal, concomitant with use of genetic information in science, law and the media, was clearly now seen as a major factor (Van Dijck, 1998).

Where certain biomedical journals saw the *Moore* outcome as closure on ownership, others remained uneasy (Curran, 1991). The denial of property was only binding in the state of California; so many believed that future claims were inevitable. The biomedical press in UK certainly followed the case with interest. In Britain, though, questions regarding ownership only surfaced during *Moore*. While the election in 1979 of a 'family-value' oriented Conservative government had put pressure on foetal research, this centred on legislative tightening and not on property in tissue – so questions of patient or family ownership were seen as novel and troubling. *The Lancet* noted that governance of UK tissue research was 'vague', and that practice here may well be exposed as 'neither ethical nor lawful' (Brahams, 1988, 1990). Rather than reject ownership, it too called for investigation.

In light of this, a number of bodies undertook surveys of patient and general public opinion. These are notable for the way they undermine the prior, and future, bioethical construction of a seeming broad resistance to work on human tissue. In 1986 the Fund for Replacement of Animals in Medical Experiments (FRAME) – devoted to promoting human tissue as alternative – issued a questionnaire on its use in research. Amidst those forms returned, 54 per cent of respondents stated they *would* support biomedical research on their tissues (Anon, 1987). In a bid to support and encourage such support, FRAME argued that all UK researchers should seek consent and recognize patient property rights (Gurney & Balls, 1993).

But, again, views on ownership remained muddied. Throughout the 1970s, UK biomedicine continued to police itself; only with Thatcherite commercialization in the 1980s did space open for external policing of research practice (Vincent, 1998). One such review body, the newly-formed Nuffield Council on Bioethics, issued a report in 1995, entitled *Human Tissue*. This argued that cases such as *Moore* were unique – that in 'the general run of things, a person from whom tissue is taken has not the slightest interest in making any claim to it once it is removed' (The Nuffield Council on Bioethics, 1995). *Human Tissue* argued that public ambivalence rendered consent and ownership unnecessary. Though the Council supported the status quo, this was not a case of medicine guarding its own interest; the report was written by a balanced mix of lawyers, biomedical researchers and philosophers.

A 1996 study of patient opinion, printed in the *British Medical Journal*, purported to verify *Human Tissue*'s findings. However, the evidence obtained was again ambiguous. When 384 patients were asked for views on who owned excised tissue, 27 per cent said the hospital, 27 per cent said no-one, 20 per cent said the laboratory it was transferred to, and 10 per cent believed they did (Start et al., 1996). Though supportive of the Nuffield report, this article did note that the 10 per cent of people who believed in patient ownership was a 'considerable minority' (Start et al., 1996, p. 1368).

Any hint of the complex views patients and the general public may have held disappeared in the wake of the scandals which erupted in Britain during 1999, following the exposure of the widespread retention of childrens' organs after post-mortem in numerous UK hospitals.[24] During the protracted media and ethical discussion of this controversy, a seemingly coherent and negative 'public opinion' reared its head. Certain British analysts argued that the public *did* see extant tissues as extension of 'the self', and that introducing systems of consent and ownership was the only way to confront this perception (Mason & Laurie, 2001; Mason, McCall Smith, & Laurie, 2002). Following negative press, researchers held press conferences to try and persuade a seemingly hostile public of the need for tissue research (Boseley, 2002). But another survey of public and professional opinion, commissioned by the UK Medical Research Council and the Wellcome Trust, proved that recent scandals had changed little; views on ownership traversed professional biomedical and public boundaries, and neither social world held consensus (Wellcome Trust and the Medical Research Council, 2000).[25] Public respondents varied in their views on consent, ownership and tissue itself. While some deemed consent an absolute requirement, others saw it as unnecessary, viewing excised tissue as waste.[26] Notably, concern over ownership was restricted to a distinct minority, represented in the report by a sole contributor from Liverpool, where organ retention had been most contentious.[27] Health professionals too continued to hold differing opinions on ownership: though the report did not give exact data, it noted that a majority believed patients should retain control of samples used in research, even after initial consent.[28]

Irrespective of such ambiguity, the need to maintain a seemingly uniform public opinion motivated the UK government to propose a Human Tissue Bill in 2003, which initially mandated that *all* excised tissue must be obtained with consent. Quickly though, resistance from the medical establishment forced an amendment whereby now, as in the rest of Europe, acquisition of post-operative tissue for research is governed by a system of *presumed* consent, with initial consent for surgery sufficient (Hinsliff & Mckie, 2004). The situation in US remains similarly unstable; whereas some institutions allow patients to consent to, or refuse, use of tissue in commercial research, others do not (Josefson, 2000). A National Bioethics Advisory Commission report issued in 2000 revealed professional and patient ambiguity similar to *Public Perceptions* (Wells & Kerr, 2000). There has also been another US legal challenge to scientific ownership, this time involving a group of patients demanding withdrawal, at the behest of their physician, of 'their' samples from a prostate cancer tissue bank. The tensions embodied in this case – and statements about how patients supposedly value their tissue – were reported in the *New York Times* in 2006 (Skloot, 2006).

Ongoing controversy and constantly changing legislature reflects owner-ship's continued currency. Today, it is an increasingly visible concept, resonating in biomedicine, government and in the media: applicable not only to tissue samples but also now to the information that may be gleaned from them, thanks to increasingly refined analytical and sequencing technologies. That the parameters of debate now include such intangible, often encoded, data as well as tangible bodily material is as much testament to increasingly geneticized and informational conceptions of identity as it is to the rate of technological change and the rise in patents (Parry, 2004; Rose, 2001). Given how entrenched both this conception of personhood and biomedicine's reliance on raw human materials are, the difficulty scientists and ethicists have in reconciling the issues I have outlined here are likely to persist for the foreseeable future. But whether or not ownership is a material concern in the day-to-day lives of the patients and research conscripts both seek to represent is another matter.

CONCLUSIONS

In this article, I have historicized questions of ownership in extant tissue. I argue that they first emerged in the 1970s, as part of US debates regarding abortion and research ethics. By highlighting the broad cultural roots of this issue, I have problematized the prevalent bioethical construction of its origins as external to science in the 1980s. Issues that become framed as 'ethical' are clearly not monolithic or divisive. As Clarke and Montini note, social worlds and arenas theory teaches 'that there are not two sides, but rather *N* sides or multiple perspectives' on any given object or concept (Clark & Montini, 1993). As we have seen, ownership was a multivalent concept; it always embodied some wider cause or context, such as anti-abortion politics, scientific self-interest, financial inequity or a means of ensuring public trust. Rather than refer to 'science' and 'public' with regard to ownership, then, it is better to recognize the *diversity* of varied sciences and publics – helping shift analysis, to quote Bauer and Gaskell, from 'science versus public to comparisons among different publics of science' (Bauer & Gaskell, 1999, p. 166; Sturdy, 2000). Conceiving of both 'science' and 'the public' as aggregates of diverse, interacting, bodies cautions against reading too much into particular representations. For bioethicists to do otherwise and frame select cases as evidence of what 'the public thinks' is an approach Bauer laments as a 'deplorable operationalism' – and is one that is increasingly open to criticism by social scientists (Bauer, 2005; Belkin, 2004; Hedgecoe, 2004).

Clearly then, like many other issues pertaining to biomedicine in the mid-1970s, debates regarding ownership did not simply follow from exposure of tissue-based research to a hitherto unaware, homogeneous 'public', as some accounts allege (Kimbrell, 1997; Nelkin & Andrews, 1998). Ownership was, and remains, derived at the intersection of emergent ethical discourse, cultural representation of bodily identity and biomedicine, institutional regulation of biomedicine, and biomedicine itself. Insofar as philosophers and lawyers acted with scientists to formulate consent for and possible ownership in tissue, we see what historians identify as the mediating role of bioethics; it is, to Charles Rosenberg, 'a conglomerate of experts, practices, and ritualized and critical discourse in both academic and public space' that works *with* the biomedical establishment as much as it works against it (Rosenberg, 1999, p. 40). This, then, is a case of an emergent ethical discourse *creating* and *harnessing* problems, not solving them. Ownership issues were a symptom of questions regarding patient autonomy, abortion, research practice and, later, commerce. They were never reactions to a general public sentiment.

Rosenberg states that we need to see ethical concepts as *products*, not goals – as system-specific outcomes of interaction between the microcosm of interlinked issues and the macrocosm of the larger society in which they play out. Situating concepts as historically and culturally contingent constructs helps us better understand their development and their limits (Wolpe, 1998; Rosenberg, 1999, p. 32; Kleinman, 1999). There can be, Rosenberg warns, 'no decontextualized understanding of bioethical dilemmas' (Rosenberg, 1999, p. 41). In this light, it becomes hard to conceive of tissue ownership as a universal standard that transcends local, cultural and historical contexts. Authors who argue for a social and historical reflexivity in bioethics claim that paying heed to this more 'bottom up' approach demonstrates that those whom bioethicists seek to represent often have standpoints at odds to those presented in philosophical and legal tracts (Hedgecoe, 2004, p. 136; Lopez, 2004). Certainly, the evidence from opinion polls I have studied shows that patients surveyed are far more concerned with therapeutic pay-offs from research than they are of retaining ownership over the samples used. Rising public engagement with biomedicine – which some see as a decisive shift in the location and exercise of biopower – generally centres on more material concerns than the overriding emphasis on individual autonomy that grounds bioethical analysis of patient ownership (Rose, 2007; Rabinow and Rose, 2006; Foucault, 1998). As many are now arguing, if bioethics can profit from the social sciences, it is by undertaking this commitment to root ethical ideas in a social reality and, when representing 'public opinion', to acknowledge the complexity and diversity contingent in that reality. As historians have long recognized, consensus is a construct, not a fact.

NOTES

1. See, for selected examples, Waldby & Mitchell, 2006; Weir & Olick, 2004; Wilkinson, 2003; Nelkin & Andrews, 2000; Weir, 1998; Gold, 1997.

2. Nelkin and Andrews' *Body Bazaar* and Kimbrell's *The Body Shop* are written predominantly for popular audiences. Nelkin and Andrews have aimed their arguments at biomedical practitioners, in a 1998 *Lancet* piece.

3. Exactly *what* these techniques were is beyond my scope. See Rabinow, 1996b; Kevles, 1998. The United States Office of Technology Assessment noted a 300 per cent increase in patents derived from human tissue from 1975–79 to 1980–84. See *Ownership of Human Tissue and Cells* (Office of Technology Assessment, Congress of the United States, 1987).

4. On embryology, see Clark, 1987. On pathology, see Wright, 1985. On Endo-crinology, see Pfeffer, 2001. On tissue culture, see Landecker, 2000.

5. As part of the US drive to conquer cancer, George Gey, who developed the human HeLa cell line, publicly presented it as a powerful weapon in the fight against cancer morbidity. See *The Way of All Flesh* (BBC television documentary, screened November 1997).

6. The most visible UK body that campaigned for research on human tissue was the Fund for the Replacement of Animals in Medical Experiments, or FRAME, founded in 1969. FRAME regularly briefed Parliament and the media on alternatives to vivisection.

7. On increasingly negative science coverage in this period, see Gregory & Miller, 1998, p. 44; Turney, 1998.

8. "Unborn Babies: Doctors May Get New Code of Practice" (1970). Emphasis in original.

9. Department of Health and Social Security, Scottish Home and Health Department, Welsh Office, *The Use of Foetuses and Foetal Material for Research: Report of the Advisory Group* (HMSO, 1972).

10. *The Use of Foetuses and Foetal Material* (1972), p. 12.

11. On the cultural, institutional and theoretical origins of US bioethics, see Fox, 1990; Wolpe, 1998; Tina Stevens, 2003.

12. On the early religious bent to bioethics, and its preoccupation with abortion, see Cooter, 2000.

13. Bookchin & Schumacher, 2004 details the endorsement of foetal tissue in popular media.

14. On Tuskegee, see Jones, 1981. On research practice, generally see Lally, Makarushka, & Sullivan, 1979.

15. For pro-research arguments see, amongst many, Enders, 1974; Edwards, 1974. On the Boston legal case, which was eventually dismissed, see Chedd, 1974; Culliton, 1974.

16. Contribution by George Hill, made during National Academy of Science symposium (18–19 November 1975), appears in *Experiments and Research with Humans: Values in Conflict* (National Academy of Science, 1975), p. 86.

17. This edition of *In Vitro* contained the proceedings of a Tissue Culture Association meeting on 'Human Tissues for In Vitro Research', held on 22–23 January 1976.

18. Prof B. D. Davis, responding to Steinberg, 1975.

19. Dr Wasserstrom, responding to Shapo, 1977, p. 628. Emphasis added.

20. On the first case, see Wade, 1980. On the Hagiwara case, see Sun, 1983.

21. Ivor Royston, cited in Sun, 1983.

22. This edition of *Clinical Research* holds the proceedings of an American Federation for Clinical Research symposium on 'The Legal, Ethical and Economic Impact of Patient Material Used for Product Development in the Biomedical Industry', held during May 1985.

23. Thomas Murray, cited in Otten, 1986.

24. This controversy deserves, and will no doubt receive, further historical analysis. For existing discussion see Richardson, 2001; Squier, 2004.

25. For more on this report, see Tutton, 2004.

26. Wellcome Trust and the Medical Research Council, 2000, pp. 22–34.

27. Male respondent, age 22–30, cited in Wellcome Trust and the Medical Research Council, 2000, p. 32.

28. Wellcome Trust and the Medical Research Council, 2000, p. 85. Rather frustratingly, *Public Perceptions* does not provide all respondent's views – nor does it detail their relative frequency in either the professional or patient cohorts. For this reason, I am unable to provide statistical data as I did for the Start et al., 1996 survey.

ACKNOWLEDGMENTS

I owe a great debt of thanks to my colleague Elizabeth Toon, for her great insight and constant advice. The research on which this piece is based was supported by the Wellcome Trust.

REFERENCES

Andrews, L. B. (1986, October). *My body, my property*. Hastings Centre Report, pp. 28–38.
Anon. (1970a, 18 May). *Unborn babies: Now doctors may get new code of ethics*. Daily Express.
Anon. (1970b, 19 May). *Use of live foetus backed*. The Times.
Anon. (1987). Human tissue as alternative in biomedical research. *ATLA, 14*, 375–385.
Bauer, M. W. (2005). Public perceptions and the mass media in the biotechnology controversy. *International Journal of Public Opinion Research, 17*(1), 4–22.
Bauer, M. W., & Gaskell, G. (1999). Toward a paradigm for research on social representations. *Journal for the Theory of Social Behaviour, 29*(2), 163–186.
Belkin, G. S. (2004). Moving beyond bioethics: History and the search for medical humanism. *Perspectives in Biology and Medicine, 47*(3), 372–385.
Blake, S. (1984). Patient sues to title to own cells. *Nature, 311*, 198.
Bookchin, D., & Schumacher, J. (2004). *The virus and the vaccine*. New York: St. Martin's Press.
Boseley, S. (2002, 17 December). *Alder Hey scandal has hampered child cancer research says charity*. The Guardian.
Brahams, D. (1988). A disputed spleen. *The Lancet, 332*, 1151–1152.
Brahams, D. (1990). Ownership of a spleen. *The Lancet, 336*, 239.
Caplan, A. L. (1985). Blood, sweat, tears and profits: The ethics of the sale and use of patient derived materials in biomedicine. *Clinical Research, 33*(4), 448–451.
Casper. (1998). *The making of the unborn patient*. New Brunswick.
Chedd, G. (1974). Whose grave? *New Scientist, 63*, 91–92.
Clark, A. (1987). Research materials and reproductive science in the United States, 1910–1940. In: G. L. Geison (Ed.), *Physiology in the American context, 1850–1940* (pp. 323–350). Baltimore: American Physiology Society.
Clark, A., & Montini, T. (1993). The many faces of RU486: Tales of situated knowledges and technological contestations. *Science, Technology and Human Values, 18*(1), 42–78.
Cooter, R. (2000). The ethical body. In: R. Cooter & J. Pickstone (Eds), *Medicine in the twentieth century* (pp. 451–69). Amsterdam: Harwood Academic Press.
Culliton, B. J. (1974). Grave-robbing: The charge against four from Boston city hospital. *Science, 186*, 420–423.
Culliton, B. J. (1984). Patient sues UCLA over cell line. *Science, 225*, 1458.
Curran, W. J. (1991). Scientific and commercial development of cell lines: Issues of property, ethics, and conflict of interest. *New England Journal of Medicine, 324*(1), 998–1000.
Department of Health and Social Security, Scottish Home and Health Department, Welsh Office. (1972). *The use of foetuses and foetal material for research: Report of the advisory group*. London: HMSO.
Dickens, B. M. (1977). The control of living body materials. *University of Toronto Law Journal, 27*, 142–198.
Durbach, N. (2005). *Bodily matters: The antivaccination movement in England, 1853–1907*. Durham and London: Duke University Press.
Edwards, C. C. (1974). Fetal research. *Science, 185*, 900.
Enders, J. F. (1974). Fetal experimentation. *New England Journal of Medicine, 290*, 1199.
Erin, C. A. (1994). Who owns Mo? Using historical entitlement theory to decide the ownership of human derived cell lines. In: A. Dyson & J. Harris (Eds), *Ethics and biotechnology* (pp. 157–178). London: Routledge.

Foucault, M. (1998). *The history of sexuality, volume one: The will to know.* London: Penguin Press.

Fox, R. C. (1990). The evolution of American bioethics: A sociological perspective. In: G. Weisz (Ed.), *Social science perspectives on medical ethics* (pp. 201–217). Dordrecht: Kluwer Academic Publishers.

Gold, E. R. (1997). *Body parts: Property rights and the ownership of human biological materials.* Washington, D.C.: Georgetown University Press.

Gregory, J., & Miller, S. (1998). *Science in public: Communication, culture, credibility.* Cambridge, Mass: Basic Books.

Gurney, J., & Balls, M. (1993). Obtaining human tissues for research and testing: Practical problems and public attitudes in Britain. In: V. Rogiers, W. Sonck, E. Shepard & A. Vercruysse (Eds), *Human cells in in vitro pharmaco-toxicology: Present status within Europe* (pp. 315–328). Brussels: VUB Press.

Harris, J. (1998). *Clones, genes and immortality: Ethics and the genetic revolution* (pp. 267–76). Oxford: Oxford University Press.

Hart, D. S. (1975). Fetal research and antiabortion politics: Holding science hostage. *Family Planning Perspectives, 7*(2), 72–82.

Hayflick, L. (1998). A novel technique for transforming the theft of mortal human cells into praiseworthy federal policy. *Experimental Gerontology, 33*, 191–207.

Hayflick, L. (2004, 23 December). Correspondence with the author.

Hayflick, L. (2005, 3 March). Correspondence with the author.

Hedgecoe, A. M. (2004). Critical bioethics: Beyond the social science critique of applied ethics. *Bioethics, 18*(2), 120–143.

Hegarty, T. (1995). The fund for replacement of animals in medical experiments: The first 25 years. *Alternatives to Laboratory Animals, 23*, 19–32.

Hinsliff, G., & Mckie, R. (2004, 6 June). *Doctors beat curbs on tissue research.* The Observer.

Holder, A. R., & Levine, R. J. (1976). Informed consent for research on specimens obtained from at autopsy or surgery: A case study in the overprotection of human subjects. *Clinical Research, 24*, 68–77.

Jones, J. H. (1981). *Bad blood: The Tuskegee syphilis experiment.* London: Free Press.

Josefson, D. (2000). U.S. hospitals to ask patients for right to sell their tissue. *British Medical Journal, 321*, 653.

Kevles. (1998). Diamond v. Chakrabarty and beyond. In: A. Thackray (Ed.), *Private science: Biotechnology and the rise of the molecular sciences* (pp. 65–79). Philadelphia: University of Pennysylvania Press.

Kimbrell, A. (1997). *The human body shop: The cloning, engineering, and marketing of life* (p. xi). Washington, D.C.: Regnery Publishing.

Kleinman, A. (1999). Moral experience and ethical reflection: Can ethnography reconcile them? A quandry for 'the new bioethics'. *Daedalus, 128*(4), 69–98.

Koprowski, H. (1961). Live poliomyelitis virus vaccines: Present status and problems for the future. *Journal of the American Medical Association, 178*, 1151–1155.

Lally, J. J., Makarushka, J. L., & Sullivan, D. (1979). *Research on human subjects: Problems of social control in medical experimentation.* New York: Transaction Books.

Landecker, H. (1999). Between beneficence and chattel: The human biological in law and science. *Science in Context, 12*, 203–225.

Landecker, H. (2000). Immortality, in vitro: A history of the HeLa cell line. In: P. Brodwin (Ed.), *Biotechnology and culture: Bodies, anxieties, ethics* (pp. 53–72). Bloomington: Indiana University Press.

Lawrence, S. C. (1998). Beyond the grave – The use and meaning of human body parts: A historical introduction. In: R. F. Weir (Ed.), *Stored tissue samples: Ethical, legal and public policy implications* (pp. 111–143). Iowa City: University of Iowa Press.

Lopez, J. (2004). How sociology can save bioethics. Maybe. *Sociology of Health and Illness, 26*(7), 875–896.

Mason, J. K., McCall Smith, R. A., & Laurie, G. (2002). *Law and medical ethics* (6th ed., p. 457). Edinburgh and London: Butterworths.

Mason, K., & Laurie, G. (2001). Consent or property? Dealing with the body and its parts in the shadow of Bristol and Alder Hey. *Modern Law Review, 64*(5), 710–729.

Montgomery, P. O'B., Jr., Cook, J. E., Reynolds, R. C., Paul, J. S., Hayflick, L., Stock, D., Schulz, W. W., Kimsey, S., Thirlof, R. G., Rogers, T., & Campbell, D. (1978). The response of single human cells to zero gravity. *In Vitro, 14*(2), 165–173.

Morgan, L. M. (2002). Properly disposed of: A history of embryo disposal and the changing claims on foetal remains. *Medical Anthropology, 21*, 247–274.

Morrison, R. S., & Twiss, S. B. (1973). The human foetus as research material. *Hastings Centre Report, 4*, 8–10.

Nardone, R. M. (2005, 18 February). Personal correspondence with the author.

National Academy of Science. (1975). *Experiments and research with humans: Values in conflict.* Washington: National Academy of Science.

Nelkin, D. (1984). *Science as intellectual property* (p. 10). London: Macmillan.

Nelkin, D., & Andrews, L. (1998). Whose body is it anyway? Disputes over body tissue in a biotechnology age. *The Lancet, 351*, 53–57.

Nelkin, D., & Andrews, L. (2000). *Body bazaar: The market for human tissue in the biotechnology age.* New York: Crown Publishers.

Office of Technology Assessment, Congress of the United States. (1987). *Ownership of human tissues and cells: New developments in biotechnology.* New York: Books for Business.

Otten, A. (1986, 29 January). Researchers' use of blood, bodily tissues raises questions about sharing profits. *Wall Street Journal.*

Parry, B. (2004). *Trading the genome: Investigating the commodification of bio-information.* New York: Columbia University Press.

Perley, S. N. (1992). From control over one's body to control over one's part: Extending the doctrine of informed consent. *New York University Law Review, 67*, 335–365.

Petchesky, R. P. (1987). Foetal images: The power of visual culture in the politics of reproduction. In: M. Stanworth (Ed.), *Reproductive technologies: Gender, motherhood and medicine* (pp. 57–81). Cambridge: Polity Press.

Pfeffer, N. (2000). Fertility counts: From equity to outcome. In: Sturdy (Ed.), *Medicine, health and the public sphere in Britain, 1600–2000* (pp. 260–279). London: Routledge.

Pfeffer, N. (2001). Pioneers in infertility treatment. In: A. Conway & L. Hardy (Eds), *Women and modern medicine* (pp. 254–261). Amsterdam: Rodopi Press.

Rabinow, P. (1996a). Severing the ties: Fragmentation and redemption in late modernity. In: Rabinow (Ed.), *Essays on the anthropology of reason* (pp. 129–153). Princeton: Princeton University Press.

Rabinow, P. (1996b). *Making PCR: A story of biotechnology.* Chicago: University of Chicago Press.

Rabinow, P., & Rose, N. (2006). Biopower today. *Biosocieties, 1*, 195–217.

Ramsey, P. (1975). *The ethics of fetal research.* New Haven and London: Yale University Press.

Richardson, R. (2001). *Death dissection and the destitute* (2nd edn.). London: Pheonix Press.
Risen, J., & Thomas, J. L. (1998). *The wrath of angels: the American abortion war.* New York: Basic Books.
Rose, N. (2001). The politics of life itself. *Theory, culture and society, 18*(6), 1–30.
Rose, N. (2007). *The politics of life itself: Biomedicine, power, and subjectivity in the twenty-first century.* Princeton, NJ: Princeton University Press.
Rosenberg, C. E. (1999). Meanings, policies, and medicine: On the bioethical enterprise and history. *Daedalus, 128*(4), 27–46.
Rosenberg, L. E. (1985). Using patient materials for product development: A dean's perspective. *Clinical Research, 33*(4), 452–454.
Royston, I. (1985). Cell lines from human patients: Who owns them? *Clinical Research, 33*(4), 442–443.
Sandbrook, D. (2006). *White heat: A history of Britain in the swinging sixties.* London: Little, Brown.
Schmeck Jr., H. M. (1976, 28 March). *Investigator says scientist sold cell specimens owned by US.* New York Times. Emphasis added.
Shapo, M. (1977). Legal responsibilities at issue – Emphasis on informed consent. *In Vitro, 13*(10), 613–631.
Skloot, R. (2006, 16 April). *Taking the least of you.* New York Times Magazine.
Squier, S. (2004). *Liminal lives: Imagining the human at the frontier of biomedicine.* Durham and London: Duke University Press.
Stanhope, H. (1970, 16 May). *Live Foetuses Sold for Research – MP.* The Times.
Start, R. D., Brown, W., Bryant, R. J., Reed, M. W., Cross, S. S., Kent, G., & Underwood, J. C. E. (1996). Ownership and uses of human tissue: Does the Nuffield bioethics report accord with opinion of surgical inpatients? *British Medical Journal, 313,* 1366–1368.
Steinberg, A. G. (1975). The social control of science. In: A. Milunsky & G. Annas (Eds), *Genetics and the law* (p. 314). New York: Plenum Press.
Sturdy, S. (Ed.) (2000). *Medicine, health and the public sphere in Britain.* London: Routledge.
Sun, M. (1983). Scientists settle cell line dispute. *Science, 220,* 393–394.
Tallerico, C. A. (1990). The autonomy of the human body in the age of biotechnology. *University of Colorado Law Review, 61,* 659–680.
The Nuffield Council on Bioethics. (1995). *Human tissue: Legal and ethical issues.* London: Nuffield Council.
Tina Stevens, M. L. (2003). *Bioethics in America: Origins and cultural politics.* Baltimore: Johns Hopkins University Press.
Turney, J. (1998). *Frankenstein's footsteps: Science, genetics and popular culture.* London: Yale University Press.
Tutton, R. (2004). Person, property and gift: Exploring languages of tissue donation. In: R. Tutton & O. Corrigan (Eds), *Genetic databases: Socio-ethical issues in the collection and storage of DNA* (pp. 19–39). London: Routledge.
Van Dijck, J. (1998). *Imagenation: Popular images of genetics.* Basingstoke: Macmillan.
Vincent, D. (1998). *The culture of secrecy: Britain, 1832–1998.* Oxford: Oxford University Press.
Wade, N. (1976). Hayflick's tragedy: The rise and fall of a human cell line. *Science, 192,* 125–127.
Wade, N. (1980). University and drug firm battle over billion-dollar gene. *Science, 209,* 1492–1494.

Waldby, C., & Mitchell, R. (2006). *Tissue economies: Blood, organs and cell lines in late capitalism*. Durham and London: Duke University Press.

Weir, R. F. (Ed.) (1998). *Stored tissue samples: Ethical, legal, and public policy implications*. Iowa City: University of Iowa Press.

Weir, R. F., & Olick, R. S. (2004). *The stored tissue issue: Biomedical research, ethics and law in the era of genomic medicine*. New York: Oxford University Press.

Wellcome Trust and the Medical Research Council. (2000). *Public perceptions of the collection of human biological samples*. London: Wellcome, MRC.

Wells, J. A., & Kerr, D. (2000). Mini-hearings on issues in human tissue storage. In: *National bioethics advisory commission, research involving human biological materials: Ethical issues and policy guidance* (National Bioethics Advisory Commission) (pp. 41–53). Rockville, MD.

Wilkinson, S. (2003). *Bodies for sale: Ethics and exploitation in the human body trade*. London: Routledge.

Wilson, D. (2005). The early history of tissue culture in Britain: The interwar years. *Social History of Medicine, 18*(2), 225–245.

Winslade, W. J. (1977). An overview of the scientist's responsibilities: Comments by an attorney. *In Vitro, 13*(10), 712–727.

Wolpe, P. R. (1998). The triumph of autonomy in bioethics: A sociological view. In: R. DeVries & J. Subedi (Eds), *Bioethics and society: Constructing the ethical enterprise* (pp. 38–60). London: Prentice Hall.

Wright, J., Jr. (1985). The development of the frozen section technique, the evolution of surgical biopsy, and the origins of surgical pathology. *Bulletin of the History of Medicine, 59*(3), 295–326.

Yoxen, E. (1990). Historical perspectives on human embryo research. In: A. Dyson & J. Harris (Eds), *Experiments on embryos* (pp. 27–39). London: Routledge.

FROM *CRUZAN* TO *SCHIAVO*: HOW BIOETHICS ENTERED THE "CULTURE WARS" ☆

Renee R. Anspach and Sydney A. Halpern

On the night of January 11, 1983, on a remote country road in Missouri, 25-year-old Nancy Cruzan was driving home from work when her car swerved off the road and rolled over. Nancy was thrown from the car, and paramedics found her lying face down in a water-filled ditch. Though she had no vital signs, they managed to resuscitate her. But by that time, Nancy had already been deprived of oxygen for 15 min, and the brain damage that ensued proved irreparable. Nancy, who never regained consciousness, would spend the last eight years of her life in the Missouri Rehabilitation Center in what neurologists diagnosed as a persistent vegetative state.[1]

The year of Nancy Cruzan's death, 1990, marked the beginning of another landmark case. In the early morning of February 25, Michael Schiavo was awakened by the sound of a thud. He found his 29-year-old wife, Terri, collapsed in the hall. The paramedics resuscitated her and transported her to the hospital. The cause of Terri's collapse, possibly an electrolyte imbalance from an eating disorder, was never established conclusively. Like Nancy Cruzan, Schiavo never regained consciousness.

☆The expression "culture wars" first appeared in James Davison Hunter, *Culture Wars: The Struggle to Define America*, (New York: Basic Books, 1992).

Bioethical Issues, Sociological Perspectives
Advances in Medical Sociology, Volume 9, 33–63
Copyright © 2008 by Elsevier Ltd.
All rights of reproduction in any form reserved
ISSN: 1057-6290/doi:10.1016/S1057-6290(07)09002-X

Within a year, several neurologists made the diagnosis of persistent vegetative state.[2]

The stories of Nancy Cruzan and Terri Schiavo provide the sociologist with the rarest of opportunities: a natural experiment. Both Cruzan and Schiavo were diagnosed with the same condition: persistent vegetative state. In contrast to comatose patients who are totally unconscious, patients in persistent vegetative state are "awake but not aware," able to respond to stimuli but unable to communicate (The Multi-Society Task Force on Persistent Vegetative State, 1994). Though both Nancy Cruzan and Terri Schiavo were able to breathe without life support, neither was able to eat or swallow. They survived only because fluid and nutrients were pumped into their stomachs. Although both patients had the same diagnosis, their stories differed dramatically. Nancy Cruzan's parents took their fight to remove her feeding tube to the US Supreme Court, which, for the first time recognized a right to die. By contrast, Terri Schiavo was at the center of a pitched battle between her husband, Michael Schiavo, who fought to let Terri die, and her parents, who were equally determined to keep her alive – a battle that eventually reached the Florida legislature, the halls of Congress, the White House, and the Vatican. In the Schiavo case, a mass movement developed around what activists viewed as Terri's right to life. In very different ways, both cases represent defining moments in the history of bioethics.

The dramatically different trajectories of the Cruzan and Schiavo cases are the subject of this paper. In the following section, we briefly describe the two cases. But the Cruzan and Schiavo cases also mark major transformations in the culture of ethical problems. Thus, in the next section, we explore how the cases are framed in the press. Our arguments are informed by work on framing in social movements. As this research has noted, the media are pivotal sites for activists in their efforts to win readers' hearts and minds.[3] Media accounts also tell us something about how ethical issues are viewed in American culture. Since this paper is exploratory, we focus our discussion on one of America's three largest-circulation newspapers, *The New York Times*. We examined in detail the 67 articles that discuss Cruzan from 1987 through 1991, and a total of 182 articles that discuss Schiavo, from 2001 through 2006. As we will show, the Cruzan and Schiavo cases are described with a very different language. Next, drawing on insights from the sociology of social movements, we provide a sociological explanation of the differences between the cases. In the conclusion, we examine the legacies of the cases and their implications for bioethics.

A TALE OF TWO PATIENTS

Nancy Cruzan

Let us return to Nancy Cruzan's story. Hopeful that Nancy would eventually recover, her parents, Lester and Joyce Cruzan, agreed to have doctors insert a feeding tube to deliver artificial hydration and nutrition – a decision they would one day regret. Although the Cruzans visited frequently, Nancy was unable to respond to their attention. After four years had elapsed, the Cruzans concluded that Nancy would never regain consciousness and should be allowed to die.

When the Cruzans wrote to the Director of the Missouri Rehabilitation Center requesting that Nancy's feeding tube be removed, he turned down their request. It was at this point that they asked the ACLU for legal counsel and obtained the free legal assistance of William Colby of Shook, Hardy, and Bacon (Robbins, 1989). The Cruzans then petitioned the trial court in Carthage, Missouri, to remove the feeding tube keeping Nancy alive.

In a 1988 hearing, Colby presented the testimony of three neurologists that Nancy was in a persistent vegetative state. The Attorney General, in turn, called two doctors who questioned the diagnosis and three nurses and a nursing assistant who testified that they had seen Nancy cry and look sad. On July 27, Judge Charles E. Teel of the Jasper County Circuit Court ruled in the Cruzans' favor (Robbins, 1989).

Nancy's court-appointed guardian and Missouri Attorney General William Webster bypassed the appellate court and appealed the decision directly to the Missouri Supreme Court. In a 4–3 decision on November 17, 1988, the Court forbade the Cruzans from ordering doctors to remove Nancy's feeding tube, thereby overturning the lower court's decision. Although Nancy had informally expressed her wish not to be kept alive in such a condition, the state argued that the family failed to present clear and convincing evidence of her wishes – a requirement in Missouri (Robbins, 1989).

In March 1989, the Cruzans appealed this decision to the United States Supreme Court, which agreed to hear the case, and *Cruzan v. Missouri* became the first right-to-die case to be argued before the Supreme Court. On December 6, representatives of both sides presented arguments and responded to aggressive questioning by the justices. The Court also heard arguments from then Solicitor General Kenneth Starr, who had filed an *amicus curiae* brief on behalf of the George H.W. Bush administration. Lawyers representing Americans United for Life argued that discontinuing food and water erodes the sanctity of life and the "inherent value of each individual" (Greenhouse, 1989).

On June 25, 1990, the US Supreme Court issued its landmark decision. Eight justices ruled that people whose wishes are clearly known have the constitutional right to have life-sustaining treatment discontinued, thereby recognizing that the right to refuse treatment implies the right to die. This was the first time that the Court had ruled that the Constitution guaranteed liberty from unwanted medical treatment. At the same time, in a 5–4 decision, the court also ruled that the state of Missouri *can* continue life-sustaining treatment when the patient's family does not show clear and convincing evidence of the patient's wishes. While clearly recognizing that the Constitution's 14th Amendment guaranteed liberty from unwanted medical treatment, the Court had, in effect, ruled against the Cruzans (Greenhouse, 1990; Special to the New York Times, 1990; Editorial, 1990).

This was not, however, the end of the story. In late August 1990, Colby petitioned the Jasper County Probate Court to allow removal of the feeding tube, noting that three new witnesses had come forward with evidence of actual conversations with Nancy Cruzan concerning her wish not to be kept alive on life-sustaining treatment. Nancy had married Paul Davis a year before the accident, and her friends knew her only by her married name. After the accident, the Cruzans asked for a divorce decree, and resumed using her maiden name; only belatedly did her friends realize that Nancy Cruzan was the person they had known as Nancy Davis. This time, Attorney General William Webster withdrew from the case. There were no objections from either the doctor at the Rehabilitation Center or Nancy's court-appointed guardians (Colby, 2002; Belkin, 1990). On December 15, 1990, County Probate Court Judge Teel permitted Nancy Cruzan's family to order the removal of artificial hydration and nutrition. The feeding tube was removed (Malcolm, 1990a).

Up to this point, the role of pro-life organizations had been limited to filing friend-of-the-court briefs with the Supreme Court. Only when Cruzan's feeding tube had actually been disconnected did a coalition of anti-abortion and anti-euthanasia activists move to the center of the controversy. Representatives of pro-life groups filed six motions in the courts to reconnect Nancy Cruzan's feeding tube, each denied by an appellate court, the Missouri Supreme Court, and ultimately, the Federal District Court (Associated Press, 1990a, 1990b).

Outside the Rehabilitation Center where Nancy Cruzan lay dying, between 10 and 25 protestors held a vigil.[4] Randall Terry, founder of Operation Rescue, traveled to the hospital in an attempt to meet with the

Cruzans, who declined to meet with him through their lawyer. On December 26, 1990, Nancy Cruzan died, surrounded by her family. She was buried in a county cemetery (Editorial Desk, 1990, A18). Although the Cruzan case came to national attention only in 1990 with the Supreme Court, in fact the Cruzans' quest to allow Nancy to die had lasted almost four years.

Terri Schiavo

Like the Cruzans, Terri Schiavo's parents, Robert and Mary Schindler, and her husband Michael Schiavo were initially optimistic and, over the next four years, made intense efforts to rehabilitate her. In September 1990, Terri came home to her family, but caring for her proved overwhelming, and she was returned to the rehabilitation facility. In November 1990, Michael took Terri to the University of California, San Francisco, where a thalamic stimulator was implanted in her brain – a highly experimental procedure that ultimately failed. In 1991, he began to study nursing, in order, his brother said, to care for Terri, later becoming a respiratory therapist and nurse (Goodnough, 2005a).

In 1992, Michael Schiavo sued Terri's former doctors for malpractice for failing to diagnose the bulimia that, he argued, led to Terri's collapse. A 1993 out-of-court settlement awarded Terri Schiavo $750,000 for her care, and Michael received $300,000. It was at this point that the close relationship between Michael Schiavo and his in-laws, the Schindlers, began to unravel. The exact cause of the rift is in dispute: Michael claimed that the Schindlers demanded he share the malpractice money with them; the Schindlers contended they argued over whether Michael would spend the money on Terri's rehabilitation. By 1994, Michael had concluded that Terri had no hope of recovery, but the Schindlers continued to believe she could be rehabilitated. Not only had Michael Schiavo just won a large settlement but he had also begun to date, and the Schindlers were suspicious of his motives for wanting to discontinue treatment. They filed a motion to have Michael removed as Terri's guardian, but it was denied (Goodnough, 2005a).

Between 1998 and 2002, Michael Schiavo and the Schindlers were embroiled in an acrimonious dispute in the courts. Michael filed motions in the Pinellas-Pasco court to have Terri's feeding tube removed, arguing that she would not want to be kept alive without hope of improvement. The Schindlers fought these motions on two grounds: first, that Terri, as a devout Roman Catholic, would never defy the Church's teachings against euthanasia. Secondly, they challenged Michael's guardianship, alleging as a "confirmed adulterer," who had fathered a child with Jodi Centone, he was unfit to make decisions about Terri's care. Citing a 1990 X-ray showing fractures, they alleged that Michael abused Terri and requested a hearing (Goodnough, 2005a; Sommer, 2002a, 2002b). Judge George Greer nevertheless ruled in favor of Michael and Terri's feeding tube was removed for the first time on April 24, 2001, only to be reinserted two days later as her parents appealed the decision (Goodnough, 2005a).

After their arguments about Terri's wishes and efforts to remove Michael as guardian failed, the Schindlers shifted their focus, challenging the diagnosis of persistent vegetative state. They argued that Terri was in a "minimally conscious state", (a neurological condition with a more favorable prognosis), that she made sounds like "mom" and "dad," and that new medical treatments could restore her cognitive function. The Second District Court of Appeals ordered a hearing to determine whether new treatments could help. Before going to court, however, the Schindlers made a brief, unsuccessful attempt at mediation (Sommer, 2002c). In the October, 2002, trial, the court heard from five expert witnesses. Testifying for the parents were a retired radiologist and Dr. William Hammesfahr, a neurologist, who argued Terri would benefit from a highly controversial treatment he had developed. Both physicians stated that Terri was in a "minimally conscious state." However, three other neurologists testified that Terri was in a persistent vegetative state and that her prospects for recovery were infinitesimally small (Sommer, 2002d; Levesque, 2002).

As part of the hearing, the judge watched six hours of videotape of Terri, recorded by the parents and Dr. Hammesfahr. This 6-h videotape was edited down to 4.5 min. The Schindlers presented testimony from 33 experts, who had viewed the tape and believed Terri would benefit from therapy. Only two of their expert witnesses had examined Terri. Judge Greer ultimately ruled that Terri Schiavo was in a persistent vegetative state without hope of recovery, a decision upheld by the Second District Court of Appeals. The Schindlers posted the edited videotape online, where it would carry more weight in the court of public opinion (Smith, 2005).

These four years of conflict received little attention in the national media. Feeling a lack of support from the local diocese and with their legal options dwindling, in 2003 the Schindlers began to seek publicity and broader support for their fight to keep Terri alive and hired Randall Terry, founder of Operation Rescue, as their spokesperson (Kirkpatrick, 2005a). Bobby Schindler spoke at a conference of the National Right to Life Committee

(Goodnough, 2005b). Terri Schiavo's case was transformed from a bitter family feud into an explosive national controversy.

In September 2003, the Schindlers petitioned the court to postpone removal of the feeding tube so Terri could receive therapy that would enable her to eat on her own. Judge Greer turned down the parents' request and ordered the removal of the feeding tube, which was removed for a second time. Six days after Terri Schiavo's feeding tube had been removed, the Florida legislature passed what later came to be known as Terri's Law, authorizing Governor Jeb Bush to intervene in the case (Goodnough, 2003a, 2003b). Bush, a supporter of the pro-life movement, ordered the feeding tube reinserted. Religious conservatives claimed that their prayer vigils, radio broadcasts, and thousands of emails to Representatives put pressure on legislators to support Terri's law. But Michael Schiavo, represented by the ACLU, successfully challenged Terri's law in the Circuit Court, which found it unconstitutional. Bush appealed the decision, but on September 23, 2004, the Florida Supreme Court ruled that Terri's law violated the state constitution's guarantee of a separation of powers. Governor Bush's lawyers asked the US Supreme Court to consider the case, but on January 25, 2005, the Court declined to hear arguments (Goodnough, 2003c, 2003d, 2004b; Newman, 2005).

Determined to prevent removal of the feeding tube, the Schindlers filed new motions asking that removal be delayed so that the Department of Children and Family services could investigate allegations that Terri had been abused. Terri's parents won delays, but their motions ultimately failed. Judge Greer ordered Terri's feeding tube removed on March 18, 2005, and the feeding tube was removed for the third time. That same day, the Vatican denounced the decision to "pull the plug as if we were talking about ... a broken ... appliance" (Rosenthal, 2005).

At this point, Governor Bush's lawyer, Ken Connor, took the case to Washington and lobbied senators and representatives to become involved in the Schiavo case. Senator Mel Martinez enthusiastically supported Terri's cause. Majority Leader Tom DeLay claimed that "Terri Schiavo is not brain dead; she talks and she laughs, and she expresses happiness and discomfort. Terri Schiavo is not on life support." Harvard-educated cardiac surgeon Senator Bill Frist watched Terri Schiavo on video and questioned her diagnosis (Stolberg, 2003b; Goodnough, 2005d). On March 20, 2005, Congress reached what came to be known as the "Saturday night" or "Palm Sunday Compromise" and passed a narrowly conceived bill transferring jurisdiction in the Schiavo case to the federal courts. Supporters of the bill included 156 Republicans and 47 Democrats. Interrupting his vacation,

President George W. Bush flew into Washington to sign the bill into law, commenting that "it's always best to err on the side of life." His dramatic return was hailed as a victory for the "culture of life" (Hulse & Kirkpatrick, 2005; Kornblut, 2005a).

Once again, the Schindlers filed requests for injunctions to reinsert Terri's feeding tube, but these motions were denied in the Federal District and Circuit Court of Appeals, and the Supreme Court once again declined to hear the case. Congressional efforts to transfer the Schiavo case to the federal courts had failed (Goodnough & Liptak, 2005).

On March 23, 2005, however, Governor Bush succeeded in getting a state court to hear new motions in the Schiavo case, citing new evidence that, he argued, called Terri's diagnosis into question. Dr. William Cheshire, Jr., a sleep researcher at the Jacksonville Mayo Clinic and a Christian bioethicist, visited Terri, reviewed the videotapes, and concluded that she was in a minimally conscious state. When Governor Bush intimated that he might try to take custody of Terri, Judge Greer explicitly barred Bush from doing so. The 2nd District Court of Appeals and the Florida Supreme Court rejected Bush's appeals (Goodnough & Liptak, 2005).

Meanwhile protestors held a vigil outside the hospice, reciting the Lord's Prayer and Amazing Grace. Some were arrested for trying to feed Terri. The crowd, consisting almost entirely of conservative Catholics, Evangelical Protestants, and disability rights activists became excited at the news that Terri made the sounds "ahhh" and "waaaaa." Very quickly, word spread among the protestors that she had said "I want to live." Some of the crowd's hostility was directed at Jeb Bush, who said he had done all he could to save Ms. Schiavo. During a vigil outside the Governor's mansion, some protestors carried signs proclaiming, "Don't Be a Pontius Pilate." On March 30, the Reverend Jesse Jackson joined the vigil outside the hospice (Lyman, 2005a, 2005b).

Terri Schiavo died that very day with Michael at her side. Fifteen years had elapsed since she had first collapsed in 1990, and by now she was 41 years old. More than 800 mourners overflowed the church during the mass held for Terri Schiavo (Associated Press, 2005c; Anon, 2005a).

On June 15, John Thogmartin, the medical examiner, reported the autopsy findings that Terri Schiavo had suffered brain damage so extensive that her brain had withered to half its size and that the damage had also left her blind, as is consistent with the diagnosis of persistent vegetative state. He also found no evidence of physical trauma or abuse (Grady, 2005).

With the autopsy findings, the protests lost momentum. Senator Martinez said he now realized that decisions need to be made at the state level.

Frist angrily commented that he "never made a diagnosis," while DeLay said only that his "thoughts and prayers remain with the family." According to the President's spokesperson, Scott McClellan, the autopsy findings did not change Mr. Bush's belief about the importance of erring on the side of life (Anon, 2005b; Editorial Desk, 2005b; Kornblut, 2005b).

Even the autopsy did not lay to rest questions about whether Michael Schiavo had abused Terri. Investigating numerous allegations of abuse, some filed by the Schindlers, the Department of Children and Family Services found no evidence of abuse. At this point, Jeb Bush ordered the state prosecutor to investigate the circumstances surrounding Terri's cardiac arrest, noting that the autopsy report suggested a gap between Terri's collapse and the time of Michael Schiavo's call to 911. However, the State Attorney found no evidence of criminal activity. It was only at this point that the Governor declared the case closed (Herbert, 2005; Associated Press, 2005a).

These summaries highlight the contrasts between the cases, most notably the scope and magnitude of the controversies. In contrast to *Cruzan*, the Schiavo case was ignited and fueled by a bitter conflict within the family. Perhaps the most obvious contrast was the level of involvement of religious conservatives. In the Cruzan case, the protests were small, and most occurred after Cruzan's feeding tube had been disconnected. The controversy surrounding *Cruzan* remained circumscribed, and politicians did not become involved. By contrast, the protests in the Schiavo case assumed the proportions of a mass movement. The Cruzan case took four years to reach its conclusion. By contrast, the Schiavo cased dragged out over seven years, involving myriad petitions and suits in state and Federal courts, 14 appeals, and three court-ordered removals of Terri's feeding tube. As the next section shows, these contrasts had a discernable effect on how the cases were framed in the media.

FRAMES, NARRATIVES, AND TROPES

Plot: From Right to Die to Right to Life

In the previous section, we used media stories as *primary sources* of "factual" information about the cases. In this section, we shift our analytic focus and treat these articles as narratives and texts, exploring *how* journalists tell their stories. We ask about the extent to which activists shaped media accounts. The *New York Times* is known for a liberal editorial

Activists shape media accounts

policy that extends to end-of-life issues. Its editorials clearly supported the
decision to allow Nancy Cruzan to die:

> On Friday, Dec. 14, the tube was removed, and yesterday Nancy was able to die
> the peaceful death for which her parents had long sought court permission. Connected
> to the feeding tube, she might have outlived them – or perhaps "outlasted" is more
> appropriate – for decades. Now, because of a decision from the US Supreme Court,
> Lester and Joyce Cruzan could lay their daughter to rest at last. (Editorial Desk, 1990)

Editorials on Terri Schiavo did not directly advocate allowing her to die.
Rather, politicians drew fire for their "abuse of power" in the Schiavo case
(Herbert, 2005, p. 19):

> In an abuse of power that has been widely denounced, and has even appalled many of his
> own supporters in the Republican Party, Governor Bush has tried to keep the Terri
> Schiavo circus alive by sending state prosecutors on a witch hunt against her husband,
> Michael.

Given these editorials, it would seem at first glance that the religious right
made few inroads into media framing of the Schiavo case. Only when we
compare the language used in the cases with an eye to their subtexts can we
see how much ground the right had actually gained in its discursive struggle.
    For example, there is a perceptible shift in the plots or core frames of the
cases, what the Cruzan and Schiavo stories were about. Journalists
consistently characterized the Cruzan case as a right-to-die story but often
associated the Schiavo case with the right to live. In a typical passage,
Nancy Cruzan is portrayed as a trope for the right to die:

> A once-vivacious young woman who became a national symbol for the right to die was
> buried in a country cemetery in Missouri. (Metropolitan Desk, 1990)

By contrast, some writers framed the Schiavo case neutrally as a "national
debate about end-of-life care" or as a "right-to-live-or-die debate." One
long feature actually contrasted the core debates in the Quinlan (and, by
implication, Cruzan) and Schiavo cases:

> In recent weeks, the polarizing fight over Ms. Schiavo produced a wrenching
> national debate about the rights of incapacitated people and when their lives should
> end if they left no specific instructions .... It drew religious conservatives and abortion
> opponents who took up the Schindlers' cause, saying no life should end prematurely.
> And just as the case of Karen Ann Quinlan prompted a debate nearly 30 years ago over
> the "right to die," the Schiavo case seemed to focus as much on the "right to live."
> (Goodnough, 2005c)

By focusing Quinlan's story on the right to die and Schiavo's on the right to live, this passage clearly illustrates the extent to which the discursive ground had shifted.

Characters: The Patients

At the center of both stories are the patients, Nancy Cruzan and Terri Schiavo, for it is judgments about their medical conditions that define the moral contours of the cases. Although both Cruzan and Schiavo had the same diagnosis, journalists described these patients very differently, as Fig. 1 suggests. Characterizations of Nancy Cruzan were bleak and unequivocal. By far the most common description of her condition was a "coma" (e.g., "Nancy Cruzan has been in a coma since she was in an automobile accident seven years ago" (Anonymous, 1990) and, less often, the correct medical term "persistent vegetative state."[5] Many writers also emphasized her total dependence on the feeding tube:

> Their daughter Nancy Beth Cruzan is 32 years old now and remains in a persistent vegetative state in a state hospital near here. She never regained consciousness, and has survived only because of chemical nutrition and medicines pumped into her stomach .... (Malcolm, 1990b, A14)

Following a typical script, reporters contrasted a once vibrant, vivacious Nancy Cruzan to the patient who now lay unconscious, alive in the most rudimentary sense of the term – a "permanent" state with a hopeless prognosis:

> Nancy Cruzan, once a spirited, vital young woman, lies unconscious in a Missouri hospital. She is condemned to "live" in a permanent vegetative state by a tragic accident – and by a 4–3 vote of the state's highest court. (Editorial Desk, 1989)

> ... While technological advances have made it possible to keep her body functioning indefinitely, medical science offers no hope that she will regain consciousness. No one who has lain in such a state for more than 22 months has ever emerged from it. (Robbins, 1989, B9)

In each passage, written in what John Van Maanen calls the realist mode (Van Maanen, 1988), an invisible author has invited the reader to "view" the unconscious Nancy in her hospital bed. In addition, s/he described Cruzan's medical condition without invoking the authority of medical opinion, treating the medical facts of the case as beyond dispute.

By contrast, Terri Schiavo's diagnosis and prognosis were bitterly contested, and the controversy had a subtle but discernable impact on

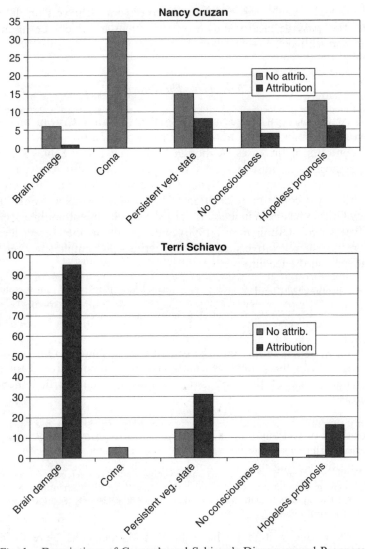

Fig. 1. Descriptions of Cruzan's and Schiavo's Diagnoses and Prognoses.

descriptions of her medical condition. As Fig. 1 shows, most writers did not
characterize Schiavo's condition as a "persistent vegetative state" – a
diagnosis the Schindlers disputed – but rather used the more neutral terms,
"brain damaged," "severely brain damaged," or "incapacitated" – descriptors

that both experts and the Schindlers could accept. Moreover – again in sharp contrast to descriptions of Cruzan – when journalists characterized Terri's condition as a "persistent vegetative state," they almost always attributed the diagnosis to "doctors," "many doctors," "most doctors," or even "some doctors."

> The brain damage Mrs. Schiavo suffered left her able to breathe on her own but not to ingest food or drink. Doctors have said she is in a persistent vegetative state, meaning her eyes are open ... but her brain is incapable of emotion, memory, or thought. (Goodnough, 2004a)

> Ms. Schiavo suffered a brain injury in 1990 that left her in what some doctors called a "persistent vegetative state." (Associated Press, 2005b)

These descriptions distance the author, who is only quoting experts, from the diagnosis, and suggest that the writer feels a diagnosis of "persistent vegetative state" requires a footnote. That journalists rarely used the term "persistent vegetative state" without invoking expert authority illustrates how pro-life activists had placed reporters on the defensive.

Running through media accounts are competing images of the same patient – images that lead to conflicting conceptions of "killing," "starving," and what is "natural." The first imagery, invoked by the Schindlers and their supporters, *personalizes* and humanizes Terri, inviting us to see her as a sentient being who smiles, suffers, and desperately clings to life. Her parents are forced to watch as their daughter is cruelly and unnaturally starved to death, increasingly "resembling a concentration camp survivor," (Schwartz, 2005) while, in the words of one activist, "they can't even give her a cool sip of water."[6]

In the second view, that of Michael Schiavo and many experts, Terri cannot think or feel anything. The "villain" in this story is modern medical technology that is keeping her alive artificially. Following this logic, removing the feeding tube is a not killing a person, but a purely medical decision to let nature to take its course. Because she lacks consciousness, Terri cannot, by definition, suffer. Perhaps not surprisingly, it is the latter view that usually dominates journalists' accounts. In a feature-length article, for example, a reporter argues that, "Neither 'Starvation' Nor the Suffering It Connotes Applies to Schiavo, Doctors Say," countering activists' opinions with scientific "facts." The account depicts the dying process in language that is resolutely clinical and impersonal:

> Once doctors stop providing the nutrient paste and fluids that flow through the feeding tube, death usually comes in about two weeks. As the days pass, organs begin to shut down, starting with the kidneys. Toxins build up in the body, and the patient slips into

what is known as a uremic coma. The balance of electrolytes like potassium and sodium is upset, disrupting the electrical system that drives muscles. The heart eventually stops. In the case of Ms. Schiavo, experts say, the potential for discomfort is nonexistent because higher functions like consciousness and the ability to sense pain were destroyed 15 years ago when she suffered the loss of oxygen to her brain. (Schwartz, 2005)[7]

The patient all but vanishes from this description, and agency is located entirely in doctors who stop providing the "nutrient paste," toxins, electrolytes, the electrical system, and the heart. Terri Schiavo is described entirely in terms of her non-existent "potential for discomfort," and "higher functions" that have been "destroyed."

Journalists did not, however, always privilege the medical voice – particularly when the disputants are not experts. As Terri lay dying in the hospice Mr. Schindler's and his supporters' impassioned pleas for his suffering daughter are juxtaposed against the belief of Michael Schiavo's lawyer that Terri is "dying peacefully."

"She is fighting like hell to live, begging for life," said Ms. Schiavo's father, Robert Schindler, red-eyed and weary as he stood outside his daughter's hospice. "She is still responding to me. She is begging for help."

Mr. Felos ... disputed that description. "Ms. Schiavo's appearance, to me, was very calm, very relaxed, very peaceful," he said. "I saw no evidence of any bodily discomfort whatsoever." (Lyman, 2005c)

Rather than counter-posing the opinions of non-professionals with scientific "facts," the reporter presented competing non-expert narratives, neither more valid than the other, leaving the reader to choose between them.

Although most journalists favored "expert" views of the medical facts, we found at least seven articles that presented both the medical and moral parameters of the case as contested and equivocal.

Mrs. Schiavo's situation is not nearly as cut and dried as some other right-to-die cases, because she is not elderly, comatose or hooked up to a respirator. And most of the facts are in dispute. Mr. Schiavo says his wife once told him that she would never want her life prolonged artificially; he believes doctors who have testified that Mrs. Schiavo is in a persistent vegetative state, unable to think or swallow food. A doctor appointed by the court supported this finding, as did those hired by Mr. Schiavo. But other doctors have testified that with intensive therapy, their daughter could eat and perhaps even speak. (Goodnough, 2003e)

Leaving aside the view, implicit in the passage, that decisions about old people hooked up to respirators are "cut and dry," the writer clearly presents medical opinions as divided. This passage illustrates the extent to which pro-life activists were able to shape newspaper accounts. However, as we have argued, even when journalists support medical perspectives on Schiavo, advocates nevertheless influenced reporters' choice of words.

Characters: The Families

Both the Cruzan and Schiavo cases began with the families. In the Cruzan case, both parents agreed that their daughter should be allowed to die; many experts agreed with the Cruzans; and there was little public controversy until the end. Thus, reporters portrayed both the Cruzans and their quest sympathetically:

> For seven years Nancy Cruzan has lain in a Missouri hospital … kept alive by artificial feeding tubes. This week the Supreme Court rejected her parents' plea to have the tubes disconnected and let her die in dignity. (Lewis, 1990)

> Nobody seriously disputes the hopelessness of her condition or the sincerity and love of her parents, whose painful decision to withdraw nourishment has been vetoed. (Editorial, 1989)

When describing the "poisonous" feud between the Schindlers and Michael Schiavo, however, journalists aimed at balance, giving both sides a chance to tell their story and distancing themselves from the protagonists' most outrageous claims and vindictive actions.

> A month later, on St. Valentine's Day, both sides say, a fight over the award signaled the beginning of their estrangement. The way Mr. Schiavo has described it, Mr. Schindler asked how much money he would receive from Mr. Schiavo's part of the malpractice settlement …. The Schindlers say the fight was about what treatment their daughter's money would go toward, with their advocating rigorous therapy and Mr. Schiavo wanting basic care. The rift quickly deepened. Mr. Schiavo blocked his in-laws' access to his wife's medical records. In July 1993, the Schindlers briefly tried to remove Mr. Schiavo as her guardian. (Goodnough, 2005a)

Yet even in this balanced feature-length article, a tilt toward the Schindlers is apparent. Note how the writer characterizes Michael Schiavo and the Schindlers, and how she struggles to explain Michael Schaivo's motives:

> Mr. Schiavo's demeanor, prickly and forceful, did not gain him much sympathy …. By contrast, the Schindlers – he affable and jokey, she quiet and melancholic – worked hard to win hearts and minds.

> It is easy for most people to assume that blinding love for their daughter drives the parents, who have begged Mr. Schiavo to give them his wife and walk away. But his motives are harder to fathom. Is it stubbornness that drives him, or fervor to commit

fully to the other woman in his life, a girlfriend of eight years with whom he has two children? Does he want Ms. Schiavo to die because she is a burden, or because, as he says time and again he promised her not to keep her alive by artificial means? (Goodnough, 2005a)

In what is the most blatant example of bias, another writer referred to Michael Schiavo as Terri's "estranged" husband, thereby treating as factual the parents' controversial claim that the Schiavo's marriage had been unhappy and faltering. Journalists' tendency to favor the Schindlers personally, even when they did not agree with them, may have a simple explanation: Michael's need for privacy led him to avoid reporters, while the Schindlers deliberately sought publicity. Once again, activists had a hand in shaping media discourse.

Characters: The Activists

There is an additional cast of characters that figures prominently in media accounts: the activists on both sides of the Cruzan and Schiavo controversies. As Hilgartner and Bosk note, advocates clamor to tell their stories to the media, and the competition can be intense (Hilgartner & Bosk, 1988). Whether intentionally or unwittingly, journalists decide whom to cover and include in (or exclude from) their stories, whom to talk to or avoid, and whom to quote (or not to quote). For this reason, a crude "measure" of a social movement's success is the degree to which activists gain media exposure.

Table 1 lists the activists who are mentioned and quoted in stories on the Cruzan and Schiavo cases. The differences between the two cases are striking. In the Cruzan case, representatives of right-to-die organizations are most often quoted, usually about living wills. Representatives of right-to-die groups are, however, absent from most stories on the Schiavo case. Instead, coverage is dominated by myriad pro-life activists and organizations. When the entire panoply of issues is considered, it is possible that right-to-die organizations had focused their energies on other controversies, such as the move to legalize assisted suicide. However, in controversies about forgoing life-sustaining treatment, right-to-die organizations, which had at one time dominated media discourse, had clearly lost control of the issue.

This discussion has avoided the question of who is to be "counted" as an activist. In media accounts of Cruzan, writers clearly identify activists and experts by their institutional and organizational affiliations, for example,

Table 1. Activists Cited in the Cruzan and Schiavo cases.

Activist	Articles in which Quoted	Mentioned	Organization
Activists Cited in Cruzan			
"Right-to-Die" Activists			
Fenella Rouse			Choice in Dying
Fenella Rouse	3		Society for Right to Die
Fenella Rouse	2		National Council for Death and Dying
Rose Gassner	2		Society for Right to Die
Karen Cooper	1		Washington Citizens for Death with Dignity
Doron Weber	2		Society for the Right to Die
Kate Michelman	1		NARAL
Pro-life activists			
Barbara Hackett	1		Missouri Citizens for Life
			Missouri Citizens for Life
Reverend Joseph Foreman	1	1	Prisoners of Christ
Patrick Mahoney	1	3	Center for Christian Activities
Ken Donhower	1		Evangelical Lutheran Church+
Mario Mandina		1	Lawyers for Life
Randall Terry			Operation Rescue (formerly)
		1	International Anti-Euthanasia Task Force
Mary Senander	1		International Anti-Euthanasia Task Force
Dr. John C. Wilke	1		National Right-to-Life Committee
Judie Brown	1		American Life League
Geraldine Oftedahl	1		Right to Life Committee, NY
Marie Dietz	1		Anti-abortion conference
Activists Cited in Schiavo			
Supporting Michael Schiavo			
Michael Schiavo		2	Terri PAC
Sunsara Taylor	1		Protestors, Revolutionary Communist
Debra Sweet	1		Youth Brigade
Paul Malley	1		Aging with Dignity
Barbara Coombs Lee	2		Compassion & Choices
Howard Simon	1	1	ACLU
Supporting the Schindlers			
Schindler family		1	Terri Schindler Schiavo Foundation
			For Health Care Ethics
Randall Terry	5	1	Founder, Operation Rescue

Table 1. (*Continued*)

Activist	Articles in which		Organization
	Quoted	Mentioned	
Phil Sheldon		1	RightMarch.com
William Saunders	3		Family Research Council
Tony Perkins	5		Family Research Council
			Family Research Council
Kenneth Connor		1	Social conservative lawyer, former president, Family Research Council
Marshall Wittman	1		Democratic Leadership Council
Wesley Smith	1		Author of books on bioethics
James Dobson	2		Focus on the Family
Carrie Gordon Earl	1		Focus on the Family
Reverend Patrick Mahoney	6		Christian Defense Coalition
Reverend Frank Pavone	3		American Life League
Reverend Jesse Jackson		2	
Reverend Al Sharpton		1	
Richard Land	1		Ethics and Liberty Commission, Southern Baptist convention
Burke J. Balch	2		Powell Center for Medical Ethics, National Right to Life Committee
		1	National Right to Life Committee
Gary Bauer	1		American Values
Ralph Nader		1	
Gary McCullough	1		Christian Communication Network
Pamela Hennesy	1	1	www.Terrisfight.org
Cheryl Ford	1		National Fight for Terri
Richard Viguerie	2		
Diane Coleman	2		Not Dead Yet
Brother Paul O'Donnell	2		Brothers for Peace
Brother Hilary McGee	1		Brothers for Peace
Carol Cleigh	1		Not Dead Yet
Joni Eareckson Tada	1		Joni and Friends (Christian disability rights group)
Jerry Fallwell	1		
Stephen Moore	1		Free Enterprise Fund
Richard Cizik	1		National Association of Evangelicals
Jay Sekulow		1	American Center for Law and Justice
Joanne Zappala	1		Protestor
Nancy Kramer	1		Protestor

"Dr. Arthur Caplan, director of the Center for Biomedical Ethics at the University of Minnesota" (Anon, 1991) or "Rev. Patrick Mahoney, director of the Center for Christian Activism" (Associated Press, 1990e). In the Schiavo case, it is difficult to tell whether some interviewees are quoted as authorities or as activists. Consider, for example, "William L. Saunders, director of the Center for Human Life and Bioethics at the Family Research Council," (Goodstein, 2005) or "Wesley J. Smith, author of books on bioethics." (Stolberg, 2003a; Benford & Snow, 2000; Gamson & Wolsfeld, 1993) These references, which blur the already elusive boundary between expert and activist, attest to the growing credibility of the religious right.

Activists are not merely concerned with media exposure: rather, they seek to influence how journalists depict them and the issues they represent (Benford & Snow, 2000; Gamson & Wolsfeld, 1993). As we have argued, even in a liberal newspaper such as the *Times*, the religious right had a notable impact on coverage of the Schiavo case. Cruzan was depicted as a right-to-die case; Schiavo as a right-to-life story. Writers portrayed Nancy Cruzan's prognosis as bleak and hopeless, but were more cautious when describing Terri Schiavo's condition. While most reporters favored the medical view of her condition, some presented Schiavo's diagnosis as contested and equivocal. Finally, accounts of Terri Schiavo's warring family depicted her parents in a more favorable light. These observations suggest that the religious right may have even a more powerful effect on media with less liberal editorial policies.

EXPLAINING THE CONTRASTS

The contrasts between the two cases are apparent. In *Cruzan*, the Supreme Court officially recognized the right to die. The Schiavo case became a rallying point for pro-life forces, a national controversy that reached from Terri's bedside to Washington.

These dramatic differences confirm the fundamental tenet of political opportunity theory that context matters.[8] *Cruzan* took place during the presidency of George H.W. Bush. Bush is a mainline Protestant and, at least in comparative terms, a centrist whose "thousand points of light" campaign promised to soften the harsh neo-liberalism of the Reagan years. During the 1970s Bush was pro-choice; only when he agreed to be Reagan's running mate did he change his stance on abortion. Although he vetoed 10 bills funding abortions during his presidency, Bush's pro-life credentials remained suspect. Given his history, it is not surprising that Bush's administration would shore up its credibility with the right by filing a friend-of-the court brief with the Supreme Court. However, Bush never fully gained the support of the right-wing base – one of many factors blamed for his failure to win a second term.[9] During this period, the pro-life movement at the time was bitterly divided between mainstream organizations that lobbied to overturn *Roe v. Wade*, and the more militant and increasingly embattled direct-action groups (Ginsburg, 1998). Given the perceived indifference from above and division within, the pro-life movement was poorly positioned to broaden its agenda to include end-of-life issues.

The Schiavo case unfolded in a very different political context. George W. Bush, who is far more conservative than his father, had recently been elected for a second term, and Republicans had gained a substantial majority in both houses of Congress. Even more important was the increasing power of the social conservatives and their growing influence on the Republican Party. The alliance between conservative Catholics and evangelical Protestants had become a potent force in American politics (Goodstein, 2005). Politicians, including President Bush, Governor Bush, and many members of Congress were beholden to the socially conservative base that had elected them. Bush had chosen Leon Kass, a noted conservative bioethicist, to head his Commission on Bioethics. Activists are much more likely to commit resources to social protest movements when they anticipate they are likely to succeed with politicians.

The right's mobilization around the Schiavo case also illustrates another tenet of political opportunity theory: networks matter. When the Schindlers called upon Randall Terry to publicize their cause, they were able to activate a vast archipelago of organizations that were politically adroit, well-funded, and, above all, interconnected. Many of these organizations had become involved in "culture of life" issues in the years between Cruzan and Schiavo, galvanized by the movement to legalize assisted suicide, and, ironically, their perceived defeat in the Cruzan case. Terry immediately involved his fellow activists, William Green and Philip Sheldon, with whom he had co-founded RightMarch.com. Sheldon is the son of Lou Sheldon, who had founded the large and influential Traditional Values Coalition. A key turning point for Jeb Bush was his choice of prominent conservative attorney Kenneth Connor to represent him. Connor, former president of the conservative Family Research Council, had ties to Washington. When the court set a deadline for removing Terri Schiavo's feeding tube, Connor called on Representative David Weldon, a Florida Republican Senator whom Connor had known for years. Weldon turned to fellow Florida Republican Mel Martinez, Connor's former college roommate, to help sponsor a bill he had

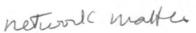

crafted with the assistance of the National Right to Life Committee. Equally important were the decisions of House Leader Tom DeLay and Senate leader Bill Frist. Frist had conferred with neurologist and Christian bioethicist William Cheshire, one of the few physicians who questioned Terri's diagnosis before crafting the "Palm Sunday Compromise Bill" that members of Congress interrupted their vacations to support.[10]

Also important was the right's coalition with disability rights organizations. Although "Not Dead Yet" had mobilized in opposition to assisted suicide, the coalition between pro-life and disability rights activists actually dates from the 1983 Baby Doe case. This alliance is important, for it enabled activists to reach across party lines and rally some Democrats to their support. For example, Democratic Senator Tom Harkin, author of the Americans for Disabilities Act, lobbied for the bill and secured the support of several Democrats. Notably absent was opposition to the bill. In the face of a Republican majority as well as strong, well-organized and, in some cases, bipartisan support for the bill, few Democratic members of Congress were willing to expend their meager political capital on the Schiavo case.[11]

One important feature of the context deserves mention: the Vatican's role in the Schiavo case. Pope John Paul II exerted a profoundly cultural influence on the right-to-life movement. In 1998, he affirmed the Church's commitment to a "culture of life" that he said is being threatened by a "culture of death," which includes birth control, abortion, and euthanasia. Support for a "culture of life" proved a rallying point for conservative Catholics, evangelical Protestants, and President Bush, and served to broaden the agenda of the pro-life movement (Kirkpatick & Stolberg, 2005). But the Vatican had a more specific impact on the Schiavo case. Prior to 2004, Catholic theologians were divided about whether feeding tubes constituted "extraordinary" medical treatment, which, like respirators, could be withdrawn when the burdens outweighed the benefits or, alternatively whether they were a form of basic care to which all patients were entitled (Johnson, 1990). In a 2004 address, Pope John settled the issue, proclaiming that "the administration of food and water, even by artificial means, always represents a natural means of preserving life not a medical act." Since then, most Catholic theologians condemn withdrawing food and fluids as a form of euthanasia (Goodstein, 2005). But the Vatican went beyond general policies and took the rare step of weighing in on the Schiavo case and lending its support to the Schindlers' cause. In a series of proclamations in the Vatican newspaper and on Vatican radio, Vatican officials explicitly condemned Judge Greer's decision allowing Terri Schiavo's feeding tube to be removed (Goodstein, 2005; Fisher, 2005).

These broader political opportunities sometimes dovetailed with some activists' personal opportunities. The *Times* questioned the motives of DeLay, who, the paper argued, used the Schiavo case as an opportunity to deflect attention from the ethical charges he was facing (Editorial Desk, 2005a). A memo by an aide to Mel Martinez detailed the political advantages of involvement in the Schiavo case (Kirkpatrick, 2005b). When leaked to the press, this memo caused considerable embarrassment, since it suggested that senators were at least partly motivated by opportunism. The intersection of political and personal fortunes is also apparent in the case of Randall Terry, organizer of the Schiavo protest. Terry is influenced by theologian Franklin Schaeffer, who viewed "secular humanism" as a threat to the social fabric (Schaeffer & Koop, 1979). He is openly committed to reconstituting society along theocratic lines – gay marriage, abortion, or euthanasia, prayer in the schools and creationism interest him only so far as they serve this broader agenda. For Terry, the Schiavo case was a "crack in the wall," a chance to begin a broader program of social change.[12] But Terry's personal fortunes also had changed. As the founder of Operation Rescue, he is credited with leading the "direct action" wing of the pro-life movement whose militant protests outside abortion clinics sometimes turned violent. By the mid-1990s, as Faye Ginsburg notes, Operation Rescue and other direct-action organizations were all but dead: they had fallen victim to a series of legal challenges by pro-choice organizations, government investigations of their finances, and the erosion of their credibility by widely-publicized murders.[13] Terry had left Operation Rescue and had turned his energies to the Internet, co-founding RightMarch.com to counter MoveOn.org (Kirkpatrick, 2005a). He was, however, an activist without a cause. For Terry, the Schiavo case was the cause he needed, an outlet for his prodigious talents as an organizer and a chance to increase his visibility. While his actual motives cannot be established, the Schiavo case was the moment in which Terry's political and personal opportunities converged.

It would be misleading to focus exclusively on political opportunities and changes in the broader context around the Schiavo case. For the Schiavo case is a story of strategy and tactics within the pro-life movement as well as social forces outside it, of narratives as well as networks, agency as well as structure. Supporters of the Schindlers deployed the full panoply of strategies and tactics, from prayer vigils to lobbying politicians to filing legal briefs. Hundreds of protestors from all parts of the country converged on the hospice where Terri Schiavo lay dying. Picket lines, prayer vigils, and attempts to cross picket lines to "give Terri water" created the visual spectacle that fed the media's hunger for drama. Conservative organizations staged a public relations drive in the mass media that rivaled an advertising campaign in its sophistication. RightMarch.com took out advertisements in *USA Today* (Kirkpatrick, 2005a). Christian radio networks throughout the country exhorted listeners to save Terri, and, perhaps most notably, millions of Americans in their homes were bombarded with images of Terri Schiavo smiling and following a balloon on the nightly news.

Ironically, the very conservative organizations that repudiated "secular humanism" and other concomitants of modernity proved remarkably adept at turning the tools of modernity to their own ends. Conservative activists who were already skilled at using direct mailing to solicit support for their causes now found that the internet provided a much more potent weapon. Websites could mobilize thousands of Americans with the click of a mouse. The web could be used for lobbying, and Florida legislators' found their computers jammed by tens of thousands of emails urging them to help keep Terri alive. For example, www.Terrisfight.org reportedly raised 40,000 signatures on a petition to Jeb Bush. Organizations such as Voice for Terri, RightMarch.com, and the Traditional Values Coalition were remarkably effective in using the web for fundraising. Video clips of Terri, scathing indictments of Michael Schiavo, and pleas to "Help Save Terri's life" were used to raise money not only for the campaign to keep Terri alive, but for other conservative causes as well.[14] Three years of challenges in the courts, attorney fees, advertising campaigns, hotels, and transportation for organizers required vast expenditures – more than the web campaign could provide. As Jon Eisenberg notes, much of the protracted legal campaign was financed by established organizations such as the anti-abortion Life Legal Defense Foundation, the Family Research Council, or the National Organization on Disability. These groups are, in turn, financed by "a consortium of conservative foundations, with $2 billion in total assets that are funding a legal and public relations war of attrition intended to prolong Terri's life indefinitely in order to further their own faith-based cultural agendas ..." (Eisenberg, 2005).

The left, by contrast, was fragmented and internally divided. It proved no match for the religious right.

THE LEGACIES OF *CRUZAN* AND *SCHIAVO*

Nancy Cruzan's case received far less publicity than the Schiavo case, but its impact may have been equally profound. The Supreme Court for the first time recognized the right to die. Implicitly, the court treated artificial food and fluids as a medical treatment that, like respirators, could be withheld. Hospitals could now withdraw treatment knowing that they enjoyed the protection of the law. Perhaps the most enduring legacy of *Cruzan* was the Patient Self Determination Act, which mandated hospitals receiving federal funds to inform patients about advance directives.[15] In the wake of the Cruzan case, right-to-die organizations were bombarded with thousands of requests for living wills (Malcolm, 1990b).

In the early 1990s, it seemed that decisions concerning adults at the end of life followed a clear progression. *Quinlan* made it permissible to disconnect respirators, the President's Commission legitimated "do not resuscitate" orders, and *Cruzan* legalized removing patients' feeding tubes.[16] As the debate now shifted to assisted suicide, it seemed that American culture was moving steadily toward increasingly permissive policies.

This progression was suddenly interrupted by the Schiavo case. The countermovement to keep Terri Schiavo alive was what its proponents called a "counterrevolution" and its opponents called a backlash designed to undo *Cruzan*.[17] The broad mobilization of social conservatives had a considerable impact on how the issues were framed in the mass media – even in a liberal newspaper such as *The New York Times*. The protests reverberated in the Florida legislature and in the Congress, as legislation designed to save Terri Schiavo was enacted.

At the same time, the legacy of the Schiavo case is more ambiguous. It did not shape public opinion: polls showed that most Americans opposed keeping Terri alive and believed Congress had overstepped its bounds (Toner & Hulse, 2005). Hospitals throughout the country continue to remove the feeding tubes of patients in persistent vegetative states. Probably the only significant change in medical practice takes place in Catholic hospitals, and the extent of change is an empirical question. The Schiavo case led politicians to propose legislation in several states. In Michigan, a proposed bill prohibited people having "extramarital affairs" from making end-of-life decisions for an incapacitated spouse. Republicans in Louisiana and Alabama introduced bills that making it illegal to remove the feeding tubes of unconscious patients who had not left advanced directives (Dewan, 2005). However, most states continue to permit discontinuing food and fluids at least under some circumstances. In fact, debates in many states concern assisted suicide rather than removing feeding tubes. Ultimately, the protests around the Shiavo case did not succeed in overturning *Cruzan*.

Perhaps the most enduring legacy of the Schiavo case was its impact on what sociologists call field formation. Bioethics emerged from the controversy radically reconfigured.[18] With the Schiavo case, bioethics had become the latest front in the culture wars. Beginning in the late 1990s, a number of well-funded conservative think tanks now made bioethics a central part of their agenda. For instance, the Family Research Council now has a Center for Human Life and Bioethics. Other conservative organizations, such as the American Enterprise Institute, which up to this time had focused on economics and foreign policy, have incorporated bioethics into their agendas. These organizations embrace a wide range of issues from abortion to assisted suicide, genetics, and cloning. Along with these developments is the emergence of what its practitioners call Christian bioethics. The Center for Bioethics and Human Dignity, based at Trinity University in Deerfield, Illinois, holds conferences, educational workshops, and programs – all designed to train practitioners in Christian bioethics.[19] While some of these groups were founded before Terri Schiavo became a public issue, the Schiavo case energized these groups and provided them with a rallying point.

In a field that issues credentials but does not license, virtually anyone can adopt the title of "bioethicist." Adopting the title of "bioethicist" enabled Christian activists to capitalize on mainstream bioethicists' credibility with the press, allowing them to speak as experts to the mass media.

These developments have radically transformed the field of bioethics. To be sure, this fusion of religion and bioethics is not new. Indeed some of the field's founders, such as Albert Jonsen, Joseph Fletcher, and Paul Ramsey, were trained in theology, although they were usually liberal Catholics or affiliated with mainline Protestant denominations. While most of bioethics has been identified with the "liberal establishment," conservatism is not entirely new to the field: in fact, both Paul Ramsey and Leon Kass were among the original members of the Hastings Center.[20] But both were, until recently, firmly tied to prestigious universities. Until recently, the major centers of bioethics were the Hastings Center and institutes attached to universities such as the University of Pennsylvania or Georgetown – organizations devoted primarily to research and teaching of bioethics. As members of blue ribbon panels and advisory commissions, practitioners of "policy bioethics" have played political roles and promulgated political positions. But, until recently they have stopped short of outright advocacy. The field of bioethics is now bifurcated into those affiliated with bioethics centers or hospitals, and Christian bioethics, usually based in conservative think [tanks]. Although both groups have adopted the title "bioethicist," the two groups have little in common and there is little exchange between them (Hinsch, 2005).

Blindsided by the religious right's dominance in the Schiavo case, some mainstream bioethicists have felt compelled to respond by becoming politicized. A conference at the Center for American Progress initiated a "progressive bioethics" movement to counter the religious right and oppose its positions on issues ranging from embryonic stem cells to national health care (Check, 2005). What will be the impact of this politicization of bioethics? Will "progressive bioethicists" relinquish some of their professional credibility as they embrace activism? Will they lose the ability to develop nuanced or balanced arguments? Or will they benefit from being forced to make explicit political positions that had remained tacit? Will "progressive bioethicists" be able to compete successfully with activists who are exceptionally well networked, media-savvy, and skilled at fundraising? Will a left deeply divided over assisted suicide and embryonic stem cells be able to coalesce around a broad-based progressive bioethics agenda? How these questions will be answered depends on the opportunities created by the broader political climate as well as the ability of "progressive bioethicists" to use these opportunities strategically. They are also questions for future research, for the last chapter of the Schiavo story has yet to be written.

NOTES

1. For Nancy Cruzan's early history, see Colby, 2002.
2. For a summary of Terri Schiavo's early history, see, for example, Goodnough, 2005a, A1.
3. See, for example, Benford & Snow, 2000; Gamson & Wolsfeld, 1993.
4. Regarding Randall Terry, see Associated Press, 1990a. Regarding protests, see Associated Press, 1990c, 1990d.
5. From a medical standpoint, it is incorrect to characterize the condition of either Terri Schiavo or Nancy Cruzan as a "coma," or a profound state of unconsciousness. Both patients were given the diagnosis of "persistent vegetative state": during the day, they were awake but unaware of their surroundings. Prior to 1972, when this condition was first described, the terms "permanent" or "unrecoverable comas" were used to describe patients such as Schiavo or Cruzan. To account for the very small number of patients who recover after long periods in a persistent vegetative state, the diagnosis of "minimally conscious state" was established in 2002. The terms are explained in an article by Benedict Terry that appeared in the *New York Times* on April 5, 2005. These distinctions notwithstanding, the majority of articles erroneously refer to Nancy Cruzan's condition as a "coma," possibly because the term "persistent vegetative state" was not widely known at the time. Only a few articles use the term "comatose" to describe Terri Schiavo, one followed by an erratum, presumably because the distinctions were more widely understood at the

time of the controversy. Very recently, some neurologists are re-examining these diagnostic categories and the very concept of consciousness.

6. Brother Paul O'Donnell, quoted in Goodnough, 2005e.

7. In this article, the author reflects upon the political use of language in the Schiavo case, particularly use of the term "starvation."

8. For a discussion of political opportunity theory, see Meyer, 2004. See also McAdam, McCarthy, & Zald, 1996.

9. For a discussion of George H.W. Bush's presidency and campaigns, see Wicker, 2004.

10. For a discussion of anti-abortion activists who mobilized around right-to-die issues in the early 1990's, see Johnson, 1990. For a detailed account of the interorganizational and interpersonal alliances that formed around the Schiavo case, see Kirkpatrick & Stolberg, 2005.

11. See the organization's account of its history at www.notdeadyet.org. It is interesting that the organization dates mobilization of disability rights activists around end-of-life issues to 1983, the year of the Baby John Doe case. For a brief account of the coalition of right-to-life and disability rights organizations in the Baby Doe case, see, for example, Anspach, 1993. For Harkin's role in the Schiavo case, see Kirkpatick & Stolberg, 2005.

12. Quoted in Goodnough, 2003c, p. 1.

13. Most of this account of Terry and Operation Rescue is taken from Ginsburg, 1998.

14. How activists used the web for lobbying and fundraising is described in Kirkpatrick, 2005a; Kirkpatrick & Schwartz, 2005; and Goodnough, 2003f. This is one of the few articles to describe Schiavo as a right-to-die case.

15. Weber, 1991. It should be noted, however, that legal recognition of advanced directives does *not* mean that they will be carried out in actual practice. See, for example, Teno, Stevens, Spernak, & Lynn, 1998.

16. For a discussion of the case of Karen Ann Quinlan, see Capron, 1976. For a discussion of "do not resuscitate" orders, see President's Commission on the Study of Ethical Problems in Medicine and Biomedical and Behavioral Research, 1983.

17. For a sociological perspective on movements and countermovements, see Zald & Useem, 1987.

18. For the role of social movements in reshaping fields, see Rao, Morrill, & Zald, 2000.

19. A comprehensive account of the emergence of these new bioethics organizations is given in Hinsch, 2005.

20. Daniel Callahan's comments on the history of bioethics made this point. He was part of a panel on "The Emergence of Politicized Bioethics" during a conference on Bioethics: Past, Present, and Future, sponsored by the Center for American Progress, April 26, 2006.

REFERENCES

Anon. (1991, November, 29). *Father battles state over comatose daughter*. New York Times.

Anon. (2005a, April 6). *Mass for Terri Schiavo*. New York Times.

Anon. (2005b, June 17). *Frist Responds on Schiavo*. New York Times.

Anonymous. (1990, January 14). *Guidelines on dying urged by both sides of case in Missouri.* New York Times, 18.
Anspach, R. R. (1993). *Deciding who lives.* Berkeley: University of California Press.
Associated Press. (1990a, December 20). *Court firm on Cruzan ruling.* New York Times.
Associated Press. (1990b, December 22). *A federal Judge scolds protestors on filing petitions in Cruzan case.* New York Times.
Associated Press. (1990c, December 20). *Court firm on Cruzan ruling.* New York Times.
Associated Press. (1990d, December 19). *Protesters fail in bid to feed dying woman.* New York Times.
Associated Press. (1990e, December 29). *Cruzan's condition downgraded to critical.* New York Times, A24.
Associated Press. (2005a, July 8). *Florida closes its investigation into collapse of Schiavo.* New York Times.
Associated Press. (2005b, December 9). *Retaliation in right-to-die case.* New York Times, A30.
Associated Press. (2005c, April 1). *Schiavo dies, ending bitter case over feeding tube.* New York Times.
Belkin, L. (1990, October 12). *Missouri seeks to quit case of comatose woman.* New York Times.
Benford, R. D., & Snow, D. A. (2000). Framing process and social movements: An overview and assessment. *Annual Review of Sociology, 26,* 611–639.
Capron, A. M. (1976). Shifting the burden of decision making. *Hastings Center Report, 6,* 17–19.
Check, E. (2005, October 12). *US progressives fight for a voice in bioethics.* Nature.com
Colby, W. (2002). *The long goodbye: The deaths of Nancy Cruzan.* New York: Hayhouse.
Dewan, S. (2005, March 30). *States taking a new look at end-of-life legislation.* New York Times.
Editorial. (1989, December 3). *Whose right to life and death?* New York Times, (4)24.
Editorial. (1990, June 27). *For the Cruzans pain for principle a triumph.* New York Times.
Editorial Desk. (1990, December 27). *Nancy Cruzan's accomplishment.* New York Times.
Editorial Desk. (2005a, April 5). *Attacking a free judiciary.* New York Times.
Editorial Desk. (2005b, June 16). *Autopsy on the Schiavo tragedy.* New York Times.
Eisenberg, J. B. (2005, March 4). *The Terri Schiavo case: Following the money.* Cal Law.
Fisher, I. (2005, March 19). *World briefing Europe: Italy: Terri Schiavo's parents meet Pope.* New York Times.
Gamson, W. A., & Wolsfeld, G. (1993). Movements and media as interacting systems. *Annals of the American Academy of Political and Social Sciences, 528,* 114–125.
Ginsburg, F. (1998). Rescuing the nation. In: R. Sollinger (Ed.), *Abortion wars: A half century of struggle, 1950–2000* (pp. 208–250). Berkeley: University of California Press.
Goodnough, A. (2003a, October 21). *National briefing South: Florida legislature enters feeding dispute.* New York Times.
Goodnough, A. (2003b, October 21). *Governor of Florida orders woman fed in right-to-die case.* New York Times.
Goodnough, A. (2003c, October 23). *Victory in Florida feeding case emboldens the religious right.* New York Times.
Goodnough, A. (2003d, October 30). *Spouse fights new law over feeding tube.* New York Times.
Goodnough, A. (2003e, October 15). *Right-to-die battle enters its final days.* New York Times, A12.
Goodnough, A. (2003f, October 16). *Tube is removed in Florida right-to-die case.* New York Times.

Goodnough, A. (2004a, September 2). *Comatose woman's case heard by Florida Court.* New York Times, A14.

Goodnough, A. (2004b, September 24). *Feeding tube law is struck down in Florida case.* New York Times.

Goodnough, A. (2005a, March 26). *Behind life-and-death fight a rift that began years ago.* New York Times.

Goodnough, A. (2005b, March 28). *In two friars family find spiritual support and more.* New York Times.

Goodnough, A. (2005c, April 1). *Schiavo dies, ending bitter case over feeding tube.* New York Times, 1.

Goodnough, A. (2005d, March 19). *The medical turns political.* New York Times.

Goodnough, A. (2005e, March 23). *US Judge denies feeding-tube bid in Schiavo's case.* New York Times, A1.

Goodnough, A., & Liptak, A. (2005, March 24). *Court blocks bid: New Schiavo tactic by Governor Bush.* New York Times.

Goodstein, L. (2005, March 24). *Schiavo case highlights an alliance between Catholics and Evangelicals.* New York Times, A20.

Grady, D. (2005, June 19). *The hard facts behind a heartbreaking case.* New York Times.

Greenhouse, L. (1989, December 21). *The right-to-die argument, personified.* New York Times.

Greenhouse, L. (1990, June 26). *Justices find a right to die, but the majority sees need for clear proof of intent.* New York Times.

Herbert, B. (2005, June 23). *Cruel and unusual.* New York Times.

Hilgartner, S., & Bosk, C. (1988). The rise and fall of social problems: A public arenas model. *American Journal of Sociology, 94,* 53–78.

Hinsch, K. (2005). *Bioethics and public policy: Conservative dominance in the new landscape.* Seattle, Washington: Women's Bioethics Project.

Hulse, C., & Kirkpatrick, D. D. (2005, March 21). *Congress passes and Bush signs Schiavo measures.* New York Times.

Johnson, D. (1990, July 31). *Schiavo case highlights an alliance between Catholics and Evangelicals.* New York Times.

Kirkpatrick, B. D. (2005a, March 25). *Conservatives invoke case in fund-raising campaigns.* New York Times.

Kirkpatrick, D. D. (2005b, April 7). *Schiavo memo is attributed to senate aide.* New York Times.

Kirkpatrick, D. D., & Schwartz, J. (2005, March 29). *List of Schiavo donors will be sold to direct-marketing firm.* New York Times.

Kirkpatrick, D. D., & Stolberg, S. G. (2005, March 21). *How a family's cause reached the halls of Congress.* New York Times.

Kornblut, A. (2005a, March 22). *After signing Schiavo law, Bush says, 'It is wisest to err on the side of life.* New York Times.

Kornblut, A. E. (2005b, June 16). *Debate over legislative actions is renewed.* New York Times.

Levesque, W. R. (2002, October 22). *Schiavo case doctor target of complaint.* St. Petersberg Times.

Lewis, A. (1990, June 29). *Abroad and at home: Conscience and the court.* New York Times, A25.

Lyman, R. (2005a, March 27). *As legal moves dwindle in the Schiavo case, the focus returns to Governor Bush.* New York Times.

Lyman, R. (2005b, March 26). *Schiavo in her last hours, father says amid appeals.* New York Times.

Lyman, R. (2005c, March 29). *Schiavo's husband says autopsy will end suspicians.* New York Times, A10.

Malcolm, A. H. (1990a, December 25). *Judge allows feeding tube removal.* New York Times.

Malcolm, A. H. (1990b, November 2). *Missouri family renews battle over right to die.* New York Times.

McAdam, D., McCarthy, J. D., & Zald, M. N. (1996). *Comparative perspectives on social movements: Political opportunities, mobilization structures, and cultural framing* (Cambridge, UK: Cambridge University Press).

Metropolitan Desk. (1990, December 29). *Farewell to Nancy Cruzan.* New York Times, 1.

Meyer, D. S. (2004). Protest and political opportunities. *Annual Review of Sociology, 30,* 125–145.

Newman, M. (2005, January 25). *Governor Bush's role is ended in feeding tube dispute.* New York Times.

President's Commission on the Study of Ethical Problems in Medicine and Biomedical and Behavioral Research. (1983). *Deciding to forego life-sustaining treatment.* Washington, D.C.: U.S. Government Printing Office.

Rao, H., Morrill, C., & Zald, M. (2000). Power plays: How social movements and collective action create new organizational forms. *Research in Organizational Behavior, 22,* 239–282.

Robbins, W. (1989, November 27). *Parents fight for right to let a daughter die.* New York Times.

Rosenthal, E. (2005, March 27). *A most personal test for the Church's rules.* New York Times.

Schaeffer, F. A., & Koop, C. E. (1979). *Whatever happened to the human race?* Old Tappan, NJ: Revell.

Schwartz, J. (2005, March 25). *Neither 'starvation' nor the suffering it connotes applies to Schiavo, doctors say.* New York Times, A14.

Smith, B. (2005, March 20). *Schiavo tapes offer powerful but misleading evidence.* Tampa Tribune.

Sommer, D. (2002a, November 23). *Judge: unhook Schiavo's tube.* Tampa Tribune.

Sommer, D. (2002b, October 23). *Parents in Schiavo case allege abuse.* Tampa Tribune.

Sommer, D. (2002c, January 19). *Failed talks send Schiavo's fate, family to trial.* Tampa Tribune.

Sommer, D. (2002d, October 23). *Doctors testify: She will not improve.* Tampa Tribune.

Special to the New York Times. (1990, June 26). *Excerpts on missouri right-to-die case.* New York Times.

Stolberg, S. G. (2003a, March 31). *A collision of disparate forces may be reshaping American law.* New York Times, A18.

Stolberg, S. G. (2003b, March 23). *The Schiavo case: Legislators with medical degrees offer opinions on Schiavo case.* New York Times.

Teno, J. M., Stevens, M., Spernak, S., & Lynn, J. (1998). Role of written advance directives in decision making: Insights from qualitative and quantitative data. *Journal of General Internal Medicine, 13*(7), 439–446.

The Multi-Society Task Force on Persistent Vegetative State. (1994). Medical aspects of the persistent vegetative state [in two parts]. *New England Journal of Medicine, 330,* 1499–1508, 1572–1579.

Toner, R., & Hulse, C. (2005, April 11). *In the partisan power struggle, a new underdog tries some old tricks.* New York Times.

Van Maanen, J. (1988). *Tales of the field: On writing ethnography.* Chicago: University of Chicago Press.

Weber, B. (1991, December 2). *Positive reaction greets 'living will' law*. New York Times.
Wicker, T. (2004). *George Herbert Walker Bush (Penguin lives series)*. New York: Lipper/ Viking.
Zald, M. N., & Useem, B. (1987). Movement and countermovement interaction: Mobilization, tactics, and state involvement. In: M. N. Zald & J. D. McCarthy (Eds), *Social movements in an organizational society: Collected essays*. New Brunswick, NJ: Transaction Publishers.

THE CHANGING CONTEXT OF NEONATAL DECISION MAKING: ARE THE CONSUMERIST AND DISABILITY RIGHTS MOVEMENTS HAVING AN EFFECT?

Rosalyn Benjamin Darling

The treatment of some newborns with disabilities has been hotly debated by both professionals and laypersons, especially since the well-publicized "Baby Doe" cases of the 1980s. These debates have involved social issues such as cost of treatment (Tyson, 1995), quality of life (Lantos et al., 1994), and the appropriate role of various decision makers, including parents and other family members, medical professionals, ethicists and ethics committees, clergy, policy makers, and society at large. Some have argued that virtually all babies should be treated, regardless of disability (Asch, 1986), whereas others have suggested that criteria based on projected quality of life be used to "draw a line" between those who should receive life-saving treatment and those who should not (Weir, 1984). This paper will focus on the decision makers.

Although the question of who should decide in these cases is perhaps as much an ethical as a sociological one, the structural conditions involved and the processes by which such decisions are reached are clearly sociological concerns. These decisions are made within an interactional context involving

Bioethical Issues, Sociological Perspectives
Advances in Medical Sociology, Volume 9, 65–84
ISSN: 1057-6290/doi:10.1016/S1057-6290(07)09003-1

participants with varying degrees of information and power. As I have suggested elsewhere (Darling, 1977; Protection of Handicapped Newborns, 1986), in the past, professional dominance played an important role in shaping parents' decisions. However, many have noted some shift in the health-care system during the past 20 years from professional dominance to consumerism (Pescosolido, Tuch, & Martin, 2001). Consumerism in health care has come to mean the increasing involvement and empowerment of patients in treatment decisions. In addition, the disability rights movement has been promoting a more positive perspective on the quality of life of people with disabilities (Shapiro, 1994). Whether these trends have changed the nature of decisions about treating neonates with impairments is an empirical question. In this paper, I review the trends in decision making from the 1970s to the present, explore the influence of the trends toward consumerism in health care and toward disability rights advocacy, and suggest the impact of these trends on treatment decisions. Finally, I present several parent accounts that illustrate the influence of professional dominance, consumerism, and the disability rights perspective on decision making during the past 10 years. I conclude by proposing a research agenda to address some of the empirical questions raised by the literature-based analysis.

AN OVERVIEW OF THE HISTORY OF DECISION MAKING

In Great Britain in the 1960s and 1970s, a physician (Lorber, 1971) developed criteria that would exclude from treatment many babies born with spina bifida ("open spine") based on what he perceived to be a poor projected quality of life. In the US, the parameters of the modern debate developed around the case of "Baby Doe," a child born in the early 1980s with Down syndrome and duodenal atresia, an intestinal blockage. Without surgery to correct the blockage, the baby would not survive. Because the infant also had Down syndrome, which typically includes some degree of intellectual disability, the parents decided not to consent to the surgery. The parents' decision was met with outrage by disability advocacy groups, as was a similar decision a few years later to forego surgery to repair a myelomeningocele (spina bifida) in the case of "Baby Jane Doe." The publicity surrounding these and other non-treatment decisions resulted in the US in the passage of the Child Abuse Amendments of 1984, largely through the efforts of then Surgeon General C. Everett Koop. This legislation effectively mandated universal treatment of newborns with disabilities. However, several court cases since have resulted in rulings allowing parents to discontinue life support based on quality-of-life issues, resulting in the establishment of state standards in addition to the federal ones (Clark, 1994). Still, the norm in the case of Down syndrome and spina bifida, two of the most common childhood impairments apparent at birth, continues to support the treatment of virtually all children born with these conditions. As a result, most post-natal decision making today involves infants with other, often more serious, impairments that result from perinatal complications or from extreme prematurity. Even in those cases, a bias toward treatment seems to prevail (Levin, 1990).

The decision-making situation has been altered to some extent by the advent of technology to detect the presence of certain impairments prior to birth. Studies indicate that prenatal diagnosis results in pregnancy termination 92% of the time in the case of Down syndrome and 64% of the time in the case of spina bifida (Mansfield, Hopfer, & Marteau, 1999). Not all women have access to prenatal diagnosis, and some choose to forego it. However, fewer parents who might choose to deny treatment to their children after birth find themselves in a position of needing to make this choice today.

Thus, the current decision-making context typically involves an infant with significant disabilities as a result of unanticipated birth complications or prematurity, who is being kept alive through artificial means in a Neonatal Intensive Care Unit (NICU). Decisions to terminate life support are being made by parents through a process of informed consent. Often, parents and hospital staff concur in these decisions. However, disagreements between various stakeholders sometimes occur. The nature of such concurrence and disagreement will be explored further in the next section.

WHO DECIDES?

The Ethical Question

Ethicists, physicians, and others have considered the question of the roles of various potential decision makers in determining whether an infant should live or die. Some have argued that parents should be the ultimate decision makers, whereas others have proposed that physicians or ethics committees should have the final say. Examples of these positions are presented below.

Many writers agree that parents are the primary stakeholders in the decision-making situation and should have the main responsibility for making life-and-death decisions regarding their children. Rothman (1986a, p. 13) wrote over 20 years ago that "parenthood is always the acceptance of responsibility for a life." She argued that mothers have the right to refuse the encroachment of medical technology into their lives because they are the ones who are most affected by the consequences. At about the same time, Kipnis and Williamson (1984) agreed that parents should not be burdened against their wishes with the care of a disabled child. However, rather than arguing for withdrawal of life support, they suggested that society assume the responsibility for care in such cases.

Weir (1984) supported the principle of parental autonomy; however, he argued that parental rights must be superseded in some cases to protect the rights of the child. He noted three circumstances in which parents should not "have the final word": "when they simply cannot understand the relevant medical facts of a case, when they are emotionally unstable, and when they appear to put their own interests before those of the defective newborn" (Weir, p. 203). In such cases, he argued that physicians may be better qualified to be proxies for the child because of their "technological knowledge, greater objectivity, and professional involvement with numerous birth-defective newborns." Because of these "qualifications," he suggested that physicians should simply override parents' wishes in "clear-cut" cases or refer "borderline" cases to an NICU committee. More recently, Tripp and McGregor (2006, p. 70) concurred that "parental autonomy must be respected – unless it clearly and unarguably contravenes the infant's rights."

In a Scottish study, McHaffie, Laing, Parker, and McMillan (2005) found that only a small minority of NICU physicians and nurses (3 and 6%, respectively) believed that parents should have the ultimate authority, whereas the majority (58 and 73%) favored joint decision making. However, 56% of the parents in the study believed that they should have the final decision, either alone or jointly.

As in all ethical questions, no absolute right or wrong answer exists in these cases. All involve weighing the interests of various stakeholders in determining the identity of the ultimate authority. However, when the question is framed simply in ethical terms, the sociological context is overlooked. All decisions are made by individuals with diverging social backgrounds, and the decision-making situation itself involves interactional processes that shape attitudes and behaviors in important ways. In other words, although ethics may address the question of *who* should decide, it does not address the related question of *how* decisions are made. The answer to this latter question, in fact, has bearing on the answer to the former, for if "informed consent" is not truly informed, the bases for ethical conclusions regarding the appropriate locus of authority may not be sound.

The Sociological Question

A consideration of the sociological issues involved in neonatal decision making requires attention to two aspects of decision-making situations. First, each of the potential decision makers is a product of socialization in a particular sociocultural environment. Prior to the birth of their children, parents have been exposed to values relating to parenting and to people with disabilities, as well as to personal experiences with a variety of people and situations. Similarly, physicians have had experiences in their professional training and practice and in their own families, in addition to their exposure to the norms and values of the larger society. Thus, all participants have *predispositions* upon which their participation is based. Second, the nature of the decision-making *situation* is important. Structural features such as status inequality may shape the outcome of interactions between parents and physicians, and the interaction that occurs in the course of the situation may influence the attitudes and behaviors of participants in important ways as well. The decisions of ethics committees also are shaped by the interactional processes that occur within them.

Parents' Predispositions
Attitudes Toward Disability. As Goffman (1963) classically noted, the prevailing attitude toward people with disabilities in our society has been based on stigma. Individuals who do not fit societal norms regarding appearance and ability tend to be devalued and sometimes shunned. Longmore (2003) and others have demonstrated how the media have long perpetuated stereotypes of the disabled based on pity and other negative attitudes. Most parents and future parents have been exposed to these stereotypes. These negative attitudes are reflected in the high percentages (noted earlier) of parents who choose to abort when receiving a prenatal diagnosis of disability.

Not all parents embrace the societal norm, however. For example, Rothman (1986b) and Zuckoff (2002) have described families who chose to bear children with disabilities as a result of personal experience with disability, interaction with supportive significant others, or strong religious beliefs. Rapp (1998) has noted that such choices are influenced by reproductive history, culture, and the interactional context as well. Moreover, during the past few decades, the disability rights movement has been promoting more positive views of people with disabilities. This movement and its possible effect on attitudes will be discussed later in this paper.

Attitudes Toward Professionals.   Freidson (1970) has classically described the position of physicians in our society as one of "professional dominance." The dominant role generally includes elements of paternalism and control: The physician determines "what is best" for the patient and provides only as much information to the patient as is deemed necessary for the clinical management of the case. Patient acceptance of professional dominance has been noted in a number of studies. In the case of decisions regarding newborns with disabilities, Brinchmann et al. (reported in Tripp & McGregor, 2006) found that the majority of parents in their sample "respected the expertise of the doctor."

On the other hand, many writers have argued that professional dominance may be declining in today's society as part of a trend toward greater consumer control in the marketplace. Haug and Lavin (1983) reported over 20 years ago that the most important variable in consumerist challenges to medical authority was the experience of medical error. Thus, parents' predispositions today are likely to include exposure to both professional dominance and consumerism. The trend toward consumerism in health care will be discussed more fully shortly.

Medical Professionals' Predispositions
Attitudes Toward Disability.   Like parents, physicians and other medical professionals have been exposed to the stigma-based attitudes that prevail in society. The following quotes from pediatricians I interviewed in the late 1970s illustrate the negative attitudes that many have had toward children with disabilities:

> I don't enjoy it … I don't really enjoy a really handicapped child who comes in drooling, can't walk, and so forth …. Medicine is geared to the perfect human body. Something you can't do anything about challenges the doctor and reminds him of his own inabilities.

> As far as having [a child with a disability], I can't come up with anything good it does …. It's somebody's tragedy. I can find good things in practically anything – even dying – but birth defects are roaring tragedies.

>   Darling, 1979, p. 214

In a quantitative study using semantic differential ratings, Gething (1992) found that a large sample of health professionals devalued individuals with disabilities, and a number of older studies (Blackard & Barsch, 1982; Haug & Lavin, 1983; Sloper & Turner, 1991) have shown that professionals tend to overestimate the negative impact on the family of a child with a disability.

Some studies suggest that professionals' views of disability may be even more negative than those of parents. Streiner, Saigal, Burrows, Stoskopf, and Rosenbaum (2001) found that in the case of extremely low-birthweight infants, physicians were less likely than parents to favor intervention to save the child's life. In a similar study in Canada 10 years earlier, Lee, Penner, and Cox (1991) had found that nurses were even less likely than physicians to favor treatment.

However, like parents, medical professionals are influenced by personal experience, as well as by professional training and societal stigma. Symbolic interaction theory would suggest that personal experience continues to play the important role in attitudes and behavior that was noted in Bosk's (1992) report of a "born again" Christian physician, whose personal views colored his decision in the case of an infant with an impairment. Similarly, in an older study, a pediatrician who had two siblings with spina bifida observed, "Maybe there is too much expectation these days that things are to be perfect. There is nothing inherently wrong with having to face problems in life" (Darling, 1977, p. 13).

Although many physicians have negative attitudes toward disability, these are overridden to some extent by medical training. Zussman (1997) notes a tendency toward overtreatment in life-and-death situations that is rooted in a medical culture that promotes treatment at all costs. In addition, fear of legal consequences may result in treatment that is in opposition to many physicians' personal preferences. Moreover, some physicians' attitudes may be changing as a result of newer training programs that promote positive attitudes toward individuals with disabilities (Darling & Peter, 1994). The current norm of treating most babies in the NICU seems to reflect these influences, rather than the personal preferences of most physicians.

Attitudes Toward Parents. Parsons (1951) classically described the role of the professional as characterized by the traits of universalism, functional specificity, and affective neutrality, among others. The parental role, on the other hand, can be characterized as particularistic, functionally diffuse, and affective. Although physicians must consider the needs of all of the children in their care, parents' concerns center on the needs of their particular child. When looking at the child, the physician may focus on the medical diagnosis and prognosis, while the parents are likely to see the child in holistic terms. As Bosk (1992, p. 109) wrote, "If physicians decontextualize infants into organ systems, parents recontextualize them as children in families." Finally, whereas physicians need to maintain some emotional distance from their patients, parents are clearly emotionally involved with their child. As a result of these differences, parents and physicians might not agree about the appropriateness of treatment in a particular case, and physicians may regard parents as being too irrational to make reasonable decisions about their children's treatment.

Training in professional dominance and a clinical perspective may also cause physicians to see parents as less knowledgeable and less competent than they are and to assume the need to take control of the decision-making situation. Paternalistic practices also derive from the belief that parents need to be "spared" the guilt that is likely to arise from taking responsibility for decision making. In older works, Gliedman and Roth (1980) and Guillemin and Holmstrom (1986) argued that the nature of the parent–professional encounter encouraged the professional to see the parent, in addition to the child, as the patient. They suggested that parents were expected to play the classic "sick role," that is, to be passive, cooperative, and in agreement with the decisions of the "experts." In a more recent study, Heimer and Staffen (1995) have suggested that in the NICU, parents who do not conform to the expectations of the staff are labeled as deviant.

However, a trend toward "family-centered care," based on consumerist principles, is also present in the health-care system today. Many physician-training programs have been attempting to educate medical students and residents to acknowledge the expertise of parents in the care of their children (Darling & Peter, 1994). As a result, more inclusive decision-making practices might be developing.

The Decision-Making Situation
As discussed above, both parents and medical staff have certain predispositions when they first enter the situation of having to make choices in the NICU. However, as symbolic interaction theory suggests, pre-existing definitions of the situation may change in the course of interaction. The interactional context in the NICU may serve to reinforce or to alter participants' initial definitions.

Although they may have certain predispositions based on their past experiences, parents commonly are in a state of anomie in the NICU environment. As my research (Darling, 1979) and that of others have shown, most parents anticipate the birth of a typical child and are not prepared for a child with disabilities. Moreover, the hospital in general and the NICU in particular are not familiar environments for most parents and, at least initially, they are not aware of the norms in those settings. Most parents of children with disabilities report experiencing either meaninglessness or powerlessness or both during the post-natal and early infancy periods, especially when a diagnosis and prognosis are not clear.

As a result of their need to define the situation and relieve their anomie, parents are likely to seek out and listen to the advice of "experts." Thus, professional dominance tends to be especially strong in these situations, and Lorber's (1971) early finding that most parents "agreed" with his recommendations *both for and against* treatment of children with spina bifida is not surprising.

A number of studies have looked directly at the interaction processes surrounding decision making in the NICU. Guillemin and Holmstrom (1986) found that physician dominance prevailed in the nursery they studied and that physicians used their authority to assure the behavioral compliance of nurses, even when nurses did not agree with a course of treatment. Anspach (1993, p. 96) found that parents were consulted only when treatment was to be discontinued, and, even then, "The actual, if sometimes unstated, aim of the conference with parents was to elicit their agreement to decisions staff had already made."

Anspach argues that the process of informing parents is one of obtaining assent rather than of informed consent. She describes various techniques for obtaining assent, such as appeal to the authority of technology. Similarly, Heimer (1999) notes medical control over the social construction of the decision-making situation. Moreover, the language used by medical staff is not always readily understood by parents, especially those with less education or from other cultures.

In addition to medical control, other aspects of the situation play a role in shaping treatment decisions. Guillemin and Holmstrom (1986) note the incremental nature of decision making; after treatment is begun, withdrawal is more difficult than continuation. Bosk (1992) suggests that the collective nature of professional decision making – decisions are made by a team rather than by an individual – enhances commitment to the decisions that are made. A team decision also creates a diffusion of responsibility, so that no staff member need "take the blame" for a controversial decision. He suggests further that the "public" nature of the nursery layout encourages treatment; babies in the NICU do not occupy private rooms out of sight of parents and staff. Thus, situational contingencies may strengthen the pro-treatment predispositions discussed earlier.

The discussion so far has focused on interaction within the NICU, especially interaction involving medical staff and parents. In some controversial cases, especially when staff and parents disagree, the case may be referred to a hospital ethics committee. Like the NICU, the meeting of an ethics committee is a social situation that takes place within a framework of predispositions and interactional contingencies. In a study done almost 20 years ago, Lo (1987, p. 48) showed how such committees "may fall victim to groupthink." Clearly, the relative status of various committee members, as well as the nature of the interaction that occurs, may play an important role in the decision-making outcome. Thus, understanding the sociological context helps to explain all aspects of the decision-making process, regardless of where it occurs.

Current Trends: Disability Rights and Consumerism

The preceding discussion included studies of attitudes and practices undertaken over the course of the past 30 years or so. During this period, two social movements relating to these attitudes and practices have been occurring. Whether these movements are having an effect on the nature of decision making in the NICU is an empirical question. In the next sections, I will describe the disability rights movement and the movement toward consumerism in health care and will speculate on the impact of these movements on the decision-making situation.

The Disability Rights Movement
The disability rights movement has been part of a shift from a medical model to a "social" model of disability (Oliver, 1996). The latter model views disability as a social construction rather than as a quality inherent in individuals. Proponents of the newer model reject the norms of the larger society that label disabilities as failings and persons with disabilities as morally inferior to "normals." Instead, they argue that disability is simply a form of human diversity, much like gender, race, or sexual orientation.

The disability rights movement has worked to change society to make it more accommodating to individuals with disabilities. In addition, the movement has promoted "disability pride" (Linton, 1998; Swain & French, 2000) in place of older, stigma-based identities and has worked to change public images of disability as tragedy. The movement regards disability as a social, not a personal, problem.

Many disability rights activists have been concerned about choices not to bear or not to treat children with disabilities (Blumberg, 1994; Asch, 1999). In their view, disability is not incompatible with a high quality of life. If this position were to become widely accepted in society, presumably more infants would receive life-saving treatment. Although the movement has achieved some notable legal successes, especially the Americans with Disabilities Act, passed in 1990, its influence on public opinion still appears limited. The high percentages noted earlier of women who choose to abort fetuses with impairments seem to attest to the failure of the pro-disability message to have reached a large audience. Even among people with disabilities, the continued acceptance of a medical model and rejection of disability pride appear common (Darling, 2003; Darling & Heckert, 2004). The disability rights movement may have more influence on the attitudes of the general public in the future; however, its message is in direct competition with that of "individualistic consumerism," which will be discussed at the end of the next section.

Consumerism in Health Care
Is Professional Dominance Decreasing?   As early as 1972, Reeder (1972) noted a shift away from professional dominance toward consumerism in health care. He attributed this shift to a number of factors, including the growth of bureaucracy in medicine and the growth of consumerism as a social movement. At about the same time, Sorenson (1974) argued that areas of uncertainty in clinical practice tend to decrease the status inequality between doctor and patient, because of the limits of medical expertise.

A number of studies in the 1980s indicated a marked decline in the public's confidence in and respect for physicians. One study (Betz & O'Connell, 1983) reported that in 1966, 72% of the public expressed confidence in doctors, but in 1975, only 43% expressed such confidence. Haug and Lavin (1983, p. 16) suggested that "in the dialectic of power relations, the increasing monopolization of medical knowledge and medical practice could only call forth a countervailing force in the form of patient consumerism."

Rodwin (1994) argues that several modern social movements, including the patients' rights, medical consumerism, women's health, and disability rights movements, have decreased professional dominance in some areas through the use of "voice" and "exit." Perhaps, as a result of the women's health movement, Zadoroznyj (2001) found strong evidence of patient consumerism in the form of expressed preferences for various treatment modalities in a sample of women receiving maternity care.

A number of writers have suggested that newer managed care plans have contributed to an erosion of trust in physicians (Glass, 1996). In the past, patient–physician relationships were more personal and holistic; patients may be more willing to challenge their doctors when their relationship is more externally controlled, time-limited, and anonymous.

As noted earlier, another trend that has promoted consumerism in the health-care system has been the movement among health-care providers toward "family-centered care" (Darling & Peter, 1994). The US Maternal Child Health Bureau and the American Academy of Pediatrics have been actively involved in initiatives to promote physician–family partnerships. Many medical education programs now include such consumerist elements as lectures by patients and visits to homes of families of children with disabilities.

Although many physicians have embraced patient (and parent) autonomy, some backlash against consumerism has occurred (Darling, 2000). Coulter (1997) notes several criticisms of shared decision making, including the argument that patients do not want to participate in decisions and that they may demand unnecessary or costly procedures, undermining the equitable allocation of health-care resources. Thus, some physicians today may still discourage parents from playing a consumerist role.

Whether consumerism in health care has in fact increased during the past two decades is an empirical question. Based on an analysis of data from large samples, Pescosolido et al. (2001) found some decrease in confidence in physicians between 1976 and 1998. However, over 90% of the 1998 sample still expressed confidence in their doctors. The authors did note some socioeconomic status (SES) differences, with respondents of higher status expressing less confidence than those of lower status. Hibbard and Weeks (1987) had reported similar findings in an earlier study. Most of their respondents had a high degree of faith in and dependency on their physicians and did not exhibit consumerist behaviors. However, the younger they were and the higher their education level was, the more likely their respondents were to be consumerist. Although the relationship was weak, Rosenthal and Schlesinger (2002) also found an association between education and consumerism, with college-educated individuals more likely to blame their physicians for error than those with less education. In a review of several studies, Hall, Dugan, Zheng, and Mishra (2001) found that age had a modest, positive association with trust in physicians.

Thus, the literature suggests that the trend toward medical consumerism is limited in modern society and that professional dominance is still common. However, among demographic groups, younger people of higher

SES, especially those with higher levels of education, appear to be somewhat more likely to espouse consumerist attitudes and practices. Thus, with some notable exceptions, most life-and-death decisions in the nursery probably continue to reflect the wishes of the physicians involved.

Recent Examples of Parental Decision Making. A review of parental accounts written during the 1990s and 2000s provides evidence for the existence of both reliance on professional dominance and consumerist entrepreneurship undertaken to challenge professional authority.

A decision to challenge the termination of life support: A recent case that has received media attention is that of Charlotte Wyatt, a child born prematurely in Great Britain in 2003. A website created by friends of the family (http://charlottewyatt.blogspot.com), which includes entries by the parents and their friends, describes the case and the parents' ongoing battle with medical professionals to reverse a "do not resuscitate" order. The parents' consumerism in this case seems to result from strong religious faith (prayers are periodically requested), physical evidence of medical error (Charlotte's development has clearly surpassed the early, negative prognosis), and strong social support, largely as a result of media attention. Significantly, the family and friends appear to have been exposed to and to have come to espouse a disability rights perspective, as this February 25, 2006 posting in response to a judge's non-treatment decision suggests:

> After all, she was Charlotte, and Charlotte ... Charlotte might always be a disabled child. She might never be quite normal, and her joys might never be quite the same as ours. Disabled people aren't like the rest of us, and when they are sick ... they have to be allowed to die .... What has our grand world come to when we can do this and still walk the streets without shame?

Charlotte's case appears to be quite unusual, as most parental reports in the case of a prognosis of poor quality of life suggest that accepting the professionally made recommendation to terminate life support is more often the norm.

Decisions to terminate life support: With one notable exception, most parental reports of decisions to terminate life support suggest that these parental decisions were made with the blessing of the professionals involved. In a blog entitled, "Patriside" (http://fatherknowsnothing.blogspot.com, 2004, p. 3), a father reports making a decision to end the life of his newborn son, Noble, after receiving this prognosis:

> I asked [the doctor] ... was there any chance at all he could be rehabilitated in the future if we decided to keep him on life support, and what kind of care we'd be looking at if we held out for that hope.

His demeanor was grim. Constant care, he said, 24/7, millions of dollars over the course of his lifetime, a lifetime, he added, that would never be assured certain survival and no rehabilitation would ever improve his condition. If we decided to pull life support, he would not suffer, he said: Noble's brain was far too damaged for that.

Noble's family's decision was based on his predicted poor quality of life. Other parents who make similar decisions after receiving a negative prognosis justify their actions as "ending the suffering" of their children:

Because if I ever went back to that moment I would have done the same thing over .... That was my baby boy there ... suffering ... I'm sure any mother would do that. (www.shareyourstory.org/webx?14@609.LkpiaHv2ItL.6@.eedbe6b/6, p. 1, posted March 13, 2006)

Late Tuesday morning, we had a heart to heart with Lauren's doctor and we came to the decision to take her off of life support. We could not prolong her life if she were going to be suffering just because we couldn't bear to let her go. Remarkably, this was not a difficult decision to make. We felt we were making our decisions with her best interest in mind. (www.shareyourstory.org/webx?50@609.LkpiaHv2ItL.50@.eedb342, p. 1, posted March 10, 2006)

Given the likely persistence of professional dominance in the NICU, the analysis of a case in which a parent challenged a professional decision can help to elucidate the factors that promote consumerism. The case is taken from an autobiographical account written 10 years ago by a mother (Alecson, 1995). Because the case is presented in a book-length account, more information is available about the decision-making process than in similar accounts found in blogs. The parents, Deborah and Lowell, are college educated and appear to be from upper middle class families. They live in Manhattan. The child, Andrea, is in a NICU as a result of perinatal asphyxia (oxygen deprivation during delivery). Tests indicate a high degree of brain injury. Believing that Andrea's projected quality of life is poor, the parents request the withdrawal of nourishment in order to hasten her death. The hospital ethics committee refuses to honor the parents' request, and the parents engage in various activities to secure the outcome they desire. Deborah clearly had a consumerist orientation even before Andrea's birth. She explains her decision to use a midwife: "Why should I pay an obstetrician four thousand dollars when we could pay a midwife half that and, most important, be the ones in control?" (p. 4).

Eventually, on the advice of her father, Deborah stops visiting Andrea to decrease her attachment. Her father's wife says, "Andrea doesn't exist ... the Andrea you wanted, who moved inside of you, is already dead" (p. 102). She and Deborah's father encourage Deborah to "get on with [her] life." Deborah describes her reaction after talking with a mother in a similar situation: "My sympathy was more for Jeanie [the mother] than for Kelly [the baby]. It was the same pity I had felt for myself, the self I had been when I, too, felt compelled to see my baby" (p. 155). In addition to support for her position from family, Deborah reads books like *Playing God in the Nursery* that reinforce that position.

The doctors' prognosis for Andrea, if she lives, is that she would be "severely to moderately developmentally delayed." Deborah clearly does not envision such a life as one of quality. She writes, "Andrea was fated to an existence of utter impoverishment" (p. 76). Even in her discussion of the Baby Doe case, which involved a child with Down syndrome, a disability generally associated with a better quality of life, Deborah expresses her support for the parents who refused treatment. When Andrea finally dies, Deborah's therapist says to her, "Well, her dying was something she did for you and Lowell, to pave the way for the next baby" (p. 177).

Deborah's consumerism clearly arose from her predispositions regarding professional dominance and the negative aspects of disability. As a well-educated, urban, middle-class woman, she no doubt had been exposed to feminist ideas as well. Her predispositions were reinforced through her interactions with supportive significant others, resulting in an increasing commitment to her non-treatment decision.

Yet, another theme emerges from this case as well, one of individualistic consumerism. Certainly, Deborah's dread of life with a severely disabled child is understandable. However, her desire to "get on with her life" (and have a "normal" baby) seems at times to be her most salient concern. In this respect she is like many modern (typically upper-SES) women who view children as they view other consumer goods – as perfectible commodities, a phenomenon Rothman (1986b) described as "commodification." Today's media are filled with stories about sperm selection to produce "designer babies" and wrongful life suits when children are born with disabilities. The quest for perfectible parenthood is reminiscent of the individualistic consumerism described by Schor (1998), which is characterized by seemingly insatiable demands for more and better products of all kinds. Schor argues that consumerism of this nature pervades modern society and is spreading from the upper classes to those of lower SES.

Although recent research is lacking, some early studies (Holt, 1958; Mercer, 1965; Darling, 2000) suggest that upper-SES parents are less accepting of children with disabilities than those of lower status. Khoshnood et al. (2006) report lower rates of prenatal diagnosis and pregnancy termination among lower-SES parents than among those of higher status, but suggest that both access issues and preferences may contribute to this finding. At least some well-educated parents have embraced the parenting of children with major disabilities. For example, Landsman (1998) describes her life with a child whose impairments are similar to Andrea's, in positive terms, and Berube (1996) writes about the joys of living with a child with Down syndrome. Ironically, the parents who are perhaps best able to care for children with disabilities, at least in terms of financial resources and knowledge, may be the least likely to be willing to do so.

CONCLUSION

As in the past, whether future babies with disabilities will be treated or not will be contingent on the predispositions of the various stakeholders, as well as on the interactions that take place between stakeholders and others, both within and outside of the nursery setting. The preceding analysis suggests that the major predispositions that have played a role in decision making have been professional dominance/consumerism and attitudes toward disability.

Recent social movements have led some to suggest that consumerism is increasing and that attitudes toward disability are becoming more favorable. However, empirical evidence indicates that professional dominance in health care is still strong in most sectors of society and that disability is still viewed negatively by many people. Such findings suggest the potential for conflict in the decision-making situation. Studies have shown that a pro-treatment norm exists in the NICU today. Yet, that norm stands in sharp contrast to prevailing attitudes about disability, which are shared by both parents and NICU staff.

Because of the level of parental anomie that prevails in the neonatal period, even "informed" consent to treatment or non-treatment will continue to be heavily dependent on past experience, coupled with interactions following the birth of the child, which take place within a relatively short time frame. Such parents are rarely well informed about the true nature of day-to-day life with a child with a disability. The strength of professional dominance may result in the acquiescence of most parents to intervention to save their children's lives. At the same time, a minority of well-educated, consumerist parents may continue to challenge professional authority. In our individualistic society, the desire for fulfillment defined in terms of personal achievement may be strong enough to withstand any challenge from a disability rights movement that promotes the value of life with "imperfection." If, as Schor has suggested, individualistic consumerism is "trickling down" to all segments of society, pro-treatment norms may be challenged more frequently in the future. Furthermore, this trend may be magnified by the tendency of younger people to be more consumerist than older ones. However, as the case of Charlotte suggests, consumerism may also result from a strong *anti*-individualistic value orientation that appears to characterize a minority of the population.

These conclusions about decision-making trends are based on limited empirical evidence and are, hence, quite exploratory. Continued large-scale research is needed to document whether a trend toward consumerism in health care in general and in NICUs in particular, in fact, exists. Future large-scale studies need to include physicians as well as consumers as respondents, in order to determine whether their attitudes and practices are changing as a result of recent trends toward family-centered care. Because of the continuing importance of professional dominance, understanding the attitudes of physicians may be even more valuable in predicting outcomes than understanding the attitudes of patients and their families.

Updated qualitative studies are needed as well. Because of the nature of the decision-making process, cross-sectional studies cannot provide insight into the interactional factors that operate when parents are actually in a decision-making situation. Although the cases described on the Internet and in Alecson's book suggest some interesting hypotheses about the influences on decision making of both pre-existing definitions of the situation and interactional contingencies, research with demographically diverse populations is needed to clarify the processes through which these decisions are made. Because of the importance of sociological research in providing insights into ethical decision making, research of this nature is urgently needed.

REFERENCES

Alecson, D. G. (1995). *Lost lullaby*. Berkeley: The University of California Press.
Anspach, R. R. (1993). *Deciding who lives: Fateful choices in the intensive-care nursery*. Berkeley: University of California Press.
Asch, A. (1986). On the question of Baby Doe. *Health/PAC Bulletin, 16*(6), 8–10.
Asch, A. (1999). Prenatal diagnosis and selective abortion: A challenge to practice and policy. *American Journal of Public Health, 89*(11), 1649–1657.
Berube, M. (1996). *Life as we know it: A father, a family, and an exceptional child*. New York: Vintage.
Betz, M., & O'Connell, L. (1983). Changing doctor-patient relationships and the rise in concern for accountability. *Social Problems, 31*, 84–95.

Blackard, M. K., & Barsch, E. T. (1982). Parents' and professionals' perceptions of the handicapped child's impact on the family. *TASH Journal*, *7*, 62–70.

Blumberg, L. (1994). Eugenics and reproductive choice. In: B. Shaw (Ed.), *The ragged edge* (pp. 218–229). Louisville, KY: The Advocado Press.

Bosk, C. L. (1992). *All god's mistakes: Genetic counseling in a pediatric hospital.* Chicago: The University of Chicago Press.

Clark, F. I. (1994). Intensive care treatment decisions: The roots of our confusion. *Pediatrics*, *94*(1), 98–101.

Coulter, A. (1997). Partnerships with patients: The pros and cons of shared clinical decision-making. *Journal of Health Services Research and Policy*, *2*(2), 112–121.

Darling, R. B. (1977). Parents, physicians, and spina bifida: A study of values in conflict. *Hastings Center Report*, *7*(4), 10–14.

Darling, R. B. (1979). *Families against society: A study of reactions to children with brith defects.* Beverly Hills, CA: Sage.

Darling, R. B. (2000). *The Partnership model in human services: Sociological foundations and practices.* New York: Kluwer/Plenum.

Darling, R. B. (2003). Toward a model of changing disability identities: A proposed typology and research agenda. *Disability and Society*, *18*, 881–895.

Darling, R. B., & Peter, M. I. (Eds). (1994). *Families, physicians, and children with special health needs: Collaborative medical education models.* Westport, CT: Greenwood.

Darling, R. B., & Heckert, D. A. (2004). Disability and opportunity: A preliminary test of a typology of orientations toward disability. Annual Meetings of the American Sociological Association, San Francisco.

Freidson, E. (1970). *Professional dominance.* Chicago: Aldine.

Gething, L. (1992). Judgements by health professionals of personal characteristics of people with a visible physical disability. *Social Science and Medicine*, *34*(7), 809–815.

Glass, R. M. (1996). The impact of managed care on patients' trust in medical care and their physicians. *Journal of the American Medical Association*, *275*(21), 1693–1697.

Gliedman, J., & Roth, W. (1980). *The unexpected minority: Handicapped children in America.* New York: Harcourt Brace Jovanovich.

Goffman, E. (1963). *Stigma: Notes on the management of spoiled identity.* Englewood Cliffs, NJ: Prentice Hall.

Guillemin, J. H., & Holmstrom, L. L. (1986). *Mixed blessings: Intensive care for newborns.* New York: Oxford University Press.

Hall, M. A., Dugan, E., Zheng, B., & Mishra, A. K. (2001). Trust in physicians and medical institutions: What is it, can it be measured, and does it matter? *The Millbank Quarterly*, *79*(4), 613–639.

Haug, M., & Lavin, B. (1983). *Consumerism in medicine: Challenging physician authority.* Beverly Hills: Sage.

Heimer, C. A. (1999). Competing institutions: Law, medicine, and family in neonatal intensive care. *Law and Society Review*, *33*(1), 17–66.

Heimer, C. A., & Staffen, L. R. (1995). Interdependence and reintegrative social control: Labeling and reforming "inappropriate" parents in neonatal intensive care units. *American Sociological Review*, *60*(5), 635–654.

Hibbard, J. H., & Weeks, E. C. (1987). Consumerism in health care: Prevalence and predictors. *Medical Care*, *25*(11), 1019–1032.

Holt, K. S. (1958). Home care of severely retarded children. *Pediatrics*, *22*, 744–755.

Khoshnood, B., De Vigan, C., Vodovar, V., Bréart, G., Goffinet, F., & Blondel, B. (2006). Advances in medical technology and creation of disparities: The case of Down syndrome. *American Journal of Public Health*, *96*(12), 2139–2141.

Kipnis, K., & Williamson, G. M. (1984). Nontreatment decisions for severely compromised newborns. *Ethics*, *95*(1), 90–111.

Landsman, G. H. (1998). Reconstructing motherhood in the age of "perfect" babies: Mothers of infants and toddlers with disabilities. *Signs: Journal of Women in Culture and Society*, *24*(1), 69–99.

Lantos, J. D., Tyson, J. E., Allen, A., Frader, J., Hack, M., Korones, S., Merenstein, G., Paneth, N., Poland, R. L., Saigal, S., Stevenson, D., Truog, R. D., & Van Marter, L. J. (1994). Withholding and withdrawing life sustaining treatment in neonatal intensive care: Issues for the 1990s. *Archives of Disease in Childhood*, *1*, 218–223.

Lee, S. K., Penner, P. I., & Cox, M. (1991). Comparison of the attitudes of health care professionals and parents toward active treatment of very low birth weight infants. *Pediatrics*, *88*(1), 110–115.

Levin, B. W. (1990). International perspectives on treatment choice in neonatal intensive care units. *Social Science and Medicine*, *30*(8), 901–912.

Linton, S. (1998). *Claiming disability: Knowledge and identity*. New York: NYU Press.

Lo, B. (1987). Behind closed doors: Promises and pitfalls of ethics committees. *The New England Journal of Medicine*, *317*(1), 46–49.

Longmore, P. K. (2003). *Why I burned my book and other essays on disability*. Philadelphia: Temple University Press.

Lorber, J. (1971). Results of treatment of myelomeningocele. *Developmental Medicine and Child Neurology*, *13*, 279–303.

Mansfield, C., Hopfer, S., & Marteau, T. M. (1999). Termination rates after prenatal diagnosis of Down syndrome, spina bifida, anencephaly, and Turner and Klinefelter syndromes: A systematic literature review. *Prenatal Diagnosis*, *19*, 808–812.

McHaffie, H. E., Laing, I. A., Parker, M., & McMillan, J. (2005). Deciding for imperilled newborns: Medical authority or parental autonomy? *Journal of Medical Ethics*, *27*, 104–109.

Mercer, J. R. (1965). Social system perspective and clinical perspective: Frames of reference for understanding career patterns of persons labeled as mentally retarded. *Social Problems*, *13*, 18–34.

Oliver, M. (1996). *Understanding disability: From theory to practice*. New York: St. Martin's Press.

Parsons, T. (1951). *The social system*. New York: Free Press.

Pescosolido, B. A., Tuch, S. A., & Martin, J. K. (2001). The profession of medicine and the public: Examining Americans' changing confidence in physician authority from the beginning of the 'health care crisis' to the ear of health care reform. *Journal of Health and Social Behavior*, *42*(1), 1–16.

Protection of Handicapped Newborns. (1986). *US Commission on Civil Rights* (Vol. II, pp. 180–202). Washington, DC.

Rapp, R. (1998). Refusing prenatal diagnosis: The meanings of bioscience in a multicultural world. *Science, Technology, and Human Values*, *23*(1), 45–70.

Reeder, L. G. (1972). The patient-client as a consumer: Some observations on the changing professional-client relationship. *Journal of Health and Social Behavior*, *13*, 406–412.

Rodwin, M. A. (1994). Patient accountability and quality of care: Lessons from medical consumerism and the patients' rights, women's health and disability rights movements. *American Journal of Law and Medicine, XX*(1 and 2), 147–167.

Rosenthal, M., & Schlesinger, M. (2002). Not afraid to blame: The neglected role of blame attribution in medical consumerism and some implications for health policy. *The Millbank Quarterly, 80*(1), 41–95.

Rothman, B. K. (1986a). On the question of Baby Doe. *Health/PAC Bulletin, 16*(6), 11–13.

Rothman, B. K. (1986b). *The tentative pregnancy: Prenatal diagnosis and the future of motherhood.* New York: Viking.

Schor, J. B. (1998). *The overspent American: Why we want what we don't need.* New York: Harper Perennial.

Shapiro, J. (1994). *No pity: People with disabilities forging a new civil rights movement.* New York: Times Books.

Sloper, P., & Turner, S. (1991). Parental and professional views of the needs of families with a child with severe physical disability. *Counseling Psychology Quarterly, 4*, 323–330.

Sorenson, J. (1974). Biomedical innovation, uncertainty, and doctor-patient interaction. *Journal of Health and Social Behavior, 15*, 366–374.

Streiner, D. L., Saigal, S., Burrows, E., Stoskopf, B., & Rosenbaum, P. (2001). Attitudes of parents and health care professionals toward active treatment of extremely premature infants. *Pediatrics, 108*(1), 152–158.

Swain, J., & French, S. (2000). Towards an affirmation model of disability. *Disability and Society, 15*, 569–582.

Tripp, J., & McGregor, D. (2006). Withholding and withdrawing of life sustaining treatment in the newborn. *Archives of Disease in Childhood, 91*, F67–F71.

Tyson, J. (1995). Evidence-based ethics and the care of premature infants. *The Future of Children, 5*(1), 197–213.

Weir, R. F. (1984). *Selective nontreatment of handicapped newborns: Moral dilemmas in neonatal medicine.* New York: Oxford University Press.

Zadoroznyj, M. (2001). Birth and the 'reflexive consumer': Trust, risk and medical dominance in obstetric encounters. *Journal of Sociology, 37*(2), 117–139.

Zuckoff, M. (2002). *Choosing Naia: A family's journey.* Boston: Beacon Press.

Zussman, R. (1997). Sociological perspectives on medical ethics and decision-making. *Annual Review of Sociology, 23*, 171–189.

PART II: THE SOCIOLOGY OF A WORKING BIOETHICS: PRIVATE NARRATIVES

The four papers in this section offer a sociology of 'bioethics at work', the ways that bioethics as a discipline or approach comes into medical care. One of the concerns we, as editors of this volume, bring to the issue is the appropriateness of the export of American 'bioethics' both in its form and its content. It is not only the creation of 'ethics committees', but also the rewriting of practice in accord with American principles that we find troubling. One of the nurses in Kohlen's study talks about 'learning the language of bioethics'. Brought into committee rooms to 'do ethics' requires of practitioners a certain way of defining both biomedical practice and ethics, reflected in the 'language' one has to learn.

Two of the papers in this section focus on the growing institutionalization of hospital ethics committees, and it is probably no accident that those are both German papers. American-style bioethics are being exported around the world, along with American-style biomedical practice. Germany has its own troubled relationship to biomedical ethical practice and is particularly self-conscious about that. While Americans largely ignore their own unsavory history of bad behavior by medicine, in research and in practice, Germany has not had the luxury of doing so, but must confront it at every turn. The German-speaking world takes issues of bioethics seriously and somewhat self-consciously.

Helen Kohlen's work is based on research in three German hospitals, where she did both participant observation and interviews. The paper begins by offering, particularly for those not well versed in bioethics, a good review of issues of nursing care, and the history of 'an ethics of care', which has developed separately from bioethics.

While most of bioethics focuses on what Guilleman and Gillam, in their paper in this section call 'the big ticket items', the dramas of new technologies and 'new questions', the reality of hospital life and medical practice are usually far removed from all of that. Sociologists who go 'into the field' to do their research see the daily-ness of medical practice, not the drama, but the simple things. While bioethicists may worry about tube feedings, doctors, and particularly nurses, as Kohlen shows, are looking at problems of ordinary eating. Bioethicists are drawn to new machines and technologies: Nurses worry about the ethics of using the sleeping patient's belly to warm blood. Hospitals clamor for money and space for new machinery and technology – but a cardboard box with a cloth cover, pulled out of a closet, becomes a makeshift sacred space for care of the dying. New wings may be built for elaborate new machinery, but in hospitals all over the world, patients and families are shunted into corners, even bathrooms for dying. It is the nature of bioethics to trivialize these problems, while focusing on 'new dilemmas'.

At the same time, bioethics has not been spectacularly successful in 'resolving' the new dilemmas, in uncovering answers to the questions it raises. Armin Nassehi, Imhild Saake and Katharina Mayr, also of Germany, make a rather startling claim in their paper: This absence of success *is* the success.

Nassehi, Saake and Mayr combine a very data-rich presentation with a deeply theoretical approach. They are looking at the hospital ethics committee as a microcosm of postmodern society. Rather than seeking an integrative vision, a systems theory that explains the interlocking workings of the system as a whole – be it the hospital or the larger society – these authors argue for the disconnect, the disintegration of the whole *as being itself* the system. It is precisely the ability to separate out, to create a specific time and place for a discussion of 'ethics' that is not integrated into clinical practice, that makes the ethics committees work. They work by creating their own little world, their own culture, separate from clinical practice. A 'society of presents' is able to disconnect presences and do without a strong idea of integration.

Wildly divergent views, they show us, are presented and celebrated within the ethics committee. The goal is not to reach consensus, not to decide what is right, but precisely to avoid that. The celebration of difference, whether religiously, occupationally or 'personally' based, mitigates against a notion of a "right" decision.

Ethics committees serve as a place where the authenticity of each perspective – medical, religious, nursing, patients, ethical, economic or other – is what really matters. In the space of the committee, decisions can be reached, papers written, 'fictions of consensus' achieved. What makes one a good member of the committee team, we see in these papers, is being flexible, being able to see other perspectives, and acknowledge other points of view. Within the space of the committee, different power dynamics are supposed to open up. The lovely description of the different physical spaces that Kohlen offers in her paper shows the significance of, for example, having an actual 'round table' for so-called round table discussions. The committees work *qua* committees, if all are heard, if all are equalized. But that equality, of patient and nurse and doctor, of theologian and patient representative and surgeon – all that equality stops at the committee room door.

And then clinical practice picks right up in another space, another present, apparently unaffected by the work of the committee.

Issues of 'communication' arise in all four of these papers. It is almost as if simply not being able to communicate, not being able to 'hear' all of the varied perspectives, was the ethical problem, and communication itself the solution. The naïve view would have us think that reaching the 'right' decision was the goal of ethical discussion. What we see in the work in this section, research on these various 'ethics committees', is that the very idea of a 'right decision' needs to be dispensed with quickly in favor of 'hearing all the voices', opening up the discussion.

Within ethics as a discipline or, as Nassehi, Saake and Mayr prefer to call it, a 'science', certain kinds of problems are permitted to arise; others are entirely outside of the imaginable realm. The naïve view would also see the apparent lack of function as the problem: What *are* we doing here, Kohlen's paper asks. But perhaps, as her work shows and as Nassehi, Saake and Mayr drive home, that lack of function may well be the solution. By moving the discussion away from good or bad decisions and practices to a focus on process, on hearing different perspectives, the committees serve their function.

Any look at hospital committees is bound to uncover the power dynamics between occupations within the hospital. Hospitals are remarkably hierarchical institutions. And as within most hierarchies, people at the top tend not to see the structural forces which benefit them. Doctors may see the lesser power of nurses as if the problem were located within nursing, even within the personalities of the nurses themselves. In the Nassehi paper, we hear a doctor describing nursing staff as having a 'lack of competence' to position themselves as speakers. But we also hear him describe the committee as consisting of an assortment of "Professors" and "poor Mrs. Bauer," the only nurse, implicitly recognizing the structural power issues.

These are not simply the issues of gender and power one deals with repeatedly in hospital settings, as Kohlen's paper shows us. These issues are also deeply entwined with the different values and practices that nursing brings as a discipline. An 'ethic of caring' is itself a kind of ethics that has little place in conventional ethical discourse, that is to say, the work of 'biomedical' ethics as it has been captured by the philosophers, scientists and physicians who dominate the discussion.

And it is not just doctors vs. nurses – ordinary, front-line workers include doctors as well as nurses and a wide assortment of technicians who do caring work, or perhaps even more fundamentally, who do *daily* work, the ordinary work of practice far removed from the 'big ticket' ethical issues. A hospital or a society might feel the need of convening a committee to decide what to do with some elaborate new technology, but ethical issues confront workers in a far less dramatic way every day, perhaps every moment, in medical settings.

While the other papers in this section use the sociological methods of ethnography and other qualitative techniques, Marilys Guilleman and Lynn Gillam, in their paper, take the newer approach, increasingly used within bioethics, of narrative analysis. In a more standard sociological work, Hannah's story would have been put together out of interviews and observations. In this research approach, Hannah is clearly the author of her own story. That does not mean that the researchers and Hannah would necessarily agree on just what the story is, just what it is that Hannah is saying. Interpretation and analysis remain in the hands of the sociological researcher/writer: Theirs is the voice of authority. But the data they analyze are neither the raw experience of Hannah, as observations would try to stick closely to, nor the mediated responses to an experience as an interview would seek to draw forth, but the story, the narrative, as composed by Hannah herself.

Guilleman and Gillam provide us a framework for practice: sociological practice and perhaps bioethical practice as well. Narrative analysis is a research approach. But using it provides a focus for bioethical work, as does their use of 'ethical mindfulness'. In this sense, narrative analysis is very much part of the 'giving voice' project that the hospital ethics committees are engaged in. Whose narrative do we request? By asking Hannah, a technician in a radiology department, and getting from her a narrative of her earlier years, a voice from 'below' is brought forth: a junior member of a relatively subservient team. A newly qualified technician in radiology cannot shape patient care; her only option would be to withdraw from the scene if she felt deeply that what was happening was wrong.

By giving us a retrospective story, one that is quite a few years old, we are learning not only about the positioning of junior workers in health care, but also the process of socialization and acculturation that occurs. Rather than becoming more solidly a 'member of the team', Hannah becomes more reflective, more open to different voices: Acquiring precisely the 'flexibility' that Nassehi, Saake and Mayr claim mark the work of 'good' bioethics committee members.

Narratives, Guilleman and Gillam claim, and we feel they demonstrate nicely, are pathways to ethical mindfulness: By creating a story, by narrating our lives, we pull the thread of ethical concerns through the tale. How else do individuals shape their understanding of bioethics in their work?

It would be impossible, at least in the American context, to discuss bioethics for five minutes, let alone for several hundred pages, without bringing up Beauchamp and Childress, and the four 'principles' they use to discuss bioethical decision making. This is an approach to bioethics that has become so widely used as to almost parody itself. Every decision, every conflict, every ethical discussion can be placed on a 'grid' of the four principles: respect for autonomy, nonmaleficence, beneficence and justice. But like a well-worn joke, the punch line is clear as soon as the set up has been made: Each principle will be considered, and autonomy will be decisive.

Daniel Morrison, in his study of genetic counselors, the final paper in this section, rightly points out that Beauchamp and Childress did not intend that autonomy would be used as a trump card, but it has most assuredly worked that way. It often seems to be the case, if one goes to bioethics meetings, or reads the literature of bioethics, that if the patient has made a decision, if the patient is acting 'autonomously', then all is right with the world.

Nowhere is this more true than in reproductive genetic counseling. Acting in accord with the larger project of prenatal genetic testing requires being willing to abort affected fetuses. If no women aborted, or even if most women did not abort affected fetuses, it would be hard to imagine how or why genetic counseling would continue to occur in pregnancy, and because abortion is (in the American context most certainly and dramatically) an 'ethically fraught' decision, the client must come to that decision on her own. Any individual patient/client/pregnant woman can 'opt out', can refuse the counseling or the testing, or refuse the abortion – and the very presence of some women refusing attests to the autonomy of the clients.

But people do not necessarily arrive in medical settings, even in genetic counseling offices, ready to act autonomously. They often arrive uncertain of why they are there, frightened, intimidated, hoping for help. The task then of the genetic counselor is to transform that client into someone ready to exercise her autonomy. Morrison, in his interviews with 10 genetic counselors, shows the techniques that they use to accomplish the necessary transformation. The session must end with the client 'making a decision'. The counselor shapes the interaction towards that end, with a series of tasks, from 'contracting', or setting goals for the session, through providing information and options, translating between medical and lay language, reflecting, providing empathy and support – support, of course, for the decision that the client has arrived at autonomously.

The intense manipulation of the client through these stages is ironic at root: to create an autonomous being should not, one would think, require a lot of manipulation. Yet of course any parent knows that it does. The 'paternalism' that is required to create an independent, autonomous person who is beyond paternalism is echoed in this situation of genetic counseling. The counselor shapes the session, and thus shapes the role available for the others, creating the autonomous client she needs to have.

These four papers, taken on their own, hew closest to one of the most traditional uses of sociology: to gain an understanding of the larger contexts in which individuals live their lives and do their work. That itself is valuable and good work. But these papers do not stand on their own in this volume: They grow out of the historical development of bioethics and bring us towards the uses of bioethics in reshaping both public policy and biomedical practice.

Barbara Katz Rothman
Editor

"WHAT ARE WE REALLY DOING HERE?" JOURNEYS INTO HOSPITAL ETHICS COMMITTEES IN GERMANY: NURSES' PARTICIPATION AND THE(IR) MARGINALIZATION OF CARE

Helen Kohlen

"... You do not only have to learn in any case,
what needs to be said about a subject matter,
but how you can talk about it. You always
have to learn the method how to approach it."

— Ludwig Wittgenstein, Colours

1. INTRODUCTION

The tradition of medicine has until now been characterized by an aspiration to provide as complete as possible a service of care to the populations to which it owes responsibility. The same holds for nursing and caring practices, but the tradition is loosening. Despite the collective assumption that medical and nursing practice rests on solid grounds of knowledge and is

Bioethical Issues, Sociological Perspectives
Advances in Medical Sociology, Volume 9, 91–128
Copyright © 2008 by Elsevier Ltd.
ISSN: 1057-6290/doi:10.1016/S1057-6290(07)09004-3

framed by a caring ethos, change in practice not only has typically come about in a complex and diffuse fashion, but has also come along with sacrifices, losses and deficits.

Managed care, evolved and developed in the United States, recently implemented in Germany, provides one example that promises efficiencies by eliminating assumed "wasteful" and "unnecessary" care. Charles Bosk and Joel Frader remark: "Other wholesale changes in practice follow changes in fashion among leaders in health-care professions prior to concrete demonstration of benefit" (1998, p. 94). What the authors once remarked for the situation in the United States can now be said for the changing processes in German health care.

The growth of ethics committees is another new phenomenon in Germany. Ethics committees were created in the United States in order to discuss not only ethical research questions but also problems in clinical care. The need for ethics consultation is generally explained by technical progress that has changed health care. Whether these changes refer to medical research or to clinical work cannot simply be explained by technical progress, but they are often reactions to external economic and socio-political forces as well as to ethical manoeuvres themselves.

In her work *Moral Boundaries: A Political Argument for an Ethics of Care*, Joan Tronto has reminded her readers of the fact that caring issues are discussed as if they were only of trivial concerns, although "... humans need to be cared for, like human infants are not capable of caring for themselves, and the sick, infirm, and dead humans need to be taken care of" (1994, p. 110). Within professional health care, nurses are the ones who do most of the care work. Liaschenko (1993, 1997) and Rodney (1993, 1997) have investigated the ethical concerns of practicing nurses and noted in their separate empirical research the invisibility of their conflicts when doing care work. Do these conflicts and concerns find a place within the bioethical debate? And more precisely, are issues of care presented in hospital ethics committees?

Before answering these questions based on empirical findings of this research project, the broader context as well as the way this matter of concern is approached, needs to be clarified first.

1.1. Changes in German Health Care and Modern Bioethics

In Germany, along with economization processes in health care, modern bioethics as a discipline as well as a practice has become established within the last 15 years. With regard to burning issues, one impulse for the evolution of applied ethics in German health care arose from a widely spread discussion of moral problems with regard to reproductive technology, gene therapy, embryo research or intensive care at the end of life.

In the dark light of German Nazi history, euthanasia has been an incessantly crucial issue of bioethical discourse and has just become the dominant point at issue in governmental committees within the context of the use of living wills. The fact that difficult end-of-life questions are now answered by a demand for written forms of living wills to secure patients' autonomy is a remarkable change in medical and nursing practice. The fact that the debate on the use of living wills has now prompted governmental intervention is another remarkable turning point: Ethics at the bedside has never been regulated by political authorities before.

On a micro-political level, the new regulations are now discussed by local ethics forums, termed Institutional Ethics Committees (IECs), Clinical Ethics Committees (CECs) or Hospital Ethics Committees (HECs), as they have evolved in the United States in the 1970s. Such committees have been rapidly growing, especially since the German Accreditation Organisations of Health Care have demanded that hospitals should have policies and procedures to cope with ethical issues.

1.2. Understanding the Idea and the Model of Hospital Ethics Committees

Besides taking responsibility for staying informed on major bioethical issues with clinical relevance like living wills, HECs serve to develop, review and apply the ethics policies or guidelines in, and of, the institution. In hospitals, the most common form of ethics policy is the "Do Not Resuscitate" (DNR) policy, which sets out the institution's guidelines for withholding or withdrawing life-sustaining treatment (Cranford & Doudera, 1984; Ross, 1986). Moreover, HECs are responsible for case reviews. The kind of review varies. The committee can be directly involved in prospective case review and becomes a consultant to assist in the ongoing management of care of patients. Committees usually also offer retrospective case review. Then the goal is to determine whether and how the case could have been better coped with. In addition, these committees play an educational role. Education involves mediation techniques and learning theoretical frameworks as well as the training to use a special "model of ethical decision-making" in order to discuss an ethical issue reasonably (Bartels, Youngner, & Levine, 1994). With regard to actors, such committees consist of small groups of people, professionals as well as laypersons, who meet on a regular basis to address so-called ethical issues that emerge within the health-care institution. Those people are mainly clinical professionals, such as physicians, nurses, chaplains and social workers. Among them, there is sometimes a lawyer and at least one person who is in the position of being an "ethics expert," usually a philosopher or a theologian. The group acts behind closed doors at a special place and time, and may serve themselves, the patient, relatives of the patients, a special unit or the entire hospital. What is generally noticeable about organizational forums for ethical discussion?

Establishing HECs implies that there is a given space for reflection within a hospital setting. This is unusual for daily clinical work since nursing as well as medical practice is action-orientated. The criterion of urgency shapes the communication culture, not the play on elaborate words, if possible, based on theoretical frameworks. Dealing with critical situations of ill or dying patients is part of the everyday practice of nurses and medical doctors. An interdisciplinary ethical consultation while sitting around a table – away from the patients' bedside – is in some way odd, since it implies the transformation of an original non-verbal act, highly shaped by sensitive competencies, into a discursive matter-of-fact talk. Therefore, HECs represent a new way of coping with conflicts in clinical practice as well as of consultation and participation.

1.3. Design and Purpose of the Study

"What are we really doing here?" is a question raised in this paper due to the current scientific knowledge of HECs in Germany. They appear to be empirical black boxes. Published research has been limited to surveys which mostly provide quantitative data, e.g. about the numbers of committees that have been established. A second written resource is reports about local experiences.

HECs are the locus of this social science work which is not primarily concerned about bioethics as a discipline, but about its effects *in* and *on* practice. I will use these committees as a vehicle to shed light on a part of the process – transformations in clinical practices and the way caring issues are dealt with.

Since mainly the nurses carry out caring practices, they are the actors of interest here. The way of nurses' participation and the presentation of caring issues in HECs will be analysed.

The aim of this work is to understand the phenomenon of ethics consultation by committee practices in hospital settings, historically as well as within its current situational local context in Germany. While the analysis of the historical context is based on a literature review and expert interviews in the United States, the inner workings of local HECs in Germany are explored by field research: participant observations in three HECs (Catholic, Lutheran and Municipal which has recently turned into Private) over 20 months (2004–2006). This article presents key parts of a larger project.

2. HISTORICAL BACKGROUND AND CONTEXT

There is no doubt that contemporary HECs evolved in the United States, but

> Origins are difficult to trace with precision. How beginnings are located, what counts as an institutional antecedent to IECs, and what forerunners are ignored to us more about the intent of the analyst than it informs us about IECs. If the analyst tells the story in such a way that IECs are seen as an extension of earlier organizational forms, then one can expect a Whig history of medical ethics. (Bosk & Frader, 1998, p. 96)

In the United States, HECs can be traced back to Catholic Medical Moral Committees that were established in the 1950s to deliberate abortions. And another forerunner could be seen in Kidney Dialysis Committee in 1960: When Belding Scribner, a medical doctor at the University of Washington, Seattle, invented a medical device called shunt; it revolutionized the treatment of chronic kidney disease, which is also known as end-stage renal failure.[1] Since there were by far more patients than the equipment could handle, interdisciplinary committees were formed to resolve this "ethical" problem by case deliberation (Katz & Proctor, 1969).

2.1. Historical Traces of Bioethics and the Development of Institutional Review Boards

Modern bioethics is usually dated back to the events of the 1960s, when the kidney dialysis machine first came into service. However, I maintain that its history is rooted in Nuremberg Military Tribunal and its aftermath.

> The Nuremberg medical trials bared the contradictions between expectable medical practice and ethical standards of European and American culture. The trials provided a wedge which allowed wider negotiations about the medical moral order to occur and were integral conditions for the construction of bioethics. (Flynn, 1991, pp. 147–148)

The Military Tribunal in Nuremberg, which tried the Nazi physicians, formulated a code of ethics that has shaped the ethos of experimental aspects of post–World War II medical research. One major contribution of the code was to make the voluntary consent of the human subject absolutely fundamental.

The duty and responsibility for ascertaining the quality of the consent rests upon each individual who is in any way involved in the experiment. This personal responsibility may not be delegated to somebody else. Surprisingly, at that time, it was not the government in Germany demanding institutional bodies to secure safe research, but the government in the United States.

Since the early 1960s, the federal government has required institutions that receive federal research support to have in place an Institutional Review Board (IRB). These committees must include at least seven members, including a scientist, a practicing physician, a nurse and one community "representative" (Bosk & Frader, 1998, p. 95). They were expected to ensure that the proposed experimentation would fall safely within professional as well as community norms for acceptable conducts.

> Operationally, this often means a limited review in practice. IRBs focus on risk-benefit ratio of proposed research and the extent to which consent forms are both understandable and complete ... in (reviewing protocols) these committees expanded a circle of those who can legitimately participate in the collective oversight of biomedical and behavioral research. (Bosk & Frader, 1998, p. 95)

In 1979 the German Physicians' Association recommended to establish IRBs and formulated in 1985 that every experimentation involving a human being as research subjects should be checked by an IRB. The 1988 European Council converted the German "should" into a must. Since then, every university hospital has established an IRB. The composition is quite similar to the one in the United States, usually you also find a lawyer. Nurses as participants are rather an exception than a rule.

In contrast to IRBs, which are concerned with medical research that involve the human being, HECs deal with ethical problems that arise in daily treatment and care of patients. In Germany as well as in the United States, they have a far broader and less well defined scope of authority than IRBs which are the product of federal mandates. While IRBs are based on legal and professional grounds and consultation is located within physicians' authority in the regional medical association, the majority of CECs are located in non-university hospitals.

2.2. Evolution and Development of Contemporary Hospital Ethics Committees in the United States

An early American advocate of contemporary hospital ethics committees was Karen Teel, a physician who wrote an article on the difficult legal and ethical issues surrounding denial of treatment to severely impaired newborns. She argued that HECs could bear some of the burden of morally challenging medical decisions, thus freeing physicians to act and keeping such cases from becoming legal disputes (Teel, 1975). In 1976, *In the Matter of Karen Quinlan,* in which physicians and the family struggled for authority of medical decision in the case of a persistently unconscious patient, the New Jersey Supreme Court took up Teel's idea of committee consultation and endorsed it. This was the official beginning of the growth of contemporary HECs in the United States.

After the Quinlan decision, the talk about ethics committees subsided. In many hospitals, however, some doctors, nurses, hospital administrators and social workers continued worrying about increasing problems inherent in high-technology care. Some rather small groups began to meet regularly to discuss clinical problems they were facing. They attended conferences on ethical problems in health care and addressed the problems to their colleagues. They called themselves *bioethics study groups* (Ross, 1986, p. 6). In a few hospitals they conducted meetings which served as a forum where health-care professionals could discuss specific cases and treatment decisions. These groups, including the ones established by nurses, worked mostly unknown.

In an expert interview (2005), the ethicist Ruth Purtilo declared herself to be "a piece of the history of ethics committees in the United States," and explains that to those unknown groups, belonged a group of nurses at the Massachusetts General Hospital (MGH) in Boston:

> A group of nurses came to me telling 'We need an informal ethics committee', what they needed was a room and time to talk about daily conflicts and dilemmas in clinical practice. We established an informal forum to discuss nursing ethical issues. ... One effect of the forum was the reduction of moral distress.

Like other *bioethics study groups,* after some time, they took on a more formal role in the hospital, began to provide education programs within the institution and worked on guidelines that would help to make decision making less traumatic. A few hospitals were known for their early establishment of committees. In 1988, Boston Massachusetts Hospital published the experiences of their type of committee. Their formation of an HEC had coincided with the decision of *In the Matter of Karen Quinlan.* It was called *Optimum Care Committee* (OCC) and was dominated by physicians. It dealt with end-of-life care and intervention (Brennan, 1988). The committee was made part of a decision-making-process "... in situations where difficulties arise in deciding the appropriateness of continuing intensive therapy for critically ill patients" (Rothman, 1991, p. 230).

In 1978, the President's Commission for the Study of Ethical Problems in Medicine and Medical and Bio-Behavioural Research was created and authorized by Congress. In its 1983 report, *Deciding to Forego Life-Sustaining Treatment,* the President's Commission recommends five possible roles for HECs: (a) diagnostic and prognostic review; (b) staff education by providing forums for the discussion of ethical issues and methodological instruction in resolving ethical dilemmas; (c) institutional policy and guidelines formulation with regard to specific ethical issues; (d) review of treatment decisions made by physicians, patients or surrogate and (e) decision making about specific cases. With respect to the educational task of HECs, the commission stresses the importance of diverse membership and shared perspectives. The committee should "... serve as a focus for community discussion and education" (President's Commission, 1983, pp. 160–163). According to the President's Commission, courts should generally be used as decision makers only as a last resort. The hope has been that CECs develop an ability to facilitate local, consensual decision making.

The commission was especially criticized for including the error made by the Quinlan court and for the suggestion that committees themselves can make decisions about a patient's treatment. Moreno opposes: "It is naïve ... to think that small groups do not already play an important role in medical decision making, as the sociological research attests, and surely the Commission was not recommending a role for ethics committees in technical medical decisions ... this was the error in Quinlan" (Moreno, 1995, p. 100). Another point of criticism he sees is the ambiguous treatment of committees as advisory panels or as decision makers.

Another external motivating factor for the establishment of these committees was the promulgation of the "Baby Doe" regulations in 1985 by the U.S. Department of Health and Human Services (Hoffmann, 1993, p. 678). These regulations did not mandate, but they encouraged, that hospitals caring for newborns establish *infant care review committees* to review cases where the withholding of life-sustaining treatment of a newborn was being rethought.

Since the *Quinlan* case, courts have started mentioning the positive role that ethics committees can play in coping with complicated medical treatment issues. The state of Maryland mandated the establishment of ethics committees by statute, and New Jersey mandated the establishment of either an ethics committee or a prognosis committee by regulation (Hoffmann, 1993, p. 679).

A 1992 action by the Joint Commission on the Accreditation of Healthcare Organizations (JCAHO) formalized the institutionalization of clinical ethics.

For accreditation, hospitals and other health-care institutions are now required to have in place "mechanism(s) for the consideration of ethical issues arising in the care for patients" (Joint Commission on Accreditation of Healthcare Organizations, 1992).

Since some legislatures and courts, as well as a powerful body like JCAHO, have embraced these committees, they have continuously been growing despite a paucity of data on their impact or effectiveness, and an overall tendency of ignoring their risks. Carol Levine remarked: "... their presence does not guarantee that they will be used constructively or that the most appropriate decision will be made" (Levine, 1984, p. 9).

The idea of interdisciplinary involvement of individuals as decision makers in the practice of medicine and nursing is not a new one, but organizing committees to address ethical concerns in the clinical setting is a relatively new practice.

Within the context of bioethics, HECs are institutionalized forms of bioethics qua practice. They can be seen as a part of a process transformation, the phenomenon of what Fox (1989) has called the "Bioethics movement." This move of bioethics from an academic setting to the hospital setting can be described as a move from the "periphery to the center ... a movement into another's space" (Chambers, 2000, p. 22). Rothman (1991) analyses this move as a history of how law and bioethics transformed clinical medical decision making. Thus, he identifies clinical bioethicists as *"Strangers at the Bedside."*[2] He notes that the era in which bioethics came to prominence was also a time of declining trust in physicians.

Besides the series of external events which have strongly influenced the formation of HECs, the growth of HECs were also interpreted from the actors' and institutional point of view. Judith Ross has described these committees as an extension of long-established patterns of peer oversight and a mechanism for educating people working in the institution and for generating institutional policy (Ross, 1986). Daniel Chambliss suggests that medical ethicists and ethics committees first served the interest of medical organizations. He remarked that over time, Clinical Ethics Committees, at least in the United States, had tended to become somewhat dominated by legal, rather than ethical, considerations[3] (1996, p. 93). The feminist sociologist Betty Sichel is convinced: "No matter what articles about ICEs state, a primary purpose for these committees is to protect health care institutions and personnel against malpractice claims" (Sichel, 1992, p. 116).

HECs are also understood as a new response to difficult painful existential dilemmas of contemporary medical care (Bosk & Frader, 1998, p. 94). "The motivation for establishing these committees has been mainly internal: Nurses, social workers, and physicians initiated the committees as a better way to deal with cases that involved the withholding or withdrawal of life-sustaining treatment" (Hoffmann, 1993, p. 677). Daniel Chambliss's one-decade-long observations in hospitals have revealed something different: Ethics committees are useful as anticipated allies of occupational group conflicts in the hospital. For the most part, he suggests that ethical problems are symptoms of such conflicts "... in which moral arguments are weapons of fight, usually decided in favour of the greater power" (1996, p. 93). And he continues by arguing from a nursing perspective:

> Debates rage, not within one's own mind but between nursing and administration, nursing and medicine, nursing and society. In the complex hospital organisation embedded in a complex society, nursing finds itself at the intersection of competing occupational groups and moral ideologies, and this is the source of its ethical problems. (p. 93)

2.3. The Development of Contemporary Hospital Ethics Committees in Germany: A Re-make of the U.S.-American Model

What are we really doing here in Germany? is a question to ask after tracing back the U.S.-American history of HECs.

The answer is that the implementation of HECs after the U.S.-American model of the 1980s has been favoured since its inception and is still supported by leading organizations with regard to ethics in health care. For example, the Academy for Ethics in Medicine (AEM) serves as an advisory body for clinical practice and education. The establishment of HECs has constantly been put in a bright light in publications, speeches and flyers, by its manager, a philosopher. The Center for Ethics in Health Care (ZfG) at the Lutheran Academy, Loccum, is especially active in offering educational classes on the establishment and inner workings of HECs. The educators are philosophers, medical doctors and theologians. Some of them were not convinced by the model academically, but they got to know it by visiting the States. They are the same persons who have published most of the German articles on HECs (Simon, 2000; Neitzke, 2002, 2003; May, 2004; Wernstedt & Vollmann, 2005; Dörries & Hespe-Jungesblut, 2005). All publications refer to the U.S.-American model of HECs of the 1980s and describe three functions: education, policy development and case consultation.[4]

The following historical steps of German HECs show some similarities with the historical steps of U.S.-American contemporary HECs: (1) When the first HECs were established in 1997, the German Lutheran and Catholic Church Association published a joint recommendation brochure to establish such committees, explicitly according to the U.S.-American model (Deutscher Evangelischer & Katholischer Krankenhausverband, 1997). In 2000 a survey revealed that among 795 members of the Christian churches' association, 30 hospitals declared to have an ethics committee or a comparable arrangement to offer consultation (Simon & Gillen, 2000). (2) Along with the installation of quality management instruments and since the Accreditation Organisations of Health Care have demanded that hospitals should have policies and procedures to cope with ethical issues, the number of institutions that declare to have HECs has been growing fast (Kettner & May, 2002). It is still a voluntary decision to build up HECs, but it is obligatory to have some kind of organized structure to address ethical questions. (3) The German Physicians' Association has just published a call to establish HECs. A diversity in structure and practices is explained by a lack of standards and the individual history of the hospital. The association would like to see a standard as soon as possible (Weising, 2006).

In medical terms, reasons for the development are interpreted in the framework of medical progress and technology. That these committees could also help in protection of hospitals and personnel against malpractice claims has not been articulated yet. Seeing the development as part of a transformation process in medical as well as in nursing practice has not been a question of interest either.

According to an analysis by the philosopher Kettner (2005), German HECs serve as a helpful instrument to meet a so-called moral insecurity due to technological progress and a plurality of values, not only among professionals at the bedside, but also among people in public.

Moreover, HECs offer new jobs for philosophers and are establishing a marketplace for medical ethicists who are selling more and more classes on applied ethics. Thereby, their own ideas, concepts and interests that serve their status quo (in medicine, philosophy and law) are stabilized.

While HECs are rapidly growing in Germany, we must ask, what will be the criteria for a good practice in CECs and who is going to define them? Questions such as what these committees are actually doing, who they are serving, what issues they arc addressing, in which way they are accessed, and what is the degree of satisfaction of the users of the service have not been empirically addressed yet. The questions of interest here are whether and how caring issues are addressed, and in which way this is linked to the participation of nurses.

3. CARING AND NURSES' PARTICIPATION IN HOSPITAL ETHICS COMMITTEES

From birth, life starts in interdependency. In order to grow and develop, care is needed. At least in some parts of life, all humans need to be cared for. Human infants are not able to care for themselves, nor are sick, handicapped, frail elderly, and dying people. Since the work of care has been more and more institutionalized over the last century – at least in Western society – care is no longer only a private activity, nor is nursing care.[5]

3.1. Caring as a Practice and Nursing

Care might best be conceptualized as a practice.[6] Care, thought as a practice, is alternative to conceiving care as a principle or as an emotion. Calling care a practice implies the involvement of thought *and* of action: Thought and action are interrelated and they are directed towards some end (Tronto, 1993, p. 108).

Exercising care work is a matter of creating and strengthening relations with people who are dependent, children, the elderly, or ill and dying patients, regardless of whether they are freely entered or socially or professionally prescribed. Therefore, in doing care work, normatively grounded and interactively recognized needs play a decisive role. Through needs, the intentions and attention of the carer are put into a spotlight.

Can caring be practiced without a disposition of care? Of course, checking vital signs of the ill newborn might be just exercised as a job, but then caring would not be an end in itself. Gadow (1985) has described that caring entails a commitment to a particular end. That end, she proposes, is the protection and enhancement of human dignity. "The caring relationship is a good in itself, the good by which other goods are measured" (Vezeau, 1990). The caring relationship has intrinsic value, not an instrumental one.

Agreeing with Tronto, I will use care in the restrictive sense, to refer to care when both, the activity as well as the disposition of care, are present. Joan Tronto and Berenice Fisher have identified different phases of care in order to understand its necessary dimensions. As an ongoing process, care consists of four interconnected phases that can be analytically separated (Tronto, 1994, pp. 105–108):

• caring about is attention to the need for care;
• caring for is assuming responsibility;

- care-giving is the practical attention to, and satisfaction of, need(s);
- care-receiving is the response of those obtaining the attention and care.

From these four elements of care, Tronto develops four ethical elements of care: attentiveness, responsibility, competence and responsiveness (1994, p. 127).

Care, of course, is not always a well-integrated process, but it involves conflict.

While ideally there is a smooth interconnection between these phases, in reality there is likely to be conflict within each of these phases as well as between them (1994, p. 109).

> Nurses may have their own ideas about patients' needs; indeed they may 'care about' patients' needs more than the attending physician. Their job, however, does not often include correcting the physician's judgement; it is the physician who 'takes care of' the patient, even if the care-giving nurse notices something that the doctor does not notice or consider significant. Often in bureaucracies those who determine how needs will be met are far away from the actual care-giving and care-receiving, and they may well not provide very good care as a result. (1993, p. 109)

In U.S.-American nursing literature, it is the notion of "caring" that is mostly used to describe the work of nursing in relation to the patient. It is the central term in its definition provided by the nurses, and it is also the key concept of what nurses believe is their task (Chambliss, 1996, p. 63).

Since the mid-1980s the concept of caring has been discussed in the realm of ethics. Gilligan's (1982) work *In a Different Voice* motivated the demand for a women-oriented ethics, and thus nursing ethics. There are authors who define caring as a *moral stance* (Benner, Tanner, & Chesla, 1996), some see it as *ethical (feminine) behaviour* (Noddings, 1984) and others consider it be a *reciprocal, mutual relationship between individuals* (Watson, 1990). Much that has been written about caring and nursing has been critically responded by critical voices.[7] Joan Liaschenko remarks: "Making a voice for care but failing to attend to the realities of institutional life would be disastrous" (1993, p. 49).

3.2. The German Perspective

In Germany, caring as a concept has been discussed by several service disciplines, including nursing, law and medicine. In general, the literature on caring approaches is very scarce, especially in nursing. There are only three articles concerned explicitly with caring and nursing (Schnepp, 1996; Dahlmann, 2003; Stemmer, 2003). Not a nurse, but the philosopher and political scientist Conradi (2001) has worked on the ethics of care in its relevance to the practice of nursing.

Although nursing has become an academic discipline within the last 20 years in Germany, its lobby is weak in comparison to the medical profession. Nurses are still struggling for more political power, institutionally as well as academically. In the 1970s and 1980s, ethical issues of nurses were dominantly discussed by theologians and psychologists. Within the rise of bioethics in health care, nursing ethics has become a sub-discipline of medical ethics. Nurses have hardly expressed their own position on bioethical issues within their academic discipline and do not show up in the public debate. Even though the decisions will have a strong impact on their practice, they lack participation in the current discussion on living wills. They hardly raise their voice and are even less listened to (Giese, Koch, & Siewert, 2006). Yet, with regard to the establishment of HECs, they appear to be in a rather active role. In one of the first conferences (Kettner & May, 2002) on HECs in Germany, the leaders told about an "interesting observation" they had made during their survey of the current number of HECs: Nurses turned out to be the ones who took the main initiative in establishing such committees.

Although this may be true for the initiating part of building up such committees, it does not answer the question whether this sort of activity accounts for their participation in HECs and the way caring issues are presented and addressed. Since there has been no German data published on the participation of nurses in HECs and their brought-in issues of care yet, the material of use for the field research in Germany is based on U.S. literature and expert interviews.

3.3. What Can Be Learned from U.S.-American Social Science and Nursing Research?

Chambliss's literature review of the basic texts of bioethics in the early 1990s shows that nursing is very seldom mentioned. He draws the conclusion that medical ethics is primarily focused on physicians and that nursing: "… which will carry out many of the decisions (made by somebody else), has no place in the discussion" (1996, pp. 4–5). Nursing research reveals that nurses have tended to view ethics within the realm of highly charged medical situations, while not addressing the ethical tensions and issues that lie within their daily experiences (Liaschenko, 1993; Benner et al., 1996; Nortvedt, 1996).

Nurses' stories identified in the literature are similar. The following struggles could be identified: *respect for human dignity*, especially in end-of-life care; stopping medical treatment; *commitment to individualized care* which is responsive to unique needs of the patient (commitment to patient advocacy); *responsibility for continuity of care;* and scope *of authority and being listened to* (Taylor, 1997).

Nurses are often the ones in the health-care team who are familiar with all the players of the conflict. "The nurse can alert the committee to various factors that may confuse the situation and conceal the major ethical issues. For instance, fear of legal consequences rather than ethical principles may threaten to guide decision making" (Murphy, 1989, p. 555). Nurses are seen to have expert knowledge in the *communication process.* As members of an ethics committee, nurses are the ones who (can) primarily collect data and express questions, viewpoints and perceptions of patients and families. Their membership provides a formal channel to communicate their observations. The handling of communication can be seen as the most important competence since it has been commonly acknowledged that clarifying the facts and fostering communication comprises 80% of an ethics committee's work (Youngner et al., 1983). Murphy is convinced that "Gathering facts and communicate them is what nurses do best" (Murphy, 1989, p. 555).

Patient advocacy is mostly mentioned with regard to nurses' role from an ethical perspective. Patricia Murphy remarks:

> Nurse members who act as *patient advocates* must articulate and defend the autonomy rights and interests of the patient. To be an advocate involves informing and supporting. Nurse advocacy occurs when the committee promotes effective communication; learns the reactions of patient, family and staff; increases patients' knowledge about their illness; and encourages more participation by nurses in the informed consent procedures. (Murphy, 1989, p. 554)

As social and nursing research at an international level has shown, ethical conflicts and critical situations in the practice of nurses are often sidelined, dismissed as ordinary or not actually seen or named as "ethical" (Liaschenko, 1993; Benner et al., 1996; Nortvedt, 1996). The dominant concerns found in stories and narratives of everyday nursing practice are the ones about caring, responsiveness to others and responsibility (Benner et al., 1996; Kohlen, 2003). One empirical study showed that nurses often feel unable to define and exemplify a conflict related to their practice in terms of right and justice (Holly, 1986).

The standards issued by the Joint Commission on Accreditation of Healthcare Organizations in 1991 had required that structures be in place within institutions to enable nurses to participate in ethical deliberations (Erlen, 1993). This standard is also included in the Standards of Clinical

Nursing Practice developed by the American Nurses Association in 1991. Erlen concludes: "If nurses are to be effective advocates and fulfil their professional responsibilities to patients, then resources for nurses have to be developed and made available within each health care agency" (1993, p. 71). The literature has not yet revealed anything specific about these structures which would facilitate nurses' participation.

The U.S.-American studies on participation of nurses in HECs between 1980 and 1994 (Edwards & Haddad, 1988; Oddi & Cassidy, 1990; McDaniel, 1998) show that nurses participate most in discussions that pertain to patient care review or to particular clinical situations. Nurses are less active in discussion regarding policy formation and even less active in discussion on topics pertaining to education.

When the number of HECs had drastically risen, the U.S.-American nurse ethicists Edwards and Haddad (1988) remarked that the specific and unique ethical concerns of nurses had not been adequately addressed by these multidisciplinary committees. Their issues were not framed as ethical issues and were therefore excluded. They further remarked: "In institutions with established Hospital Ethics Committees, nurses are routinely included as members; however, the number of nurses able to participate at this level is small and not proportionally representative of nurses in clinical practice" (Fleming, 1997, p. 7).

As told in an expert interview (2004), the nurse ethicist Diane Bartels who co-chaired an HEC in Minnesota in the 1980s, is convinced: "I do not think hospital nurses have trouble speaking up, they just need a place to show up ... you need a place to convene, and then, once you are there, people don't have trouble ... representing their issues." She also thinks that the co-chair model equalizes power, expands interaction in the committees and increases the comfort of nurses to be able to speak up. Moreover, nurses need to "learn the language" to be able to discuss the issues. The nurse ethicist and nursing manager Hanns de Ruyter who has 10 years of committee experiences in two different hospitals remarks in an interview (2004):

> Nurses' issues get addressed if they present them the way that the people, the physicians and the kind of the leadership sees it. So, you have to present it in a certain way, and if you go outside of that model, ... so if you bring up an issue that they do not classify as being an ethical issue, you don't get listened to. But people and nurses, I think, we are very adaptable, so there is always nurses that will learn the language and you get listened to ... But then you cannot truly bring up the issues that you think are ethical issues because it's very much I think with ethical issues which issues are classified as ethical issues and which ones aren't. And, I think that the nurses who do that and I can't talk about ... their mind, but for me, the quandary is: Do I want to be a part of the leadership

and then I have to adapt, or do I speak what I think should be spoken, and that automatically makes me an outsider.

Traditional theorists' exclusions operate forcefully to set boundaries between those questions and concerns that are central and those that are peripheral. Caring issues usually belong to the peripheral matters of concern. While current feminist concepts could be extended to include concerns of care, the boundaries that circumscribe how moral concepts might be used in the current style of "ethical" thoughts foreclose such thinking.

With the inclusion and exclusion of voices, certain issues and conflicts are brought to a head while others are left outside and become invisible. There might be issues that get discussed because they can be framed ethically and fit into a rational model of decision making. Caring and social issues might get excluded, because they do not fit the model and therefore cannot be framed as ethical. Does this account for HECs in Germany? And which kind of organizational structure blocks and which enhances nurses' participation?

4. JOURNEYS INTO HOSPITAL ETHICS COMMITTEES IN GERMANY: NURSES' PARTICIPATION AND CARING CONCERNS

The selection of three different organizational forms of HECs is based on a survey[8] of ethics committees in Germany, which helped to identify the hospitals that had started the implementation of their ethics committee nearly at the same time (preliminary research phase). Out of five that had started in 2003, access to field research was finally given by three door-openers of the following hospitals: Protestant (525 beds), Catholic (400 beds) and Municipal non-university hospital, now Privatized (570 beds). The Privatized[9] (hospital A) and the Lutheran (hospital B) hospital are both located in the north of Germany, and the Catholic one (hospital C) is located in the south. While the Privatized and the Catholic ones are HECs in the classical U.S. form, called CEC, the Lutheran hospital has established an open forum (without standing membership), called "Round Table Dialogue Ethics." Besides being open for everybody's participation in the hospital, its tasks are also structured along the U.S. model.[10]

The main research began with a first visit to the hospital that involved the introduction of the project to the members, who were participants of the committees. All the written material documenting the prehistory of the committee, its initiating phase and the working procedures of the ethics committees (standing orders, protocols) were given to the researcher under confidentiality. The first contacts with the door-openers (via telephone and e-mail), the first entrances into field and the hitherto written documents allowed a first situational analysis of each committee. Trust building had been decisive during this first step of the main research phase in order to make sure that the planned sequenced participant observations of the HECs' meetings could then take place over two years (2004–2006). While the detailed protocols of 20 participant observations provided the central material for the analysis, the informant interviews served in getting additional information. During the whole field research, a continuous communicative contact through e-mailing and telephoning was kept to the committee chairpersons. Questions with regard to additional information and explanations that would help to clarify confusions and understand the collected data in their situational context were answered either by this form of communication or by interviewing committee members. Nurses' participation were analysed with regard to structural elements as well as with regard to the communication practices of discussions, especially when caring issues were raised.

4.1. Organizational Structures

While looking at the different organizational structures of the committees, such as membership and leadership, the distinction was made between commonalities and differences as the table shows:

Municipal, Privatized	Protestant	Catholic
Membership		
Physicians (2), nurses (4), ministers (3), hospice care representative (1), psycho-oncology retired lawyer (1), patient representative (1)	Open: "Everybody working in the hospital can participate in the meetings." Usually about 12–16 people attend.	Physicians (4), nurses (5), ministers (2), technical service (1)
Leadership		
Male nurse (management), male physician (internist)	Male theologist (ethics expert), female lawyer	Male physician, female nurse (both palliative care), clinical pastor
Meeting monthly	Meeting 4–6 times a year	Meeting monthly

When the written papers are viewed from the *outside* of these committees, they all look alike. Documents created during their design phase, such as standing orders or preambles as well as the minutes of the first meetings, refer mainly to membership and functions which are taken over from the U.S.-American model. But a look *inside* the committees reveals different practices, including diverse procedures and techniques of dealing with the issues raised.

In the *Municipal, recently privatized, hospital* the initiative to establish an ethics committee was born within the dynamics of its preceding working group, called "pastoral care and quality management." The female minister played a decisive role to "get people again around a table to discuss what really needs to be discussed"; this was how she put it. A male physician (internist) and a male nurse (intensive care) who had been in the preceding group, were the ones who asked people in the hospital to become members of the ethics committee. Most of the people agreed. The male nurse, who had just finished his college degree at that time, and the physician announced themselves chairpersons of the committee. While the nurse was the first chairperson, the physician took the position of his deputy. During the meeting in the so-called House of the Ministers, the members of the committee sit around two small round tables with no assigned seats. The atmosphere is relaxed, and people like to drink tea during the meeting. Three out of four nurse committee members have been regularly present. In comparison to other committee members, they are the ones who have mostly participated in educational classes on ethics and moderation techniques. Therefore, they voluntarily take over the role of moderating discussions during committee meetings. They praise the educational programs on ethics[11] and try to convince other committee members to participate.

The history of the ethics forum in the *Lutheran hospital* goes a couple of years back to an "ethics project" (Wehkamp, 2004), and its results had a strong influence on the structure. Taking special care of communicative effects is an idea that can be directly related to the findings of the preceding research project in the hospital: Interviews with physicians and nurses had revealed that the perceived lack of communication between professionals had negative effects on patient care (Wehkamp). Therefore, the leader of the hospital, a minister, has strongly been supporting the committee idea of fostering a "dialogue-culture" in the hospital.

The name "Round Table Dialogue Ethics" of the open forum in the *Lutheran* hospital signifies (1) Dialogue ethics: everybody should feel invited to get involved in a dialogue of ethics and (2) Round table: while talking to each other, you can see each other, there is no formal hierarchy of seats.

Nevertheless, the observations in the committee meetings revealed that the name "Round Table Dialogue Ethics" turned out not to be real, but rather symbolic. The conference rooms actually do not have round tables, but long tables instead, where the two chairpersons (a male theologian and a female lawyer), always sit at the top. Consequently, the participants do not look at each other, but their eyes constantly move toward the chairpersons. When questions are asked, their reactions are focused on the chairpersons' while the moves made by the others remain rather unseen. Therefore, committee members who feel neither addressed nor really involved in the conversations take the time to do "other things," like communicating through messages on their mobile phone. Calling and being called have been constant interruptions during the meeting.

The number of nurses who participate varies from meeting to meeting. There is one staff nurse who has always been present. In an interview, she articulated the following reasons:

> I was invited by the hospital director and chairpersons to participate in the committee and I thought ... because that will make me think and helps keeping pace what is going to change, because otherwise, here, in this hospital you are usually the last one who knows what the people in power have decided. ... (SN: Staff Nurse, 2005)

The nursing director explains the absence of nurses and physicians:

> ... we do not want to waste our time any more ... there were so many ethical initiatives within the last years, and nothing has changed ... the ministers are finding nice words for unbearable situations, and we are trying to put possible solutions into actions ... the ministers do not like to structure a real plan, they like to talk. ... and physicians have enough stress, they go straight forward to get their work done, they are actually in a much more terrible situation than we are ... with all these problems, most of them structural, of course ... physicians are not used to suffer, we are, so it is harder for them ... and I do not think that they will really participate in the committee. (ND: Nursing Director, 2007)

In the *Catholic hospital* the building of an ethics committees is strongly connected with the prior existence of a palliative care unit. After attending a conference on CECs, the palliative care physician took the initiative to talk to people in the hospital about the idea. He said that talking to people over a long period of time had given him the feeling that questions about end-of-life issues had been growing. Especially for those questions raised by people working in intensive care and the associated elderly home, an ethics committee could be helpful. His idea was supported by the head of the hospital, other physicians and the nursing manager. He asked the nursing leader of the elderly home as well as the head nurse of the palliative care unit to co-chair with him. They agreed and the three people along with the nursing manager made a list of who to ask to join them. People who were asked were willing to participate. The meetings take place in a room of the palliative care unit. The chairpersons do not take seats at the head of the table, but in every meeting, everybody changes seats.

According to their standing orders, the educational role of the committees consists of educating the committee itself as well as those people working in the hospital. The question who is going to participate in what kind of classes or programs has been a minor issue raised within the committee meetings.

The following findings are based on the participant observations during the committee meetings as well as information gathered through constant leadership contact, and selected individual interviews with other committee participants.

4.2. Committee Functions and Practices: Education and Policy Making

The Privatized Municipal hospital's ethics committee and the Lutheran hospital have engaged in a continuous educational program including retreats, sending people to conferences and having speakers to come to talk about ethical issues. In the Municipal hospital especially, education is seen as the most important task. The members of Catholic hospital prefer finding "their own way," which means they read about ethical issues and then talk about it during the meeting in a rather informal way. Some attend conferences and then talk about it. This happens rather accidentally in the Municipal hospital and there is certainly not any kind of educational plan for ethics, as I would call it.

Policy construction can be a very influential process as the literature as well as the expert interviews revealed. However, none of the committees had started with this task in the beginning of their work. Compared to bioethics committees in the United States, the committees observed have rather shown a reservation and hesitation with regard to policy making surrounding *DNR orders*. Currently, only the ethics committee in the Catholic hospital has started to work on a DNR order. The head nurse of the intensive care unit has kept asking for it since the committee started its business. The committee in the Catholic hospital also feels the need for a policy surrounding the withdrawal and withholding of treatment as well as surrounding nutrition by *tube feeding.* These were the issues mostly raised, and nurses asked for consultation. Nevertheless, this expressed need has not been put into action yet. The Lutheran hospital's committee has developed a policy to provide procedures on the handling of living wills, which have just been presented to the head of the hospital to give consent for implementation. One physician in the Privatized hospital tried to build up a working group that would work on policy guidelines with regard to *tube feeding.* The group of physicians met once and since they were not able to find consensus, they never met again. The physician remarks: "It is a pity, I really thought that this is important, but since we spend more time arguing with each other than being constructive on this issue ... we failed" (PC: Physician and Co-Chairperson, 2005).

In general, the field study, including the interviews, reveals that the committee members thought policy making to be rather "uninteresting" and "tedious" for the most part. What they are really excited about are the cases. The task of advising on cases (retrospective or concurrent) which are brought to the committee for consultation or reflection is seen as the most meaningful to the committee members. This is actually what the literature tells, and this is also shown in all of the three committees included in the study.

4.3. Committee Discussions: Patient Care Review

"At bioethics committees and conferences and discussions people start off talking about moral wrongs and end up talking about regulatory oversight" (Katz Rothman, 2001, p. 36). This is also true for my observations during committee meetings. The following empirical part of the research aims to examine the way caring issues are presented. The questions are as follows: What counts as an ethical problem? Who defines it? Which issues get attention and which ones are sidelined and dismissed? How do the different members of the committee cope with concerns of care and how much space for discussion is given to them? What kind of caring issues are raised by whom, and what kind of responses are given? Do the attended issues of care change in the course of a discussion, and how are they framed? What conclusions are drawn when caring issues are discussed, and how are they put into action? Who feels responsible, and what are the conflicts revealed in the discussion? The following three examples are taken from discussions during HECs' meetings. I have chosen one example for each hospital. They all appeal to the questions raised.

5. EXAMPLE A

5.1. "A Petit Ethical Problem": Using the Warmth of an Old Patients' Belly to Warm Up a Blood Bottle

A retrospective case consultation in the Privatized hospital:

A nurse had written down a concern in order to consult the committee. The female minister took the paper to the committee meeting and read it aloud. The nurse had experienced a situation two years ago that was still bothering her: An elderly female patient was in need of a blood bottle. When the blood bottle arrived from the lab, it was still very cold, and the physician on shift asked the nurse to put the bottle on the old lady's belly, so that the blood bottle would warm up easily for her. The nurse, who knew the patient, could not imagine doing it. The patient had been sleeping and was not in an alert condition at all. The female physician then told her to ask another nurse to do it, someone who would be more professional than her.

The discussion in the ethics committees developed as follows:

Female minister:	"That is really uncomfortable to get a cold something on your belly!"
Physician A:	"This is absurd from a medical perspective. There are, of course, other technical aids that can help to warm up blood bottles."
Nurse A:	"This nurse feels as an advocate for the patient, and wants to take care of her autonomy."
Physician A:	"This is really a mini ethical problem!"
Physician B:	"I think the problem emerged from hierarchy!"
Minister A:	"I think they have some communication problems on the ward."
Physician C:	"But this is really a petit ethical problem!"

The discussion ends after some minutes, declaring that this is really a minor problem. The minister explains that she will have to talk to the nurse who has revealed her concern.

Female minister:	"What should I tell her?
Physician A:	"You can tell her that she did not do anything wrong within the current knowledge of practice."

Physician B:	"And you can add that the problem had to do with hierarchy and failed communication.
Physician C:	"Well, the more I think about it, the more I feel instrumentalised by this nurse, because this is not an ethical problem at all!"
Nurse B:	"You can tell that she did not do anything wrong, and you can tell her about the possible hierarchy and communication problem behind, but never tell her that this is no or a small ethical problem."

The meeting abruptly ends, people rise from their places and leave the room. The minister keeps sitting there and takes some notes.

5.2. Interpretation

The first reaction is given by the minister who states "that it is really uncomfortable to get a cold something on your belly." And this actually collides with a practice of care that does not allow putting somebody into an uncomfortable state for the use of something for somebody else. The lady who is ill and sleeping cannot defend herself and therefore needs protection.

The physician explicitly speaks from a medical perspective that "this is absurd" and that this is not the right way to warm up blood bottles, because there are technical aids. He clarifies that this is obviously not a medical dilemma in which physicians do not know how to make an adequate decision.

Nurse A shows empathy for the nurse who has opened her concern. She identifies the role of the nurse who cared for the old lady as an "advocate for the patient" who wanted to take care of her autonomy. Caring for her autonomy from a nursing understanding could mean that the patient cannot articulate herself and therefore needs protection, here given by the nurse. This is nurses' mandate. It is different from the mandate of a physician who is interested in getting a warm blood bottle for a medical intervention. Nursing care for patients who are sleeping implies keeping them in a state as comfortable as possible while protecting them from disturbing noises and interventions that can be postponed like "taking the blood pressure," as well as putting a cold blood bottle on their warm belly.

Although the patient is in a state of not being able to verbally interact, the nurse sees that her autonomy still belongs to her and cannot be taken away.

She uses the principle of autonomy to justify her nursing care, namely her responsibility to take care of the patient's sleep.

When the physician defines the situation as "a mini ethical problem" without giving any reason, no questions or controversial points are raised. The question why this is only a small ethical problem is left open. The physician does not feel a need for explanation, and nobody else asks for it. Then the commentaries that lack explanation go on: Physician B declares it as a problem that has to do with hierarchy, and minister A remarks that the problem might be linked to "some communication problems on the ward." Since these are exclamations which follow after the non-rejected definition of a "mini ethical problem," one could ask whether hierarchy and communication are categories that can be put under the umbrella of small ethical problems or whether they are indicators of difficult situations that cannot simply be framed as ethical. Framing them in the context of small ethical problems minimizes their potential for conflicts and understanding the situation in its complexity which, of course, can not only harm patients but also disrupt professional identities, here nursing care.

When physician C repeats the remark of physician A that this is a "petit ethical problem," the conversation is ended. There seems to be a hidden consensus on how much time should be spent on what kind of issues. That the discussion of the concern does not deserve much time could have been evoked by the minimization of the problem. The minister, realizing that the discussion is ending, asks the rather pragmatic question: "What should I tell her?" and the first answer is given by physician A who started commenting on the concern. "You can tell her that she did not do anything wrong ...," he authorizes the minister to tell. Does this mean that the nurse acted correctly according to a medical perspective? What are finally the criteria to distinguish between wrong and right in this situation? And who has the power to define it?

Physician B adds that the nurse should be told that "the problem had to do with hierarchy and failed communication." What does this message of this information signify? What can the nurse take out of this kind of analysis? This is difficult to tell, because there is no explanation. With regard to interrelationships, especially in between different professions, you can narrow down and contextualize nearly everything with hierarchy and communication problems in a hospital. Physician C "feels instrumentalized" by the concern of the nurse. This is a strong reproach. "This is not an ethical problem at all!" is the explanation for his feeling. Does a discussion of problems which are not defined as ethical ones instrumentalize disputants? Again, it is not clear what counts as a "real ethical problem" in comparison to a "petit" ethical problem, or a different kind of a problem, e.g. of competence and communication? Criteria are not given. What is the legitimization to minimize the nursing concern at all?

It was the physicians who had the power to declare what counts as a "real ethical problem" and what counts as a petit ethical problem. Nobody in the group asked for an explanation why the problem is declared to be a petit ethical problem. Nobody talked about the physician who told the nurse to use the warmth of a patient's body to warm up a blood bottle. What is her part in the story? What can be said about her clinical expertise and responsibility? Did she behave in a correct manner? Did she possibly think that this might be a "petit ethical problems" that counts less than the outcome of having a blood bottle warmed for another patient in need? Then putting somebody in an uncomfortable situation is justifiable, because this serves somebody else. And in this case, even when the patient is not able to reject, and is silent.

The nurses' professional role is to take care of the patient's sleep. The nurse theorist Nancy Roper has developed a conceptual framework for nursing practice. One component of the model is called the "Activities of Daily Life" (ADL). Relaxing and being able to sleep is one element of these daily activities nurses have to care for. This involves having an eye on the duration of sleep, times of sleep, day- and -night rhythm, sleeping quality, rituals of falling asleep, habits, and aids to fall asleep. Knowing the patients involves knowing their sleeping habits and also knowing what special patients need to get the kind and duration of sleep that helps them to recover and gives them comfort, especially when they are in pain and are dying.

The more dependent the patient is due to the situation of illness or disease, the more *comfort* the patient needs. For nurses, comfort implies a moral stance, clinical knowledge, and the tangible, practical skills in which they have developed expertise.[12]

6. EXAMPLE B

6.1. "How Do People Die in 'Our' Hospital?" A Spatial Problem: No Rooms for the Dying and Relatives

The following example is neither a retrospective nor a concurrent case discussion in the Lutheran hospital, but an issue raised (unplanned) at the end of a meeting.

Close to the end of the meeting, the chairperson of the ethics forum explains that more than three people working in the hospital had turned to him to raise the issue of care for dying people in the hospital. He explains that he does not want to ignore questions of staff people in the hospital with regard to difficulties in the care of the dying and asks the participants of the committee to name the positive as well as the negative forms of behaviour towards the dying.

First, the director of the hospital who is present in this meeting informs about one observation he made.

Hospital director:	"A patient in bed was taken out of his room on the floor, and then a patient died in this room. Then the patient who died was taken out of the room and the one on the floor could be taken back to the room. The director showed his surprise about this "strange behaviour" as he called it."

There is silence in the committee.

Female nurse A:	"In such situations there is only one last resort, we have to put the dying patient into the bathroom. This is what we very often have to do."
Male nurse B:	"I am glad that we do not have such kind of situations on the intensive care unit any more. When they re-constructed the unit, I had a hard time to convince the planners that we do need a separate room for people who are dying and also a room for relatives. Finally, I had to tell them that I would leave the hospital if they wouldn't do it ... although I had just been there from Berlin ... then they did what we as nurses wanted. We are really happy about it."
Nurse A:	"Yes, you can be really happy about it, but this is an exception."
Female minister:	"Since we have these room problems, we have started to attend the dying with the help of *Dying Boxes*!

The committee members (including me) look astonished when the name *dying box* was dropped in. The female minister realizes the astonishment.[13]

Female minister:	"A *Dying Box* is a box with a candle, a tablecloth and a prayer written on a piece of paper. This is what we can simply catch when somebody is dying, and this is what we can do ... at the least."
Female nurse A:	"We have the problem on our ward that we usually do not know who is the responsible physician for a patient who is dying in pain. Sometimes it takes me for hours to find him!"
Male minister A:	"We have a chapel and we could put the people there when they have died. Then there is room where the relatives can say good-bye."
Male minister B:	"But this counts only for the ones who have already died, we are talking here about the once who are not dead yet, they are dying!"
Female minister:	"I think this is really a bizarre situation when dying people are pushed into the bathroom. Imagine you are a relative and then you are sitting in a bathroom when your loved one is dying."

The male chairperson is watching the time.

The male chairperson:	"I think it is best to establish a working group that will tackle this issue further."
Nurse A:	"This has something to do with administration! And this has something to do with physician practitioners with hospital-cottage affiliation."

The nursing director (female) has not participated up to this point. She looks nervous and furious.

Nursing director:	"What can we do and actually change in a working group when there are only nurses and ministers? Nurses cannot solve the problem!"
Hospital director:	"This a matter of diaconia!"

There is a short silence.

Male chairperson:	"Time is running out, we have to postpone the issue to the next meeting!"

6.2. Interpretation

This discussion reveals the phenomenon of invisibility and the unsaid. The issue of care for the dying is not on the agenda. The issue of concern has been approached by hospital staff who are not present at the committee meeting. Since this committee has an open forum, they could have raised the issue themselves. Why they chose this indirect way of getting the caring issue discussed can only be answered by speculation: They feel that the chairperson is in a more powerful position. He is in a leadership role, and he is also a highly respected theologian in the field of bioethics. Due to this authority, the issue of care for the dying might get attention and be taken seriously. Another structural reason might be found in a simple lack of time. The issue is not put on the agenda, but the chairperson raises it at the end of the meeting. This handling gives the impression that he feels a duty to tackle the issue somehow and at some place, but not as an official point of discussion. Since the agenda is sent out to the hospital via intranet, this issue as an official matter of discussion could have had the following consequences: (1) People who are involved in the care of the dying could have felt motivated to participate in the meeting; (2) it could have given rise to the possibility to prepare oneself on this issue for the meeting; and (3) staff who had originally raised the issue could have been informed that their concern was actually given attention to. Care for the dying then would have been a visible concern with a readable line on a piece of paper that would have taken official space and time. But instead, there is silence.

When the chairperson starts the discussion, he asks the committee participants to distinguish between the positive and the negative forms of behaviour towards the dying, but as the course of the discussion reveals, except one remark by the intensive care nurse, nobody can talk about a *"positive behaviour."*

The hospital director starts giving an example of a *"strange behaviour"* he has observed. He does not say who took the patients forth and back to the room. Usually, this work is done by nurses, but he does not say it. Maybe he wants to make the situation as neutral as possible so that nobody should feel directly addressed. The question is, what could have been the kind of alternative to the described "strange behaviour?" This is answered by a nurse who possibly felt she was addressed. She talks about "the last resort" for the dying: the bathroom. Hereby she has answered the mode of behaviour when there is a problem of space: Is there room for the dying? If not, either they can take the place of somebody else, or they can be put into the bathroom. The intensive care nurse (B) remarks how glad he is about having the necessary space for dying patients as well as for their relatives.

He had to fight for these rooms and finally was successful after he threatened to leave the job he had just got. Of course, this is not a convincing argument based on professional nursing care competence and responsibilities, but rather a strategic threat. What are the (nursing) standards in the care for the dying? Are they disregarded or have they not been established in the hospital yet? Is dying in dignity an issue that goes without saying? These questions are not a matter of the discussion.

When the female nurse (A) declares the situation in the intensive care unit as an exception, the female minister reveals how the hospital ministers solved the problem: They invented a *dying box*.

When the box is named, the committee participants are astonished. Most of the people seem to have never heard about it before.[14] Nobody seems to know what the meaning is and what is inside the box. Although this name could make you think of somebody who is dying in a "box," nobody reacted on its possible connotations. Not only the talk about the "box," but also the name itself has a symbolic meaning: The *dying box* is a black box since nobody knows what is inside. Moreover, there is no visible shared understanding about the practice of care for the dying.

Nurse A continues to complain about unclear responsibilities. She remarks that it takes nurses' time to find the responsible physician for a dying patient in pain. Besides the question of responsibilities, the care for people in pain is another issue raised, but not discussed further. Minister A, who seemed not have listened to the problems just raised, talks about the chapel that could offer a place for the people who have died. His colleague (minister B) tells him that this is not an answer to the problem they are facing.

The female minister takes up the fact anew that people are *dying in the bathroom*. She challenges the committee members by putting them into the role of relatives who might sit in a bathroom when their "loved one is dying." Hereby, she is trying to show the impossibility of the situation, mainly from the emotional perspective of a relative. Putting oneself into the perspective of the patient, one would have to imagine oneself dying in a bathroom. Here, the impossibility has reached such a dimension by violating a person's dignity that the question is probably beyond the powers of imagination and therefore not asked despite its reality.

The male chairperson who is watching the time does not leave the female minister's remark to any reactions by the participants, but thinks it best to tackle the issue by the establishment of a working group. There is a German saying: If you do not know how to go on, then establish a group who will work on it. This solution is, in fact, not taken seriously, at least not from a nursing perspective. Nurse A reacts first to this suggestion. Instead of picking up the idea, she wants to put the attention back to reasons for the problem she had referred to earlier in the discussion. Repeatedly, as it happened before, her concern is not picked up. However, the nursing director raises her voice for the first time during the meeting and takes up a position on the question of what could actually be changed in a working group consisting of nurses and ministers. Hence, she questions the power of nurses and ministers in resolving the problem. Her reaction can be explained on the following background revealed in an interview:

> There had been more than one working group established to cope with the deficits of care for dying people in the hospital. Those groups were mostly attended by nurses and ministers. And: there had also been a separate nursing group activity who developed a standard for the care of the Dying. But, nothing got implemented ... we are giving up."
> (ND: Nursing Director, 2007)

When the nursing director finishes her stance (in the committee discussion) with the exclamation "Nurses cannot solve the problem!" the hospital director reacts determinedly by claiming, "This a matter of diaconia!" By making it a matter of *diaconia* at this point of the discussion, caring as a professional practice is reduced to a religious service. It appeals to the nurses' conscience and is morally laden. Thereby, he excludes the explanation that nurses are being impeded in their care for the dying.

The male chairperson, a theologian, reacts as if this is asking too much of him, and closes the meeting without any substantial comment or outlook on the controversy.

7. EXAMPLE C

7.1. "What Are We Actually Doing Here?" A Nameless Problem: An Old Lady Does Not Want to Eat and Drink

This last discussion presented here is a reflection of a retrospective case consultation in the Catholic hospital. The Catholic hospital is associated with the elderly home, and if there is a need for an ethics consultation, it is taken over by people of the ethics committee. One passed consultation is reflected during an ethics committees' meeting:

The chairpersons (palliative care physician and nurse) were asked by a nurse of the elderly care home to give consultation to the following situation: An old lady, born in the 1920s, had not been willing either to eat or to drink. The nurses in the elderly home felt helpless and had no idea what to do about it. In accordance with the nursing personnel, the consultation team (physician, nurse and pastor) arranged a meeting with the old lady; the nurses in charge gathered.

The physician recalls:	"When we got to her room, in the elderly home, she was caught by surprise" and asked: "Am I ill?" "Do I have to die now?"
And he explains:	"I understand that *we*, the people coming from the hospital irritated her, because we entered her room in white clothes. We answered to her question. No, we are not here because we think you are ill. We want to ask you: whether you are hungry? Then the lady explained 'It is really nice that you care about my eating, but I have never eaten much in my life!'"
The nurse tells:	"Then I offered different meals to the old lady, but every idea was rejected. Finally, there was one meal when she said: 'Yes'. The nurse in charge felt quite uncomfortable and said she would arrange getting the meal. Then we (consultation team) could leave."

While talking about the consultation, the physician and the nurse smiled. The other committee members neither asked nor questioned anything. They listened carefully, some of them smiled too.

Closing their report on the consultation, the physician and the nurse remarked: "What are we really doing here?" Then they moved on to the next issue to be discussed in the meeting.

7.2. Interpretation

The nurses in the elderly home cannot cope with an old lady who is refusing to eat and drink. They are possibly afraid of letting the old lady die in case she continues rejecting food. They might also be afraid of being blamed for it, because taking care of the intake of food belongs to their professional responsibilities. Since the old lady does not seem to respond to the care-givers, they probably feel unsure whether their care has been attentive enough and whether they might have overlooked anything. As a way out, the nurses ask for the ethics consultation by calling the chairpersons of the ethics committee, and the head nurse agrees to a meeting with the old lady.

When the consultation team including the head nurse comes into the lady's room, she is self-confident and asks her question right away. The old lady, seemingly needy for food, but without willing to eat, is the one who reveals the situation as a grotesque comedy: She is surprised that people in their professional white coats are visiting her and spontaneously asks: "Am I ill? Do I have to die now?" Since she has reached the last part of her life, dying is not that far away from her imagination. Why should she expect that hospital personnel would come over to ask her, what she would like to eat? She has never eaten much in her life, and as a matter of fact, getting older implies that the need for food and drink decreases.

The physician realizes the reason for her irritation and expresses it in the ethics committee. Both he and the nurse smile about this situation because they are irritated themselves. One question in their mind probably was, did four people really had to go to an old lady who is fully competent to articulate her needs? And, of course, the following questions are relevant to understanding the problem: What does this old lady really need? Have the nurses responded to her needs besides caring for her food? Is there not at least one nurse who knows the old lady well and knows how to respond to her? What is really known about her eating habits? How much food does she really need at that time? What is "enough" for this old lady who has not eating much in her whole life? This is not clear. Does she finally decide for a meal, because she really likes the suggested dish, or does she just want to get rid of these "strange" people visiting her? While reporting on this case consultation, neither the consultation team nor any other committee member including nurses raise questions of care. The only question put here is, "What are we really doing here?" This question is repeated several times, but not answered. The reaction is a smile that renders the passed consulting situation a humorous tune.

Although this behaviour, at first sight, fits the way the conflict has been dealt with, at second sight, it conceals questions of care practices and sharing responsibilities, procedures and effectiveness of ethics consultation. The ignorance of questions from a caring perspective releases the nurses of a confrontation with their professional duties and challenges and the reflection on their unique conflicts of care.

8. CONCLUSION

The discourse of HECs in Germany has strongly been influenced by the U.S.-American committee model, and even events like the story of Karen Quinlan have been taken over to Germany as the historical starting point of these committees. In the United States, the rapid growth had been caused by the Joint Commission on the Accreditation of Health Care that demanded to have some structure available to meet ethical questions in hospitals; now, the same development takes place in Germany: Accreditation is speeding up the number of HECs.

U.S. studies on nurses' participation in HECs have revealed that they are included as members of these multidisciplinary forums. Yet, their number is rather small and not proportionally representative of nurses in clinical practice. At the same time, their active involvement is limited. While they are mostly involved in discussions that pertain to patient care review or specific clinical situations, their ethical nursing concerns are not adequately addressed. On the contrary, their issues are not framed as ethical issues and are therefore excluded. The necessity of "learning the (ethics) language" as one nursing professor in an expert interview remarks then implies that nurses' issues might get transformed into ethically acceptable problems that do not hit the point of caring conflicts.

Although the findings of the empirical research in Germany are not generalizable, they support this assumption: Conflicts in delivering professional caring practices, such as watching patients' sleep in quantity and quality (example A), protecting the dying from uncomfortable actions (example B) and finding out the patients' eating habits (example C), are not seen as such. Hence, in the case of framing it as an ethical problem, it is framed as a "petit ethical problem," thus minimizing its importance for attention and consideration. Conflicts over care for the dying are related to "spatial problems." Responsibilities are moved away from professional groups and individual persons, because they feel powerless to solve it. Their suggestions for solving the problem has not been put into action, but instead, has been answered by starting a second or third working group that should face the problem anew. Solving problems by ethical discussions and not by deeds has been frustrating for the nurses and ministers in the Lutheran hospital. Therefore, the nurses do not see any sense in participating in the committee work.

Caring is marginalized, nurses are marginalized, and they further marginalize themselves as the issues of concern for them are systematically ignored: declared to be, at best, "petit" ethical problems, and not part of what we are really doing here.

NOTES

1. Normally, the kidneys remove toxic substances from the blood. If the kidneys fail, the person is slowly poisoned and dies. Dialysis machines were invented earlier.

They could cleanse the blood, but the purification had to be performed several times each week. Every time, entry had to be made through the person's veins. After a while when a vein collapses, another vein must be used. The body has a limited number of veins that are large enough to accommodate the dialysis needles. When the veins are used up, dialysis is no longer possible and death follows. The newly developed plastic shunt could be more or less permanently implanted in the patient's vein. Since the tubes of the dialysis unit could enter the patient's veins over and over again through the shunt, dialysis could be performed repeatedly as long as the patient would need it. And the patient would need it as long as he lived.

2. "Bioethics proceeds in a largely deductive manner, formalistically applying its mode of reasoning to the phenomenological reality it addresses. An array of cognitive techniques are used to distance and abstract bioethical analysis from the human settings in which the questions under consideration occur, to reduce their complexity and ambiguity, and to control the strong feeling that many of the medical situations on which bioethics centers can evoke in those who contemplate them, as well as those live them out" (Fox, 1990, p. 207).

3. 2006-7-20 written as e-mail.

4. With regard to historical events, some texts mention that the starting point of HECs traces back to the U.S. American case story of Karen Quinlan.

5. The historian Susan Reverby suggested that nursing evolved from women's historical role in caring for vulnerable people in the community. She asserted that caring was imposed as a (moral) duty first on women, and then, as society's needs increased and changed in times of war and epidemics, on a paid nursing force. In her terms, nurses were "ordered to care" in a society that ignored to value caring (Reverby, 1987).

6. I am aware of the ideology of caring and the criticism that feminist ethics of care has been facing: the inability to address problems: the problem of exploitation as it threatens caregivers, the problem of sustaining caregiver integrity, the dangers of conceiving the mother–child dyad normatively as a paradigm for human relationships and the problem of securing social justice on a broad scale among relative strangers (Carse & Nelson, 1996), but since the practices of care are my focus, I will bypass this debate.

7. See note 5.

8. The survey was mostly done by telephoning, e-mailing and getting into contact with people of the field due to conferences on clinical ethics committees (University of Essen, 2002; Academy of Tutzing, Munich, 2003).

9. This hospital is privatized since 2005.

10. Despite this formal difference in structure, this forum is also called an "ethics committee" here.

11. These educational programmes are offered outside the hospital, and the hospital pays for the participation.

12. See Kaufmann (2005), p. 41.

13. A week later I got to see this "Dying Box" in the hospital. I met a minister in the Lutheran hospital and she took a little bible-sized wooden box out of the cupboard. She opened it and took out an off-white candle as well as an off-white tablecloth, and a little piece of paper with a prayer written on it. She told me that the ministers of the hospital had decided to have such boxes for the hospital on each unit in order to be able to attend to the dying.

14. As their facial expression shows, some people seem to know something, but they do not talk about it.

126HELEN KOHLEN

ACKNOWLEDGMENT

I am grateful to Hanns Lilje Stiftung who has sponsored this project. I am thankful to all my colleagues, especially Prof. Dr. Kathrin Braun and Prof. Dr. Barbara Duden who have commented earlier and in different versions.

REFERENCES

Bartels, D., Youngner, S., & Levine, J. (2004). HealthCare Ethics Forum '94: Ethics Committees: Living up to your potential. *AACN Clinical Issues, 5*, 313–323.

Benner, P., Tanner, C. A., & Chesla, C. A. (2004). *Expertise in nursing practice: Caring, clinical judgement, and ethics*. New York: Springer.

Bosk, C., & Frader, J. (1998). Institutional ethics committees: Sociological oxymeron, empirical black box. In: R. DeVries & J. Subedi (Eds), *Bioethics and society: Constructing the ethical enterprise*. Upper Saddle River, NJ: Prentice Hall.

Brennan, T. A. (1998). Ethics committees and decisions to limit Care. The experience at the Massachusetts General Hospital. *JAMA*, (6), 803–807.

Chambers, T. (2000). Centering bioethics. *Hastings Center Report, 30*(1), 22–29.

Chambliss, D. F. (1996). *Beyond caring: Hospitals, nurses, and the social organization of ethics*. Chicago: University of Chicago press.

Conradi, E. (2001). *Take care: Grundlagen einer ethik der achtsamkeit*. Frankfurt, New York: Campus Verlag.

Dahlmann, H.-U. (2003). Fürsorge als prinzip? Überlegungen zur grundlegung einer pflegeethik. *Zeitschrift für Evangelische Ethik, 47*, 6–20.

Deutscher Evangelischer Krankenhausverband e.V., Katholischer Krankenhausverband Deutschlands e.V. (1997). *Ethik-Komitee im Krankenhaus*. Berlin/Freiburg.

Dörries, A., & Hespe-Jungesblut, K. (2005). *Bundesweite Umfrage zur Implementierung Klinischer Ethikberatung in Krankenhäusern*. Unpublished paper.

Edwards, B. J., & Haddad, A. M. (1988). Establishing a nursing bioethics committee. *JONA, 18*(3), 30–33.

Erlen, J. A. (1993). Empowering nurses through nursing ethics committees. *Orthopaedic Nursing, 12*(2), 69–72.

Fleming, C. M. (1997). The establishment and development of nursing ethics committees. *HEC Forum, 5*(1), 7–19.

Fox, C. R. (1989). *The sociology of medicine: A participant observer's view*. Englewood Cliffs, NJ: Prentice Hall.

Fox, C. R. (1990). The evolution of American bioethics: A sociological perspective. In: G. Weisz (Ed.), *Social science perspectives on medical ethics* (pp. 201–217). Boston: Kluwer Academic.

Flynn, P. (1991). The disciplinary emergence of bioethics and bioethics committees: Moral ordering and its legitimation. *Sociological Focus, 24*(2), 145–156.

Gadow, S. (1985). Nurse and patient: The caring relationship. In: A. H. Bishop & J. R. Scudder (Eds), *Caring, curing, coping: Nurse Physician patient relationships* (pp. 31–43). Alabama: University of Alabama Press.

Gilligan, C. (1982). *In a different voice: Psychological theory and women's development*. Cambridge, MA: Harvard University Press.

Giese, C., Koch, C., & Siewert, D. (2006). Sterbehilfe – kein thema für die pflege? *Dr. med. Mabuse, 164*, 43–46.

Hoffmann, D. (1993). Evaluating ethics committees: A view from the outside. *The Milbank Quarterly, 71*(4), 677–701.

Holly, C. (1986). *Staff nurses' participation in ethical decision making: A descriptive study of selected situational variables.* Unpublished doctoral dissertation, Columbia University, Columbia.

Joint Commission on the Accreditation of Healthcare Organizations (JCAHO). (1992). Accreditation Manual for Hospitals Oakbrook Terrace III.

Katz, A. H., & Proctor, D.M. (1969). *Social Psychological Characteristics of Patients Receiving Hemodialysis in Treatment for Chronic Renal Failure.* Public Health Service, Kidney Disease Control Program.

Katz Rothman, B. (2001). *The Book of Life.* Boston.

Kaufmann, S. (2005). *And a time to die: How American hospitals shape the end of life.* Chicago: University of Chicago Press.

Kettner, M., & May, A. (2002). Ethik-Komitees in kliniken – bestandsaufnahme und zukunftsperspektiven. *Ethik in der Medizin, 14*(4), 295–297.

Kettner, M. (2005). Ethik-Komitees. Ihre Organisationsformen und ihr moralischer Anspruch. In Erwägen Wissen Ethik. Deliberation Knowledge Ethics. (vormals: Ethik und Sozialwissenschaften (EuS) – Streitfragen für Erwägungskultur. 1/16, 3–16.

Kohlen, H. (2003). *A collection and analysis of narratives told by nursing students.* Are we really talking about ethics? Unpublished paper.

Levine, C. (1984). Questions and (some very tentative) answers about hospital eEthics committees. *Hastings Center Report, 14*(3), 9–12.

Liaschenko, J. (1993). *Faithful to the good: Morality and philosophy in nursing practice.* Unpublished doctoral dissertation. University of California, San Francisco.

Liaschenko, J. (1997). Ethics and the geography of the nurse-patient relationship: Spatial vulnerabilities and gendered space. *Scholarly Inquiry for Nursing Practice, 11*, 45–59.

May, A. T. (2004). Ethische enscheidungsfindung in der klinischen praxis: Die rolle des klinischen ethikkomitees. *Ethik in der Medizin, 16*(3), 242–252.

McDaniel, C. (1998). Hospital ethics committees and nurses' participation. *JONA, 28*(9), 47–51.

Moreno, D. J. (1995). *Deciding together: Bioethics and moral consensus.* New York: Oxford University Press.

Murphy, P. (1989). The role of the nurse on hospital ethics committees. *Nursing Clinics of North America, 24*(2), 5551–5555.

Neitzke, G. (2002). Ethische Konflikte im Stationsalltag. *Planetarium, 42*, 9–10.

Neitzke, G. (2003). *Ethik im Krankenhaus. Funktion und Aufgaben eines Klinischen Ethikkomitees.* Ärzteblatt. Baden-Würtemberg, Heft 4.

Noddings, N. (1984). *Caring. A feminine approach to ethics and morals.* Berkeley, California.

Nortvedt, P. (1996). *Sensitive Judgement. Nursing, Moral Philosophy and an Ethics of Care.* Otta.

Oddi, L. F., & Cassidy, V. R. (1990). Participation and Perception of Nurse Members in the Hospital Ethics Committee. *Western Journal of Nursing Research, 12*(3), 307–317.

Presidents Commission for the study of ethical problems in medicine and biomedical and behavioural research. (1983). *Deciding to forego life sustaining treatment.* Washington, DC: U.S. Printing Office.

Rodney, P. (1993). *A phenomenological study of emergency nurses' perceptions of the ethical issues encountered in their practice.* Unpublished paper. Vancouver, University of British Columbia.

Rodney, P. A. (1997). *Towards connectedness and trust: Nurses' enactment of their moral agency within an organizational context.* Unpublished doctoral dissertation. University of British Columbia, Vancouver.

Ross, J. W. (1986). *Handbook for Hospital Ethics Committees. Practical suggestions for ethics committee members to plan, develop, and evaluate their roles and responsibilities.* Chicago: American Hospital Publishing, Inc.

Rothman, D. (1991). *Strangers at the bedside: A history of how law and bioethics transformed medical decision making.* New York.

Schnepp, W. (1996). Pflegekundige Sorge. In Deutsche Gesellschaft für Pflegewissenschaft e.V. (Hrsg.): Pflege und Gesellschaft. Duisburg.

Sichel, B. A. (1992). Ethics of Caring and the Institutional Ethics Committee. In H. Bequaert Holmes, & L. M. Purdy (Ed.), *Feminist perspectives in medical ethics* (pp. 113–123). Bloomington and Indianapolis.

Simon, A. (2000). Klinische Ethikberatung in Deutschland. Erfahrungen aus dem Krankenhaus Neu-Mariahilf in Göttingen. In: *Berliner Medizinethische Schriften* (Vol. 36). Dortmund: Humanitas.

Simon, A., & Gillen, E. (2000). Klinische Ethik-Komitees in Deutschland. Feigenblatt oder praktische Hilfestellung in Konfliktsituationen? In: Engelhardt, Volker von Loewenich/ Simon, Alfred (Hrsg.) (2000): *Die Heilberufe auf der Suche nach ihrer Identität. Jahrestagung der Akademie für Ethik in der Medizin e.V.* Hamburg (pp. S.151–S.157). Berlin, London: LIT.

Stemmer, R. (2003). Zum Verhältnis von professioneller Pflege und pflegerischer Sorge. In: Deutsche Gesellschaft für Pflegewissenschaft e.V. (Hrsg.): Pflege und Gesellschaft. Sonderausgabe. Das Originäre der Pflege entdecken. Pflege beschreiben, erfassen, begrenzen. Frankfurt/Main.

Taylor, C. R. (1997). Everyday Nursing Concerns: Unique? Trivial? Or Essential to Healthcare Ethics? *HEC Forum, 9*(1), 68–84.

Teel, K. (1975). The Physician's Dilemma: A Doctor's View: What the Law Should Be. *Baylor Law Review, 27*, 6–9.

Tronto, J. (1993). *Moral Boundaries. A Political Argument for an Ethics of Care.* London.

Wiesing, U. (2006). Ethikberatung in der klinischen Medizin: Stellungnahme der Zentralen Kommission zur Wahrung ethischer Grundsätze in der Medizin und ihren Grenzgebieten (Zentrale Ethikkommission). *Deutsches Ärzteblatt, 103*(24), A1703–A1707.

Youngner, S. H., Jackson, D. L., Coulton, C., et al. (1983). A national survey of hospital ethics committees In Deciding to Forego Life-Sustaining Treatment: Report of the President's Commission for the Study of Ethical Problems in Medicine and Biomedical and Behavioral Research. Washington, DC, US Government Printing Office: 443–449.

INTERVIEWS

Bartels, D. (2004). *Expert Interview.* Minnesota: Center for Bioethics, University of Minnesota.

DeRuyter, H. (2004). *Expert Interview.* Minnesota: Center for Bioethics, University of Minnesota.

(2007). Nursing Director, Interview in the Lutheran hospital, Hannover.

(2005). Physician and Co-Chairperson.

(2005). Staff Nurse. Interview in the Lutheran hospital, Hannover.

Purtilo, R. (2005). *Expert Interview.* Boston: Massachusetts General Hospital (MGH).

Wehkamp, K.-H. (2004). *Expert Interview.* Hamburg: Hochschule für Angewandte Wissenschaften Hamburg.

HEALTHCARE ETHICS COMMITTEES WITHOUT FUNCTION? LOCATIONS AND FORMS OF ETHICAL SPEECH IN A 'SOCIETY OF PRESENTS'

Armin Nassehi, Irmhild Saake and Katharina Mayr

TWO COMMONPLACE ASSUMPTIONS

Before starting research in the field of ethics, a few common assumptions need to be cleared up. The first is so common that it needs very little space at all: *Ethics is a scientific discipline*. This accurately describes its location and the problems it covers in a modern, functionally differentiated society. As a branch of philosophy and a normative science, its frame of reference is initially located in a world of possible competing reasons. The basic problem is that of trying to explain good reasons – and the horizon is the sayability of ethical sentences which, even when they reflect an ethical practice, open up a *scientific* horizon. Ethics is therefore a science – and like every science it can only solve scientific problems (see Luhmann, 2002, pp. 79–93). Practical problems are also the scientific problems of ethics – and that is not a deficiency, but rather a consequence of the basic structures of modern society. A modern society cut loose from political, economic, legal,

Bioethical Issues, Sociological Perspectives
Advances in Medical Sociology, Volume 9, 129–156
Copyright © 2008 by Elsevier Ltd.
ISSN: 1057-6290/doi:10.1016/S1057-6290(07)09005-5

scientific, artistic, educational and medical problems, on the one hand, allows these disconnected spheres to relate radically to each other, while on the other hand making them logically incompatible. A modern society could not exist any other way (see Luhmann, 1998, pp. 1–21; Nassehi, 2005a). This should first be understood before venturing into research on ethics.

A second common assumption is that ethics – as a philosophical/ theological/scientific form of observation, explanation and archiving of moral intuitions and judgments – *has to have an interdisciplinary format*. This assumption about what is internationally understood as *ethics* is already clearly visible in international research and publishing practice and has become established in a variety of university faculties. The scientific reflection of ethical decisions is dependent on an interdisciplinary format and thus appears to resemble the practice of ethical decision making. It can be observed, on the one hand, in modern societies that an integration of the whole of society through ethical maxims or moral consensus is categorically ruled out. This does not, however, mean that morally motivated codices such as human rights or even professional moral standards, general forms of moral principles or even moral motives may not be valid and effective as a guide for living. Of course, an integrating function cannot be attributed to morals for the simple reason that most forms of order in modern society do not appear immoral, but rather *amoral*. On the other hand, this is exactly the prerequisite for philosophical-ethical attempts at providing universal and collectively acceptable ethical figures with reasons, which in turn can achieve a rational status open, for instance, to criticism (see Nassehi, 2001). Modern ethical reflection – irrespective of its theoretical form – with its posit of acceptability, or at least of procedural implementation of operative coordination in political processes, can be seen as a reaction to the very pluralism of world views, ways of life and basic intuitions of the 'good life', which first produced the conditions for the disintegration of morality's clear claim to validity. The disciplines involved in this discourse are themselves an expression of this diversification of ethical argumentation. They range from the philosophical reflection of the rationality of ethical judgments to figures of reasoning from applied ethics. They specialize not only in demonstrating their 'practical' efficacy, but also in theological reflections on the significance of the religious content of 'unconditional' figures of rationality under conditions of differentiated modernity. The juridical and legal theoretical assertion of the accountability of legal entities (bodies, persons) creates subjects of moral judgment. In other words, the reflective form of an ethical practice of rationality based on good reasons reacts in the final instance to the fact that hardly any undisputed good reasons can be found for these or for maxims of action found in societal practice –as far as this holds true, the reason must be separated into an ethical form of reflection, which in turn takes on a scientific form.

Thus, in the end a process is repeated which has already been seen in the form of religion: The most infallible example for the differentiation of the religious is the emergence of academic theologies, which now produce religious reasons in a manner which can be distinguished from the day-to-day religious practices of believers. In this respect, and in view of religious styles in globalized world society, the existence of an academic, religiously more or less indifferent theology is of enormous importance. Something similar could well apply to ethics. Just as in the final analysis, theology is the result of social secularization, academic ethics could also be seen as a consequence of the secularization of social morals – its reasoning is far more complex and no longer clearly accesses the practical realization of the moral.

Our argumentation uses the standard distinction between ethics and morals from the field of philosophical ethics: *ethics* as a form of *morality*, which in turn need not be conscious of itself but simply applies empirically (or not as the case may be). It should be abundantly clear that this is a heuristic distinction. It is used only to determine the different worlds we are talking about here: *on the one hand,* the moral world, in which a certain form of morality applies and which has to arm itself with rigor to gain validity; *on the other hand,* the reasoning world of ethics which does not perpetuate itself though the enforcement of moral standards, but rather through its argumentative reasoning or ability to reason. Here we follow Niklas Luhmann's characterization of morality as a form of communication which avails itself of the respect or disrespect toward individuals, in order to qualify their behavior as good or bad (see Luhmann, 1996). So it is not a question of morality as a certain substance or quality, but solely a question of moral communication in the sociological sense, i.e. it is a question of forms of communication which command moral respect or disrespect. The following point is decisive here: It is not that one is an empirical world while the other provides its reflections; rather we are dealing here with two empirical cases, with the moral regulation of actions and speech as well as with the practical business of reasoning.

PRACTICAL INTERDISCIPLINARITY

The following results from these two common assumptions: The inter-disciplinarity and differentiation of ethical reflection in theoretical and practical research concurrently reflects a *practical interdisciplinarity of ethical decision making*. Similar to the way in which the practice of academic ethics hinted at here can be determined in social terms, it is of particular relevance for ethics research to demonstrate *the empirical conditions and locations* under which and by which ethical decisions are made in modern society. Such a research perspective does not negate the possibilities and necessity to search for good reasons. But it assumes that – to paraphrase Wittgenstein – no practical ethical problem can be solved even with the final explication of the best reasons. As said before, this is not an argument against the explication of reasons, which is a very specific type of practice and not an external observation. It is rather a plea for a supplementary and truly sociological, i.e. *empirical research,* perspective. We are definitely *not* dealing here with the question of the rationality of good reasons, nor is it a question of the application of general ethical theoretical forms to concrete fields of 'applied ethics'; in other words, we are not talking about implementation questions, but rather about the *empirical conditions under which ethical decisions can be* practically *made in modern society*.

Thus, the problem of ethical *reasoning* turns up as an *object* of such research. It can be illustrated with a small example: The fact that the 'dignity' of the 'persons' and their 'responsibility' is highlighted, that they are ascribed 'rights' and they 'themselves' are allowed to decide, is just as much emphasized as the fact that only 'rational' reasons are 'good' reasons, and reasons are rational when they can be embedded in a 'structural rationality', within which they appear both temporarily and systematically 'coherent'. One should not judge such assumptions against the worst versions of ethical reflection. Rather, in the German-speaking world we take probably the best and most well-known forms as grounds, for instance the ethical writings of Nida-Rümelin (1996, 2000, 2001, 2002). They are full of such assumptions which have precisely the function of removing ambiguity and describing a world which in the final analysis is subject to a continuum of rationality. They are suffused with the idea of a harmonious placing of their parts, the realization of which is in fact only impeded by a lack of insight on the part of the actors. The philosopher assures us quite simply, as though speaking to children: 'A fully coherent way of life does not throw up any internal reasoning problems' (Nida-Rümelin, 2001, pp. 160). Nida-Rümelin's utopia consists of inaugurating a way of life in which problems of reasoning no longer arise, as a result of the insight into the necessity of rational continuity and coherent reasoning. However, this also represents its reference problem, because in the final instance it always reckons with ambiguity, irrationality and inadequate reasoning and consequently relies all the more on a coherent phantasm which at times turns into a caricature of a rationality machine. Although the philosopher knows that 'real people' are occasionally prone to wandering less-straight and narrow paths and that day-to-day decisions are sometimes made on the basis of intuition, the 'structurally rational persons' will be really free – free to gain insight into the necessity of being able to make their decisions in favor of a coherent way of life (see op. cit., p. 151 ff).

One may or may not consider this philosophically astute. In any case, it completely lacks any empirical basis as to how actions come about, how decisions are made and in which contexts persons can become accountable in this manner. And finally, such a perspective is completely insensitive to which status reasons have for forms of practice *at all*. The philosophical–scientific problem is of reasoning separated from reasons which have created a world in which actions are the consequences of action maxims.

However, sociological research must pose more relevant questions. So, to put it more clearly again, the question here is not *which* good reasons or philosophically demonstrable maxims or virtues we can use to deal with certain problems, but rather *how* ethical arguing and decision making works in practice; how the appropriate forms of practice become established and under which conditions – in which concrete locations – which forms of ethical reflection prove to be empirically plausible and who becomes established as a legitimate speaker, as well as where and how. This is the decisive question that sociology has to pose to ethics.

THE LOCATION OF THE ETHICAL DECISION

The place in which ethical decisions which have consequences for practice are made in western-type societies is not only the location of moral intuitions of a private way of life, nor is it the ethos of professionals. Rather, more than anywhere else, it is in the area of biomedical and biotechnical research and practice – by no means owing allegiance only to the new biotechnical opportunities, but also to the pluralism of ethical perspectives and the loss of the ethical justification of the classical professional role, especially in the medical sphere.

The empirical location of such ethical decisions is usually the ethical committee, in other words institutionally supported bodies. Here, under organizational conditions, a particular style of ethical reflection has become established in the shape of the following committees: clinical ethics committees and commissions, the ethics committees of professional

associations, the ethics committees of scientific associations, commissions
of enquiry in parliamentary decision-making processes, public discourses,
especially on bioethical issues, ethic committees at the federal state level and
even large companies etc. What all these forms of practice have in common
is that they do not do exactly what would be expected of fervent moralists
with fundamentalist interests. It can be observed empirically that in such
communication contexts, it is the limits of the final moral claim which
become clear in the face of decision-oriented, i.e. practice-relevant, ethical
forms of reflection (see van den Daele, 2001a, 2001b).

It is particularly interesting that in these forms of practice, ethical
decisions by no means copy the routines and patterns of arguments of
scientific and academic reflection on ethical questions. Nor do they involve
anything like a theory-practice transfer. Instead, a unique form of
communication has become established, which of itself has taken on a kind
of ethical quality. This can be witnessed for instance in public hearings
of the national ethics committee or in the proceedings of clinical ethics
committees.

The typical participants in such committees are not exclusively ethics
experts. Despite the growing need for ethical expertise and the development of
decision-making processes, an operative demarcation between ethicists and
other professions has not taken place. Rather, the ethical decision-making
process has become a genuine *interdisciplinary* process – interdisciplinary, not
in the sense of different scientific disciplines, but in the sense of different
professional groups. Their *practical interdisciplinarity* does not just decide *on*
the ethical discourse, it *is the ethical discourse*.

The aim of the research perspective being followed here is, therefore,
to research the empirical implementation conditions of ethical decisions
supported by committees, and to gain an insight into the social,
organizational, political and legal structure of the forms of decisions rather
than of the ethical decision-making algorithms and levels of reasoning.

The following perspectives will be scrutinized in the process:

• a view of modern society as a functionally differentiated society without
  a central ethical/moral perspective,
• a perspective of the status of bioethical issues for achieving public and
  political consensus,
• an empirical perspective of the real-time practice of committee-supported
  ethics which, in contrast to the academic reflection practice of the ethical
  work of the concept, must find the means to generate ethical decisions and
  reasons under different conditions involving incomplete information,

limited time, cooperation constraints, participation pressure and goal-oriented discourse.

ETHICAL SPEAKERS

Ethical forms of reflection are always linked to certain *images of human beings*, from which the status of the particular speaker's position is derived. In this case also, the perspective of our research does not become involved in the reasons for, or the invention of, human images. Rather, it views the problem of human images empirically by inquiring after the image of the subject of the ethical decision. This is usually the self-responsible, more or less autonomous and at least accountable, individual who in the western tradition may be called the subject because he or she is equipped with a kind of internal infinity which offers sufficient *requisite variety* to make the accountability credible. A perspective of the actual practice of ethical decision making in organizations raises doubts as to whether these are the type of people actually making the decisions. It seems much more to be constellations of actors propelled by the dynamics of an institutional context which give rise to speaker positions, whose practical cooperation and organizational pressures assign a curiously singular dynamic to ethical decision making. In addition to this, one will find, for instance in the communication between professionals and semiprofessionals or between professionals and clients (e.g. doctor and patient), that asymmetrical positions become established and cannot be explained away as a rational basis for communication, neither with good will nor with the philosophical norms of 'eye-level' encounter (see Saake, 2003; Maynard, 1991; Nassehi, 2004).

Even the medical-critical communications, e.g. in Hospital Ethics Committees (HECs), have become aware of just how rewarding the theoretical switch of the systems theory to communication is, in other words to the issue of generating order through the creation of connectivity (see Luhmann, 1995, p. 137 ff.). The following quote is from an interview with a patients' representative in the context of a research project on 'Clinical Ethics Committees'[1]:

Well, the main problems are communication. Communication, is, let's say -, let's start with the doctors, well they're -, it's always the patients who ask the questions, and it is always the doctor who answers, and its never actually clear what it's all about. That the doctors don't have enough time is also clear. It's very much on the communication level that it doesn't work. Of course, there are patients who are unhappy in themselves, who you can never really calm down, but for the most part it's through the discussions we have, that we can usually solve it ourselves, the problem. We have cases where the

communication between the doctor and patient is so disrupted that we conduct
mediation discussions in our rooms, in other words we invite the patient, and we invite
the doctor involved, and try in a small group usually with the Mrs. [name] from Quality
Management, we try to carry out mediation'. (E-WG-6, 41–53)

The major aspect here is not what is being reported, as that seems quite
clear. Far more decisive is the fact that it is being reported and that it seems
so clear. The patient's representative is communicating about the communication and makes clear that the practice in a hospital is such that different
perspectives confront each other, different presents and different practices
cannot be brought together through the expertise of the doctor but only by
discussing the communication itself. An oncologist formulates a similar view
when considering the difference between medical and nursing perspectives:

I think that this is the cause of the problems. If, well, -since eh, it can be forecast, that
the nurses for instance will come, we've already had that, there on Monday, you know,
this poor communication, the nurse, who: did not find out, why: what was done, for
example. You see there is obviously a communication problem again. No one tells
them, -although I did in fact raise the subject later, -certainly, it is difficult, whether we
should make these decisions together, it would be a good idea. But of course it would
have to be such, the decision, that the doctor could stick up for it because he must take
the responsibility in front of [name of the head of the medical department]. If we haven't
got this consensus, eh, then he has to like make the decision alone, against the rest of the
world if necessary. But, when they did talk about it, then the others at least knew what
the reasons where for his decision. Now whether that is subjective, justifiable or
unjustifiable pressures or whatever, but at least they knew how the decision came to be
made. And then I believe that the nursing staff can deal with it far more easily, even with
decisions that they don't have to make themselves'. (E-W-12, 848–862)

In this case too, the discussion of the crisis diagnosis does not focus
on whether the decision was right or wrong, but exclusively on the order-
generating role of communication, in other words, on a possibility to be
produced in a present that can be linked to an opinion status. Simply the
fact *that* communication took place seems to be the decisive point here,
not the deliberate dispelling of differences in perspectives. The issue is one
of respect and recognition, and in this respect it appears that the power
structure and the asymmetry between the professional and client or
semiprofessional roles are being hidden behind their communicative
relativization, without of course completely disappearing.

At a first glance, this practice of ethical communication might appear
to be a democratization of decision-making processes. What can most
definitely be observed is the *demand* for symmetrization and democratization. The whole of the discourse about clinical ethics committees and clinical
ethical consultancy is in the end determined by such demands – even when

the prime objective is not the solving of all decision-making problems, the aim is at least to relativize the medical power monopoly in favor of an internal democratization. But in fact it is exactly these democratization demands which facilitate the asymmetrical decisions.

The function of democracy is misunderstood when it is seen as a generator of consensus. The democratic program binds the holder of power – in other words, the 'sovereign' or superior – to stick to his own decisions – even at the cost of deferring his own insight to that which has been asserted. Democracy does not prove itself through consensus, but rather through the tolerance of dissent and at times through the transfer of dissent experiences to the consensus of what is to be accepted now. The political formula of 'democracy' as the central self-descriptive instance of modern political formats thus enables the people who are affected to be stylized as the decision makers. In this sense, democracy protects the powerful from the powerless rather than the reverse – and in this sense it is so attractive to extend the program formula of democratization not just to political areas in the narrower sense, but also to society as a whole, knowing full well that almost nothing in modern society can be traced back to a binding democratic decision. No decision at all, on economic figures or scientific truth, on artistic styles or love, not even on what is visible in the mass media and most definitely not on the healing relevance of religious content, is made *democratically*. The program formula is so attractive for this very reason alone. It throws up questions of legitimation – not in the sense that legitimation will be *found*, but in the sense that the function of the question in the continuing and normalizing of what in the end must always be seen as *irrational* solutions.

This also applies to day-to-day hospital politics as can be seen in our two illuminating examples of the patient representative and the oncologist. The reference to the *democratization* of day-to-day hospital life aims not only at democratizing decision making, but also at breaking the organizational/ medical routine in favor of the power *circle* which lends the medical position its *authority* in the first place. The *informed consent*[2] does nothing else than this either. It forms an interruption in the routine of the *informed* decision-making process. The *competence* dimension of the decision-making process is thus interrupted by the *social* dimension of *consent*, in other words by an *individual decision*.

Symmetrizing forms of communication serve then – almost ironically – to create mutual recognition of the speakers' incommensurability by increasing their respective authenticity. This – in this sense 'democratizing' practice – is indeed the basis for the peaceful coexistence of incommensurable practices, which thus become commensurable. The different speaker positions of the doctor, the patient representative, the patient and other speakers can, through mutual recognition, perpetuate the recognition of *their own* practice formats and thus act as if they were all involved in a mutual reference system. It is exactly for this reason that the conversion *communication* is being engineered even in the self-reflection of practice.

As will now be demonstrated, the idea of discourse, in particular, feeds on a high level of trust in the order-generating power of communication – as manifested in the institutionalized form of clinical ethics committees. It is from this perspective – we are only interested in connectivity from a systems theory perspective – that new perspectives emerge on a research issue which can be summarized as follows: The function of HECs is at best unclear, and at worst does not exist at all. Approaches to this subject begin with the findings that it is obviously not about concrete decisions (see Michel, 1993, p. 80) and not about a consensus (Moreno, 1988, p. 428). Instead of this, the process itself and the consensus about the process (Moreno op. cit.), or something like a 'narrative approach' – in contrast to ethical principalism – (Brody, 1999, p. 50; Poirier, 1999, p. 35) themselves represent a reasonable meeting, because 'While it is unlikely that an ethics committee would ever explicitly address the moral fragmentation of Western or American culture in the midst of a case review, there are attitudes that committee members might readily strike that do reflect these subtle cultural conditions. I would like to comment on two: a tendency toward ethical skepticism and relativism, and a tendency to consign ethical matters to one's 'private life' (Blake, 1992, p. 7).

What sounds here like an attempt to gain something positive out of a failed experiment is due to the tone of voice which in the ethical sense is a solution in itself. The style of Richard Moskowitz is very similar: 'It is therefore inevitable that serious ethical conflicts should occur within the hospital. The amazing thing is that HECs have succeeded so well with them, while their parent hospitals are often powerless to resolve issues of far lesser difficulty and importance. Their healing function clearly has to do with their ability to articulate moral values which are generally recognized and adhered to throughout the hospital community. But it also implies a commitment to broad and faithful representation of the diversity of interests and viewpoints in the hospital and the community at large, and to a process of dialogue and mutual respect in an attempt to reconcile them when they disagree' (Moskowitz, 1989, p. 36).

While the opponents of such an approach can plausibly accept criticism of the procedure and promise a better future for the HECs if they professionalize their procedures (see Wolf, 1992, 1993; Hoffmann, 1994;

Hayes, 1995), we would like in what follows to turn the argumentation around. The HECs' apparent lack of a function is not a problem, but rather it is a solution insofar as under the special conditions a form of address has developed which breaks precisely with the classic expectations of functionality, consistency and professionalism. While the vanishing point of a philosophical discussion always offers the possibility of agreement, group discussions on the subject of ethics, according to the statements made by participants of HECs, seem in the first place to be especially suitable to practically mediating the experience of difference.

A patient representative, also in the HEC, who had just begun her contribution, formulated it in a very similar manner to that of the ethical consultation (Saake & Kunz, 2006), saying she found it very positive to experience in the discussion that other people could see things differently:

> Well we also had the experience at congresses that cases were presented on which concrete work had been done, and that had been helpful to someone, because other people saw it quite differently, for instance. You got the chance to see the variety. I think that is very important, and I also think it is important that we, now in this group, naturally deal anonymously with cases that occur with us. It is, it has: something to be said for it too. So I think of course the case studies do help somewhat.' (E-WG-6, 516–521)

Different ways of looking at things translate into opposite opinions, and their expression, especially in the committee, can gain importance against the backdrop of opinions as is clear from the statement made by a chief physician.

> I: *'Hm, what do you wish to express specifically to the ethics committee? How would you describe it?'*
> B: 'That's just another general formulation that doesn't say anything to me, eh, I try, the things, that are being discussed simply, with what I think, what appears to me to be right, so that I can contribute something when other opinions are being aired'. (E-HT-13, 218–223)

A surgeon reports about the effects the many ways of viewing an issue have on his own perspective:

> [...] I simply say now what I feel, what is good for me, if the discussion with people who simply have another way of looking at things and who view and discuss the issue in an open discussion round, evaluation round, simply from different perspectives. That means, I listen happily when a Pastor Kern, or a Ms. Hauck, or a Ms. Lustig, or a Doctor Stein, or simply from –, or the nursing personnel, just simply in the situation, you see? The non-medical side for once, how does someone see it who sees it from the outside or from another position, how is the issue viewed, what values have a massive importance and what values do we not really take any notice of?

That means, the thing about bodily injury, that we perform every day, with the consent of our patients of course-, make, is -, we make it just something normal that we do every day. And then for example, a Ms. Hauck comes along, who became involved in the discussion about the patient who was given a PEG without her consent and asks how = how shocking, or how extreme this reaction also seems from someone who sees it really as it is: yes as bodily injury but with what a degree of emotionality, of sentimentality it was brought into the discussion by someone, emotionality that we ourselves are not aware of. Yes I find the whole thing is an expansion of my horizons, yes, what I say ethically-morally, but also my thinking horizon.

I 1: *'Mhm. That probably doesn't make it easier as a doctor, does it?'*
B: 'Yes it does make it easier'

I 1: *'It does?'*
B: 'Yes. It makes it easier, because you can recognize why someone reacts with fear in this situation, I erm-, I can recognize-, then I feel again as a normal person, as a human being who gets into such a situation and says, okay, so like now on the intensive care ward with one patient, I can understand the difficult situation people find themselves in, who normally have nothing to do with medicine in this borderline situation, who simply feel overwhelmed, literally steamrollered, you see?' (E-WG-15, 134–163)

By acknowledging other perspectives, the 'normality' of one's own view becomes relativized, one's own perspective is recognizable as one *perspective* among others. It is not the matter-of-fact things of the everyday working world which should form the basis of the situation evaluation; the asymmetry is pushed much more in the direction of a non-medical, normal perspective which must then be understood and taken on board. Accordingly, a *good* participant in the discourse – in other words, a participant who acts as one in the discourse – is less characterized by arguing consistently over a period of time than by being flexible and showing his ability to change perspectives. There will be more on this later.

The idea of interdisciplinarity, to which the composition of the ethics committees from different professions seems to be geared, appears from a discourse perspective to be a necessary prerequisite to allow a free play of the good reasons (see also Capron, 1985). In the context of the ethics committees, however, it loses some of its instrumental character, and even the production of a multiplicity of viewpoints appears to be the aim of an ethical discussion rather than being just a partial victory.

Against this horizon, being of different opinions appears almost entirely unproblematic:

That too is an experience for me, to ask someone about -, his autonomy and so on -, it's been many years, but it was a decisive point for me, so to speak, I have my opinion, the person, the person affected had a different opinion and we still get on although our opinions are the exact opposite! Well not exactly opposite, but very contrary. And I believe, that when you deal with each other like that, then I believe that you can even allow ethical problems to stand, at least if people do not explode and emotionally eh completely decompensate [...]. (E-WG-15, 663–671)

Having another opinion is not only a problem; it is actually seen as a solution since we are only dealing with *opinions*. The productivity of the discourse is measured not according to how far it contributes to a consensus, but according to how much it contributes to producing different speakers.

Seen in terms of social history, one cannot imagine a form of society in which a 'natural state' would tolerate symmetrical speaker positions in the long term. A situation where all are allowed to have their say – even should have their say – is initially a highly unlikely social situation, and the dyed-in-the-wool discourse theoreticians would not accept that the idea of a power-free discourse was anything other than an ideal, a theoretical claim rather than an empirical description.[3] However, it has been observed that in the ethics committees a discourse has become established in which the speaker positions can no longer be legitimately limited. One also sees that situations in which speakers get the chance to speak have to be repeatedly re-established.[4]

The descriptions of a former doctor and member of the ethics committee illustrate the consequences of this particular type of openness for potential speakers in the committee:

And I must say, my idea was: well, when I allowed myself, eh, eh, for example with someone who wished to speak, a dialog ensued, and I was warned again and again that there was a speaker list, but it had only been my intention to clarify some concepts with him. So, something was said, perhaps a term such as self-determination, or enlightenment, or like, oh I don't know, truth or something like that, and it was my intention to ask what was meant by these terms, in order to make it clearer for the group what was being said. Because if I just let a discussion like that: run, so that everyone around the table just presents his statement then in the end I just have a collection of statements in which the same term may be used seven times but is probably used differently seven times. (E-WG-12, 231–241)

The reference to a speakers' list in the discourse is apparently very difficult to ignore, which is why the clarification of and agreement on terms took second place to the right to be heard – to the regret of the interviewee. From the position of the sociological observers, this can not be criticized; of far more sociological interest are the consequences for the discussion of this behavior if this approach leads to a 'collection of statements' which will then have to be dealt with in later practice.

Just how much discursive decision making is interpreted as a symmetrizing event can be seen in the idea of speaking eye-to-eye, which has to be learnt in the asymmetrically structured hospital organization:

> So we try now and again to get a discussion round going, so that everyone can learn how to discuss and to get over inhibitions when speaking to the consultant, and the consultant could start looking a bit less arrogant when speaking to a nurse, well all = all these things, and if, I believe if it had been practiced a little over the long-term-you can't do it in a year, then another type of everyday behavior would become normal, and the nursing staff because they would have the space where they could speak in a certain manner, and then they would be able to do it a bit more on the ward, if the situation allowed it, but these are long-term projects that would take years. (E-HB-1, 44–53)

In the view of this doctor, a successful discussion requires competent speakers capable of contributing to the discussion. For this to happen, different persons must see themselves in the first place as speakers in order to position themselves as speakers. A lack of this competence is found particularly among the nursing staff who are, however, supposed to learn this in the protected space of the ethics committee, to present themselves as speakers and thus be able to stand up to the consultant in the future.

THE FORMAT OF ETHICAL SPEAKING

An ethical discourse is obviously a discourse which allows room for many potential speakers and to which, in principle, everyone can contribute. The contribution that a speaker can make should be associated less with his/her role in the hospital or profession and more with his/her status as an ethical speaker:

> I: *'How would you, how should I say, see your special role in these diverse working groups, as a medical ethicist? In other words, how do you see your tasks, what do you do there?'*
> B: 'Well first of all, independent of any professional background or educational background, I think everyone can contribute insofar as they have interested themselves in the subject and have gained experience, and have thought about it. It has been my experience that the roles become blurred relatively quickly in these committees so that the doctor suddenly starts talking very theoretically, the medical ethicist suddenly brings in medical aspects which he's experienced and so on. And that, I won't say that the roles completely disappeared, but that we work very soon together very fluidly [...]'. (E-HB-29, 168–179)

A medical ethicist reports here about his experience that the usual appointed roles no longer function in the discourse of the clinical ethics committee, and it appears as an ethical competence of the speakers gathered there to be able to argue flexibly and in doing so to be able take on the perspective of another discourse participant. The discussion partners are also expected to be seen separately from the anticipated professional role.

> It makes a difference because one no longer sees the role names and functions, but really the person who is sitting opposite, so that if there are five people sitting there, then I really am aware of each individually. And those hierarchically further up behave again a little differently. In the palliative medicine working group we have Professor Niemann, Professor Steinem, Professor Koch, then poor Ms. Bauer is, I believe, the only nursing staff member we have – but she contributes as well. She is a little reserved alright, she is normally able to speak in quite an excited manner, but, nonetheless, if she has something to say, she does, and she contradicts too. So we do have the imbalance that there are more of them. In the therapy limits working group Professor Arenz is the only one, we have two nurses, it is fairly well mixed, and Possner is in it too, a registrar, another registrar, it's fairly well balanced. But the nurses have the least to say here too, it's true, it all takes time. (E-HB-1, 90–102)

A member of the management describes the dissolution of expected roles in a similar manner which is attributed to the discourse itself:

> It is a recommendation, the forming of opinion and there are several people involved in it, not just one or two. There are many involved. Many different professional groups are involved, and I at least have always experienced that in the third round at the latest the discussion already has this, this, this crusted, mhm, guideline: We nursing staff see the actual patients and you as the doctor only see an object of your actions. Or the other way around: the doctor says: No, no, you always want to bring in lots of emotion. Try and be a bit more objective! At the latest by the second or third round this, this, this crust is broken, [I: *yes.*] and one learns to understand each other across professional boundaries – somehow the way of thinking – I get the impression that there is understanding for the other professional group. And that is, I think, very important. - The external members of the ethics committees play a decisive role for me also in this special area. [I: *Mhm.*] Because they simply, -I don't know whether this is getting across properly, what I mean. The externals are capable, and they do it too, they simply ask: Why this, why that, why the other? [I: *Mhm.*] And they don't just accept certain things as given, as something that just has to be accepted. (E-HT-9, 844–861)

It is rather surprising that what is being described here is the dynamics of a discourse which release the participants from their specific expertise, since it is the interplay of different professionals and professions which is generally stylized as being a part of the solutions in the decision-making process. In the practice of ethical discourse in the clinical ethics committee, argumentation with reference to one's own profession is problematical.

B: 'When something is discussed there, it also affects me emotionally, it's

I: 'Mhm'
B: 'absolutely clear on the human level too, I try not to repress that aspect but to allow it room …, but I also try then to simply view the legal aspects of the matter. In fact both, when you look at the situation and the disagreements, when we discussed, erm, the treatment of patients and eh, the alleviation of a patient's conditions in the final phase',

I. 'Mhm'
B: 'who was really very ill, erm, it was clear alright, that, eh, we could have simply on the one hand looked at the matter from the legal aspect, but then naturally the way those who were involved were affected, they were very easily left out'

I: 'Mhm'
B: 'left out, they're just in a certain relationship, in a certain context, there are dependencies, and it's obviously very important that we see this. There's no point in just saying: legally it appears like a, b, c'

I: 'Mhm'
B: 'no-one is helped by that, rather I have to look, eh, is what I'm saying of any use to those involved?'

I: 'Mhm'
B: 'I have to ask, but at the same time the aspect of eh, human feelings, of empathy has to be looked at and included, eh, what in the context are the problems, what is of particular note, what plays a role'. (E-HT-5, 674–699)

The participation of this lawyer in the ethics committee is legitimized a priori by her status as a legal expert, but in the discussion, the reference to this expertise is no longer so promising. Professions in the classic sense, such as the medical and legal experts, usually present 'good reasons' for establishing an asymmetry which is systematically chipped away at in the ethics committee. Different opinions must be heard, and every evaluation is only valid as long as it does not affect the validity of other evaluations.

A patient representative explains the rule of taking a position without 'condemning' an opposing practice:

B: 'It's often happens that we're not of one opinion in the ethics committee, there are often differing opinions, and I can say that it is certainly an interesting experience, and I often come, and when there is case to discuss and it is presented, and I read it through and I immediately have some idea, a feeling, no, that's not possible, and I'm often astonished how through the reflection of different professional groups, which I find very important, in, with this difference among the members, how then suddenly in fact other aspects come into play for me too, and I have never turned 180 degrees say, but 45 degrees yes, so that I said afterwards: I can't look at it one-sidedly, that aspect is also part of it for me, and that was really only happened through this discussion with one another'

I: *'yes'*
B. 'and I find it important because there are so many layers simply because of the existence of a'

I: *'yes'*.
B: 'group like this, and what I also find interesting is that in the hospital the people are afraid of some kind of judgment or accusations, aren't they?, we submit a case and they say no that's not possible, says the ethics committee, that's just not true because we always try to understand the different layers, and we always vote which provides an opinion but does not judge, because I think it is not the job of the ethics committee to accuse but to help in coming to a judgment or it may be important for later cases, mightn't it?' (E-HT-2, 477–498)

The process itself is of great importance for the participants of the ethics committee in which a decision is to be made. In the 'many layers' of the positions, the depth of the ethical reflection can be shown esthetically.

That does not mean that we are better than the others! That was an interesting case with the prenatal diagnostics, for instance, after we'd sorted out certain things for ourselves, one doctor came out with the accusation [quote], yes and you think other doctors at other hospitals are much less ethically responsible because you leave the ethical problem to them, because you don't carry out some abortions because of social indications, or because even that is not available. And then we had a discussion round in the town. There was a forum, I think it was organized from Friedrichsstadt, that's a larger hospital, and it turned out that the ethical problem is the same there, in other words other hospitals are just as careful and in-depth. It's just that they use different reasoning. And that really relieved us. (E-EH-1, 274–285)

Other positions are no less ethical, the rationale behind them is just different. Of key importance for this hospital pastor is the fact *that* there were reasons. With this reasoning the discussion is no longer about good or bad decisions.

In the context of the argumentation in the ethics committee, reasons lose their quasi-ontological status; they get their validity not just from their prepositional content but also through their relationship to the discourse. In what follows, a registrar explains the difficulty of not letting her own position play a determining role in the argumentation:

Well I just noticed that I personally, but this is absolutely just a personal opinion, which stems from my personal background, moral beliefs, ethics, religion, I tend personally to reject termination of pregnancy, but as I say, that is a completely personal attitude, and it is also a challenge not to allow this opinion to dominate, since it is always there, something you always have when making a decision when it's difficult, it goes without saying, only we have to approach this in a very structured and transparent manner and the pastor involved, for example Ms. S., she put it very clearly, for her it is simply killing and the value of the ... and so on and then she cannot vote and then she is against it you see? OK. I think it's good that she's said it clearly, that is naturally very difficult when someone says you can offer me here whatever you want, I will always say no because of my background alright? Then it is naturally a very difficult situation that we have there. But, when she says in the individual case, [quotes] I must point out the protection of life in my role as pastor, mustn't I? Then that is transparent isn't it? It's just this 'always', that would be difficult. (E-HB-19, 299–314)

The required openness of the discourse only appears to be assured when the arguments are not linked to specific persons or roles. It is seen as problematical that you can tell beforehand how someone is going to reason his/her position. A good discourse is not measured by the fact that different disciplines argue consistently over a period of time, but by the fact that role-typical expectancies can be systematically disappointed. Very practically, it means that a medical argument gains in persuasive power when it is postulated by a layperson. Redundancy in the argument, in contrast, weakens the value of the contribution for the discussion as can be seen from this statement by a theologian:

I: *'Mhm. We judge you then, eh, that someone is involved who is not in fact an expert in that sense, but is herself a former patient?'*
B: 'Yes, eh, in principle I find that good, ehm, however right now, eh, we have a concrete case in mind, eh, since, since this member of the committee, dwells a bit too strongly on his own position and asserts his own person a lot and it is sometimes a bit redundant, [...]'. (E-HT-6, 364–369)

An approach is put forward, which implies continuous learning and continuous revision, and which reasons but then turns round and doubts these reasons. A patient representative expresses:

B: 'Well, I find that I, eh, for me it is the case, that erm, there too, I said this earlier already, I really often am amazed at myself'

I: *'Mhm'*.
B: 'that I have to look up and look again, and have to constantly revise my opinion and that I'm always learning and I have to keep learning that everything is not so exclusive',

I: *'Yes'*.
B: 'as it appears initially, well, I find that very interesting for myself and also, erm, well that's a completely positive aspect, because you naturally start immediately, in day-to-day life: to think about, what you can really see'. (E-HT-2, 642–650)

What can be observed here is described by us elsewhere as 'ethical sensitization', and we are describing in this way a characteristic feature of this ethical discourse, the 'reversibility of any argument in favor of a *culture of the reversible argument*' (Saake & Kunz, 2006, p. 41). From a rationalistic viewpoint, this type of discourse can appear as indecisiveness (see Reamer, 1987); in the case of interest in the ethical discourse as a social practice, a specific logic can be detected behind it. Every argument and every solution appears provisional, every decision is designed to communicate the fact that it might possibly be wrong.

> Yes, that is -, I mean, an obstetric clinic is obviously another very controversial problem, the late abortion is certainly one of the most difficult decisions which the doctor has to make and there is no solution, it is a rare problem where in the end one is almost always guilty. So. And what is necessary, and what the ethics committee and this working group has to do, that such decisions, as bad as they are, are at least transparent and are subject to a certain structure, that means that it is not as if the decision is made behind closed doors in any kind of arbitrary way, but rather it is discussed by external staff or, the comm, we are not just the ethics committee making the decision, there are also geneticists and psychosomatic experts, psychiatrists, in case there is a danger of suicide, or so, so, and it is done very transparently and it has to be argued out. And I think this is an adequate procedure even though one can't actually solve the problem, in my understanding we have found the best solution, and we are all agreed, since such a procedure at least facilitates a discourse, a transparent discourse and thus the best that one can do in the situation. And the decision is then a reasoned one, a weighed up reasoned decision even though we know that it is of course possible to get it wrong. And I find that very positive even for these sometimes really terrible decisions which we can, and that came out yesterday, we can stand by our decision! (E-HB-19, 227–245)

In a similar manner to this registrar, a psychologist assumes that there can be no 'solution' to an ethical problem, but that it is the fact of dealing with this problem which makes up the ethical aspect.

> This is the debate, that it is often not black or white but grey, yes, well there is no *one* solution, but there is perhaps the best possible decision, that I am now also in this working group about dying in the hospital, where everything is simply super time and again, where one gets to know people again from other professions and where we sit down together and discuss certain subjects. (E-HB-15, 537–542)

The impossibility in some situations of forming an opinion or making a decision is expressed by a nurse:

> B: 'Well, one has great difficulty with one's own opinion and I always have serious problems. I just see both sides and feel more or less helpless, caught between the fronts so to speak. And that is the reason why I am in an ethics committee, yes perhaps, well, to find clarification, or somehow to be involved in a process which leads to clarity, I mean, if I have to choose between two terrible things, it will always be terrible and if you can do it, and decision-making mechanisms evolve and so, well, as I said, that is the main reason I participate'.
>
> I: *'Mhm. So you mean, something like, [quotes fictively] I'm not quite clear about this myself yet'*
> B: 'Is it possible to be clear about it?'

I: *'No, of course not, but –'*

B: 'one can only find a way of making a decision, which can help one, well, to more or less do justice to the subject'. (E-HB-24, 374–385)

When a solution to a problem does not appear to be possible, attention is concentrated on the procedures of the discourse, which may not appear to be suitable in helping create clarity in the sense of the discourse theory, but which must meet specific requirements to do justice [...] to the subject'.

What put me personally under pressure was the fact that I had to be involved in the decision, where I myself simply did not know what is right! We often do not know what is right, but in such a massive decision about life and death one wants to, well -, you try to make the right decision, and you can't make the decision, there is no weighing up of the different arguments, yes, there is no method of reaching the right decision, but rather one has to be aware of ones subjectivity, [...]. We must be clear about it, simply to be transparent with oneself, about which roots my decision is coming from. (E-HB-19, 593–602)

What should have been demonstrated up to now is that in clinical ethics committees, during the processing of ethical issues somehow a friendly reasoning algorithm has developed with the aid of which decisions can be demonstrated to be the right decisions, and that a certain way of speaking has established itself, an *ethical way of speaking* which shows the ethics in the discussion itself. A perspective must be able to show itself to be a perspective, and at the same time other speakers receive recognition on the basis of their contribution; positions must be reasoned, while reasons are always seen as being reversible; solutions should always be presented as being provisional.

In answer to the question by the interviewer, whether the discussion in the ethics committee simply represents a meeting of different professional perspectives, or if it gains a specific new quality, a theologian points to the discussion as a practice which one must allow oneself to be surprised by:

I 1: *'[...] Well is it, is it somehow something independent, something new, could you say, that has developed there?'*

B: 'Hm, well I think that is now more difficult to answer because, because somehow that, this meeting itself is somehow something new, but not so that one would have to invent a medical ethics, so, no, that is in a small way my point, it's more that you allow what is there to meet up in the right way and then discover how it converges. That's how I would describe it'. (E-HB-10, 366–373)

The point is not to set oneself up in a new reasoning logic, to 'invent' a medical ethics; the aim is rather to manage to deal with the concurrence of different perspectives, different presents, and *practically* to get around with the horizon of a missing central perspective.

How then does the ethics committee reach its decisions, how can clarities be produced, when every argument is expected to be presented in a gesture of self-doubt, when the non-compulsory compulsion of the better argument shortens the reasons to such an extent that the best of all the reasons have selected themselves and the discourse has come to a standstill?

A solution remains always only a provisional solution so that the discourse perpetuates into infinity as can be seen in the descriptions of a doctor:

> And that, that, that [sigh], too little progress is made, in the end too few tangible results come out in the end, since carrying on this type of debate with details, it is not very productive, or so. And I think it bored most of them a little, well I had the impression, there were always voices that said [quotes] now we have to finish up and in God's name the issue comes to a provisional end if it is not finally concluded, and what issue, particularly such subjects, is then concluded? In the end it always needs to be revised, it has to be, it needs to be developed, a solution can only ever be a provisional one and can never be conclusive. In this respect there was also a tendency simply to finish with the issue in order to turn to other topics. (E-WG-12, 507–517)

How then is the discourse ended? Through a decision being made. The discourse itself is not terminated, since it presents itself every time only as a provisional decision which is why, for instance, the discussion is often ended with a reference to the lack of time since other issues have to be dealt with.

It seems impossible to deal with truths argumentatively. Instead, there are more likely to be plausibilities which seem to almost force themselves into the discussion and can hardly be fended off, precisely because no reasons are required for them. They present themselves far more transcendentally as can be seen in the following example from a theologian:

> One cannot vote on something that is simply perceived! You see? Instead one has to-if need be – naturally – you have to wait very patiently, until everyone is gathered and until really everyone says, yes, that's it! And then there can be no more arguing. You can argue so wonderfully if the point is not grasped, the point of perception, then you just won't succeed! and there are enough examples where you can point to that, that is something I always try to make clear in my lectures, to show this point where the truth cannot be found through argument, where it simply forces itself upon you, when it somehow becomes unavoidable. For instance, the example we had earlier with parents and children.[5] You would have to push very hard indeed to reject such a powerful perception. You would have to force the issue extremely hard, you would have to dig very deeply into anthropology. (E-HB-10, 545–555)

On the one hand, there are certainties which cannot be brought about through arguments, while on the other hand, the discourse produces simple arguments which can be linked up to other arguments

A doctor:

> I: *'It is-, have you the feeling with the consultations that, -that the arguments -, well, how should I put it,-can the arguments be continued indefinitely, or are they exhausted at some point?'*
> B: 'No, no, it becomes exhausted. It becomes exhausted. It definitely becomes exhausted. And one does not find a solution, right? Well, afterwards –, also, well, when we have talked for two hours, we basically still have not got any further. In fact I can actually remember cases where I had no idea up to ten minutes before a telephone call I'd arranged, that I just had no idea what I should do. We had one case that I can remember, where I actually phoned a friend that evening, she is neonatologist and questioned her again about the disease, it certainly occupies your thoughts for a long time. And as I said, up to ten minutes before the telephone call still unsure-, and the decision smacks to a degree of arbitrariness too -, but it is still a prerequisite, I have to create a structure, that at least has the potential, that one looks at the thing from every aspect. It's a kind of thoroughness postulate in such a difficult decision. Well, even if it is not somehow instrumental in helping find a solution, the process in itself is extremely important'. (E-HB-19, 405–419)

What becomes exhausted is not the arguments, but rather the resources such as time and attention, which the discourse in this form demands as interaction. The arbitrariness of the decision which then *must* be taken is more or less obvious to the participants also.[6] Nonetheless, the discussion does not appear to have been a failure, since it was designed less as an instrument to produce a consensus and more to facilitate in the ethical form the production of speakers and reasons. And sufficient uncertainty remains, so that in the end a *decision* can be made.

CONSEQUENCES FOR ETHICS OR THE RUSE OF ETHICAL REASON

At the end of our discussion we would like to briefly consider the consequences of our results for ethical theory. Sociologists know that organizational practices such as those of hospitals, government policy, advertising, suitable treatment of animals, and investment decisions cannot be conditioned or programmed with such new philosophical–scientific labels as medical ethics, political ethics, ethics in advertising, animal ethics or industrial ethics and economic ethics. If it were possible, such ethics could not be treated scientifically. In the case of medical ethics, sure enough it can clearly be seen that there has been a marked ethical sensitization of problems. And we believe that we can say normatively with our results that HECs are indeed ethically significant, that is to say insofar as they create a form which meets one of the expectations of a culture accustomed to symmetrical communication, even in organizations which in the end functionally serve the suspension of symmetry requirements. How else are organizations to deal with the multiplicity of speaker positions other than by establishing islands inside the organizations where these may be visible *as speaker positions* – this is one of our results.

Ethical theory must, however, still continue to ask itself, how it can be in a position to *shorten* ethical arguments, i.e. to make sure that it at least offers criteria or procedures to distinguish right from wrong. Whether – as in the case of – we are talking about the discourse on evolving values and their integrative power (see Joas, 2001), whether the discourse of the ethical potential of the language can be seen as a basis on which morally integrated action coordination can be emphasized (see Habermas, 1990a), whether it can be cultivated in the sense of Rawls' justice as a basic category of adequate socialization (see Rawls, 1971), or in particulate communicative liberalism criticism, limited to patriotic universalisms (see Taylor, 1992; Sandel, 1982; Etzioni, 1993), whether a minimal morality compatible with differentiated modernity can be shaped in contrast to the communitaristic revitalization of Durkheimianism, as practiced by Nunner-Winkler (2001) for instance, whether reference is made to theoretical coherence and embedding in a structural rationality in the sense of a theory of rationality (Nida-Rümelin, 2000) or whether a general humanity is posited as the moral yardstick of the social as with Martha Nussbaum in an Aristotelian-essentialist sense (see Nussbaum, 1995), the discourse always takes the form that it, on the one hand, still emphasizes the integrative force of moral judgment, while on the other hand shortening the argumentative possibilities. Scientific ethics is not possible without such a shortening algorithm. It must at least demonstrate an intuition of a true or right ethical perception and its rationality to be ethically meaningful. Taking this as a presumption, the ethical practice in the HECs contradicts this diametrically, since it is exactly the opposite that succeeds here: Arguments, speakers and reasons are produced and multiplied, and *in this* and *only in this* is the ethical sense of communication revealed in practice. It is particularly interesting from a sociological perspective, because it is only this perspective that can see how such locations develop for the special form of 'ethical' speaking – without itself falling into the pattern of ethical speaking. To all others it will only appear to be evidence of the lack of function of HECs, who then somehow rescue themselves 'ethically' by finding it positive to get into discussion with each other.

The consequences of these results reach much further. They are an almost symbolic expression of the 'society of presents', i.e. a society which is able to disconnect presences and to do without a strong idea of integration. In that sense this description of modernity is a radically post-Parsonian systems' theoretical description. Our empirical results show that HECs are sociologically more significant than they may first appear. Two things can be observed in HECs: *On the one hand*, the recognition of the incommensurability of different forms of practice and reflection perspectives is celebrated. HECs deal with the structural impossibility of generating a total perspective from different professional and practical perspectives. In contrast, the functional meaning of HECs appears to be to accomplish communicatively and to be decidedly able to forbear the use of such a perspective.

In ethical theory this experience – in the German-speaking world at least – has been embedded in the incontrovertible prominence of the discourse ethics of Apel (1990) and Habermas (1990b) (see Kettner, 1996, 1999). It ethically and philosophically reflects what can be practically and empirically observed: The practical efficacious substance of the ethical committee does not consist of good and better reasons, but of more and more authentic speakers. For reasons of space we cannot show here how this is reflected in the philosophical-ethical discourse. Finally, we would like to point out that our empirical results have far broader sociological significance than simply in reference to HECs.

The ability of modern societies to disconnect presents from each other can be observed in the practice of the HECs. What is decided in HECs and what commitments, fictions of consensus and common papers are generated do not in any way condition clinical practice. The present of the committee meetings differs from the present of clinical decision-making practice in the wards. HECs learn mentalities in order to avoid mediating these presents. They thus form both a culturalizing and therefore, an interlocking, recognition of different perspectives: Medical, religious, nursing, patients', ethical, economic and other perspectives are communicated without being mediated. Care is taken that they can be spoken about authentically. HECs do not take the drama out of the pressure of decision making. Like all organizations, organizations in healthcare are decision machines (see Nassehi, 2005b). But they do take the drama out of the incommensurability of decision-making presents and generate a space within the clinic, in which other rules apply than those which apply in the clinic outside of the committee.

To a certain extent, HECs channel culturalizing interruptions and appoint speakers who are not explicitly found in the committees even when the 'human beings' involved in the ward and the committee are possibly the same; they are not the same 'persons' (see Nassehi, 2007). The HEC reflects how modern society disintegrates into presents in the manner of a functionally differentiated society which does not treat its incommensurability from their perspective as a problem or fault, but rather, in fact, as a potential. We call this – in systems theory terms – a *society of presents*, in which the continuity of a total perspective gives way to concrete presents (see Nassehi, 2003, 2004, 2005a, 2006). A modern, functionally differentiated society can only be in possession of political or ethically effective self-descriptions which aim at the whole and wish to produce the continuity of an integrated society showing solidarity, and which has split off from other presents – just as the HECs have broken off from standard hospital practice. In this respect, it is in fact the HECs' apparent *lack of* function which is their true *functional* feature. One can learn from the example of HECs that a modern society with a strict interconnection of its instances is unthinkable and that society's modern moral and functional disintegration is not to be treated as a structural defect, but rather that it is the pulling apart which enables the modern moment, which the theory of modernity has discovered and known for 200 years as the essential structural feature – without ever having paid sufficient attention to this potential. That this is diametrically opposed to the basic intuitions of the formation of ethical theory with its attempt to integrate the different and the plural conceals a certain irony of our results. And one can always learn from this, which is just where we started with our thesis: Ethics is only a scientific discipline, disconnected from practices which give themselves the same name.

NOTES

1. Research project at the universities of Munich and Göttingen (Germany), supported by the DFG (German Research Foundation). The interviews cited have been conducted in German language at several German hospitals.
2. See Beauchamp and Faden (1995) for more detail on the emergence and criticism of this term.
3. See Habermas, 1984/87 in general and Kettner (1996, 1999) with regard to HECs.

4. It is quite remarkable that such expectations of a symmetrical discourse can only be achieved within the context of an organization, one level of creating social order, where one always seems to recognize the asymmetry. Interestingly, self-descriptions of such discourse trust more than anything else in interaction, which – as another level of the social creation of order is also full of asymmetries – can always only be addressed sequentially and can always only focus on one subject at a time (cf. Luhmann, 1975).

5. At an earlier point, this theologian had argued that beyond the bounds of every argument it was part of the nature of humans that children need parents in order to be able to develop their personality (E-HB-10, 439–480).

6. Jonathan Moreno criticizes these decisions as blind compromises; the disconnection of reason and final decision can be understood, however, from the practice of the ethics committee (cf. Moreno, 1988).

REFERENCES

Apel, K.-O. (1990). Is the ethics of the ideal communication community a utopia? On the relationship between ethics, utopia, and the critique of utopia. In: S. Benhabib & F. Dallmayr (Eds), *The communicative ethics controversy* (pp. 23–59). Cambridge, MA: MIT Press.
Beauchamp, T. L., & Faden, R. (1995). Meaning and elements of informed consent. In: W. T. Reich (Ed.), *Encyclopedia of bioethics* (pp. 1238–1241). New York: Simon & Schuster Macmillan.
Blake, D. C. (1992). The hospital ethics committee: Health care's moral conscience or white elephant? *Hastings –Center Report, 22*, 6–11.
Brody, H. (1999). Narrative ethics and institutional impact. *HEC Forum, 11*, 46–51.
Capron, A. M. (1985). Legal perspectives on institutional ethics committees. *Journal of College and University Law, 11*, 417–431.
Etzioni, A. (1993). *The spirit of community: Rights, responsibilities, and the communitarian agenda.* New York: Crown Publishers.
Habermas, J. (1984/87). *The theory of communicative action. Two volumes.* Boston: Beacon Press.
Habermas, J. (1990a). *Moral consciousness and communicative action.* Cambridge, MA: MIT Press.
Habermas, J. (1990b). Discourse ethics: Notes on a program of philosophical justification. In: S. Benhabib & F. Dallmayr (Eds), *The communicative ethics controversy* (pp. 43–115). Cambridge, MA: MIT Press.
Hayes, G. J. (1995). Ethics committees: Group process concerns and the need for research. *Cambridge Quarterly of Health Care Ethics, 4*, 83–91.
Hoffmann, D. E. (1994). Case consultation: Paying attention to process. In: S. Spicker (Ed.), *The healthcare ethics committee experience: Selected readings from HEC forum* (pp. 257–264). Malabar, FL: Krieger Publishing Company.
Joas, H. (2001). *The genesis of values.* Chicago: University of Chicago Press.
Kettner, M. (1996). Discourse ethics and health care ethics committees. *Jahrbuch für Recht und Ethik, 4*, 249–272.
Kettner, M. (1999). Discourse ethics: A novel approach to moral decision making. *International Journal of Bioethics, 10*, 29–36.

Luhmann, N. (1975). *Interaktion, Organisation, Gesellschaft.* In: *Soziologische Aufklärung* (Vol. 2, pp. 9–20). Opladen: Westdeutscher Verlag.

Luhmann, N. (1995). *Social systems.* Stanford, CA: Stanford University Press.

Luhmann, N. (1996). The sociology of the moral and ethics. *International Sociology, 11,* 27–36.

Luhmann, N. (1998). *Observations on modernity.* Stanford, CA: Stanford University Press.

Luhmann, N. (2002). In: W. Rasch (Ed.), *Theories of distinction: Redescribing the description of modernity.* Stanford, CA: Stanford University Press.

Maynard, D. (1991). Interaction and asymmetry in clinical discourse. *American Journal of Sociology, 97,* 448–495.

Michel, V. (1993). The ethics committee as a 'Community of Concern': A reflection on the accountability of bioethcis committees and consultants. In: S. Spicker (Ed.), *The healthcare ethics committee experience: Selected readings from HEC forum* (pp. 76–80). Malabar, FL: Krieger Publishing Company.

Moreno, J. D. (1988). Ethics by committee: The moral authority of consensus. *The Journal of Medicine and Philosophy, 13,* 411–432.

Moskowitz, R. (1989). Hospital ethics committees: The healing function. In: S. Spicker (Ed.), *The healthcare ethics committee experience: Selected readings from HEC forum* (pp. 32–38). Malabar, FL: Krieger Publishing Company.

Nassehi, A. (2001). Religion und Moral. Zur Säkularisierung der Moral und der Moralisierung der Religion in der modernen Gesellschaft. In: M. Krüggeler & G. Pickel (Eds), *Religion und Moral* (pp. 21–38). Opladen: Westdeutscher Verlag.

Nassehi, A. (2003). *Geschlossenheit und Offenheit. Studien zur Theorie der modernen Gesellschaft.* Frankfurt, Main: Suhrkamp Verlag.

Nassehi, A. (2004). Formen der Vergesellschaftung des Sterbeprozesses. Paper presented at a public symposium of the Nationaler Ethikrat (German National Ethics Council), http://www.ethikrat.org/veranstaltungen/pdf/Wortprotokoll_Aug_2004-03-31.pdf

Nassehi, A. (2005a). Society. In: A. Harrington, B. L. Marshall & H.-P. Müller (Eds), *Encyclopedia of social theory* (pp. 436–441). London: Routledge.

Nassehi, A. (2005b). Organizations as decision machines: Niklas Luhmann's theory of organized social systems. In: C. Jones & R. Munro (Eds), *Contemporary organization theory* (pp. 178–191). Oxford: Blackwell.

Nassehi, A. (2006). *Der soziologische Diskurs der Moderne.* Frankfurt, Main: Suhrkamp Verlag.

Nassehi, A. (2007). The person as an effect of communication. In: S. Maasen & B. Sutter (Eds), *On willing selves: Neoliberal politics and the challenge of neuroscience* (pp. 100–120). Hampshire: Pelgrave.

Nida-Rümelin, J. (1996). *Angewandte Ethik. Die Bereichsethiken und ihre theoretische Fundierung. Ein Handbuch.* Stuttgart: Kröner Verlag.

Nida-Rümelin, J. (2000). Rationality: Coherence and structure. In: J. Nida-Rümelin & W. Spohn (Eds), *Rationality, rules, and structure* (pp. 1–16). Dordrecht: Kluwer Academic Publishers.

Nida-Rümelin, J. (2001). *Strukturelle Rationalität. Ein philosophischer Essay über praktische Vernunft.* Stuttgart: Reclam Verlag.

Nida-Rümelin, J. (2002). *Ethische Essays.* Frankfurt, Main: Suhrkamp Verlag.

Nunner-Winkler, G. (2001). Devices for identity maintenance in modern society. In: A. van Harskamp & A. W. Musschenga (Eds), *The many faces of individualism* (pp. 197–224). Leuven, Belgium: Peeters.

Nussbaum, M. C. (1995). Aristotle on human nature and the foundations of ethics. In: J. E. J. Altham & R. Harrison (Eds), *World, mind, and ethics: Essays on the ethical philosophy of Bernard Williams* (pp. 86–131). Cambridge: Cambridge University Press.

Poirier, S. (1999). Voice: Structure, politics, and values in the medical narrative. *HEC Forum, 11*, 27–37.

Rawls, J. (1971). *A theory of justice*. Harvard: Harvard University Press.

Reamer, F. G. (1987). Ethics committees in social work. *Social Work, 32*, 188–192.

Saake, I. (2003). Die Performanz des Medizinischen: Zur Asymmetrie der Arzt-Patienten-Interaktion. *Soziale Welt, 54*, 429–461.

Saake, I., & Kunz, D. (2006). Von Kommunikation über Ethik zu 'ethischer Sensibilisierung': Symmetrisierungsprozess in diskursiven Verfahren. *Zeitschrift für Soziologie, 35*, 41–56.

Sandel, M. J. (1982). *Liberalism and the limits of justice*. Cambridge: Cambridge University Press.

Taylor, C. (1992). *Sources of the self: The making of the modern identity*. Harvard: Harvard University Press.

van den Daele, W. (2001a). Von moralischer Kommunikation zur Kommunikation über Moral. Reflexive Distanz in diskursiven Verfahren. *Zeitschrift für Soziologie, 30*, 4–22.

van den Daele, W. (2001b). Gewissen, Angst und radikale Reform-wie starke Ansprüche an die Technikpolitik in diskursiven Arenen schwach werden. In: G. Simonis, R. Martinsen & T. Saretzki (Eds), *Politik und Technik. Analysen zum Verhältnis von technologischem Wandel am Anfang des 21. Jahrhunderts* (pp. 476–498). Wiesbaden: Westdeutscher Verlag.

Wolf, S. M. (1992). Due process in ethics committee case review. In: S. Spicker (Ed.), *The healthcare ethics committee experience: Selected readings from HEC forum* (pp. 243–256). Malabar, FL: Krieger Publishing Company.

Wolf, S. M. (1993). Toward a theory of process. *Law, Medicine & Health Care, 20*, 278–290.

ETHICAL MINDFULNESS: NARRATIVE ANALYSIS AND EVERYDAY ETHICS IN HEALTH CARE

Marilys Guillemin and Lynn Gillam

There tends to be a preoccupation in bioethics with 'big-ticket' ethical concerns. Discussion around issues such as euthanasia, reproductive cloning and end-of-life decision making is abundant in the bioethics literature. However, spend time with health-care practitioners and it appears that their ethical concerns have a different focus. First, what is noticeable is that practitioners tell stories – often heartfelt and complex stories. These stories are not generally about the 'big-ticket' issues but are more about the everyday ethically important moments of health-care practice: stories about when to speak up when you know something is not quite right, or how much of the truth to tell to a patient or what to say when a patient asks about your own family life. These are small moments, marked by their ordinariness, which are faced by practitioners of all disciplines in health care. Despite their everydayness, these moments are nonetheless ethically charged. In this paper, we draw attention to these kinds of concerns, which we call the 'everyday ethics' of health care, and show how a sociologically informed approach can address them in a useful and meaningful way.

In doing so, we do not dispute the value of the contributions of bioethics. Bioethics has provided us with both the linguistic and the conceptual tools

Bioethical Issues, Sociological Perspectives
Advances in Medical Sociology, Volume 9, 157–178
Copyright © 2008 by Elsevier Ltd.
All rights of reproduction in any form reserved
ISSN: 1057-6290/doi:10.1016/S1057-6290(07)09006-7

with which to identify and analyse key ethical dilemmas in health care. But ethics in health care is about more than just dilemmas. Dilemmas in ethics usually involve having to make stark choices between competing values. With ethically important moments, there are generally neither stark choices nor directly competing values and usually no dilemma as such to consider and make a decision about. With everyday ethics, the task is not to necessarily weigh up competing considerations and make a decision, but rather to recognise the ethical significance of the moment and act accordingly. Often the marker of ethical significance is a feeling of discomfort, of uncertainty and of being troubled, not always at the time of the event but often long after the actual experience. For those caught up in the hectic pace of health-care practice, it is often difficult to even recognise these moments as ethically important. They do not come pre-labelled, and they are often enmeshed within clinical concerns. Despite this blurring of clinical and ethical dimensions, we argue that it is important to first recognise these important moments in health care, and second, to acknowledge them as *ethically* significant.

Drawing from the field of narrative ethics, we propose a narrative approach to understand everyday ethics in health care.[1] This is both a methodological and a theoretical contribution which brings together bioethics, sociology and narrative analysis. This interdisciplinary approach has developed from our teaching of health ethics. Lynn is a bioethicist and Marilys a sociologist, and in our work together, we combine our disciplinary approaches. Our graduate students are predominantly experienced health-care practitioners who are seeking to understand health ethics and to learn conceptual tools with which to address the ethical concerns which permeate their experiences of health-care practice. Although our teaching includes the more traditional bioethics principles, it is grounded in a narrative approach which has arisen largely from our students, who invariably engage by telling stories – stories that are rich and powerful, and imbued with the complexities of health care. In the process of teaching, we ask students to write stories of personal, real-life, everyday ethical situations they have experienced. In addition to telling the story itself, we ask students to reflect on their story. When choosing their stories, we ask students to consider ethically important moments in their everyday practice – moments that had caused them concern or disquiet, rather than ethical dilemmas per se. More often than not, these experiences date back many years and have remained unsettling for them. We specifically direct students to write in the first person and to include themselves in the story, taking into account their emotions and responses, as well as those of the others involved.

Our approach takes seriously the work of narratives in health-care practice. We argue that through the process of storytelling and engaging with stories, we become ethically engaged, and the outcome of this ethical engagement is what we call 'ethical mindfulness'. As we go on to explain, being ethically mindful provides the potential for making sense of the everyday ethics of health care. We begin by discussing narrative ethics and situate our approach within this, before setting out our approach in more detail. We focus on the contributions of a narrative approach to ethics and reflect on the growing interest in this field. Since our approach is founded on the meaning of stories and the value of engaging with them, we present a story. With the author's permission, we tell the real-life story of Charlie,[2] a young boy undergoing radiotherapy for cancer, and his family. The story is told by Hannah, one of our students who, at the time of the experience, was a newly qualified radiotherapist. We analyse Hannah's story and point to what a standard bioethics approach offers us, but also to what gets left out. We go on to employ our narrative approach; we engage with Hannah's story, and using this process of engagement, explore its potential for producing and enhancing ethical mindfulness.

NARRATIVE ETHICS

There has been growing interest in narrative ethics over the last three decades. However, narratology, or the study of narratives, has a much longer history dating back to Plato and Aristotle.[3] Structural linguistics, and its formal study of grammar and structure of language, was a major contributor to the development of the classification and interpretation of narratives.[4] This structuralist period was followed by an increased interest in the relationships between narratives and social and historical dynamics and ideologies. Key social theorists, such as Derrida, Bakhtin and Ricoeur, have urged us to consider the relationship of the text to the way we understand ourselves and the worlds we inhabit. In summary, the study of narratives long preceded its association with ethics, and it was only recently that the interest in narratives has been adopted by the health-care disciplines, notably medicine and nursing.

Indeed, it was not until the late 1970s and early 1980s that an interest in the application of narratives to ethics developed. This was largely in response to a number of critiques aimed at bioethics. In particular, these critiques were directed at the perceived lack of usefulness of the impersonal, abstract and universal claims of moral theory (particularly the principlist approach in bioethics) to real-life, clinical situations. Principlism, or the principlist approach to ethical decision making, has been a dominant force in Western bioethics since the 1970s.[5] In their principlist model, Beauchamp and Childress (2001) put forward four key principles: beneficence, non-maleficence, autonomy and justice. Principlism argues that these principles are universal and are derived from a 'common morality'. Furthermore, Beauchamp and Childress argue that these principles should form the basis of ethical decision making, to ensure that ethical decisions are reasoned and justifiable on grounds of universally accepted norms.

In response to these claims came the argument that universal and generalised principles are not helpful in the context of individuals' lives.[6] There was a call for an approach that took into account the particularities of individuals, their histories, communities and contextual features (Montello, 1995). There was also a challenging of the notion, prevalent in bioethics, that there is a correct solution to a given ethical dilemma, or at least a best approach in trying to resolve it. These criticisms led, amongst other things, to some authors seeking to combine narratives and ethics in a variety of different ways.

Although the term 'narrative ethics' is often used today to imply a single phenomenon, there are many different approaches to narrative ethics, with different foundations, aims and ways of employing narratives.[7] Nelson (2001, p. 36) offers a useful definition of narrative ethics in stating that it 'accords a central role to stories, not merely employing them as illustrations, examples, or ways of testing our intuitions regarding moral theories or principles, but regarding them as necessary means to some moral end'. Nelson's emphasis on the central role of stories highlights an important premise of our approach to narrative ethics. Like many scholars in the field, we take seriously the claim that we are narrative selves; we do not just tell stories for the sake of it but these stories work to make sense of our lives. As Montello (1995, p. 111) states, 'All the stories we tell ourselves and each other, spoken and written, are part of our ongoing quest for a narrative structuring of our lives'.

Our approach to narrative ethics is based on personal real-life stories, rather than fictional or hypothetical case studies. In particular, we are interested in the narratives of health-care practitioners and patients, which attempt to make sense of the everyday ethical concerns that infuse so much of health-care practice. These stories are notably rich, contextual, reflective and written from a personal perspective. They stand in sharp contrast to the case studies and 'thin' hypothetical-type narratives much favoured in bioethics. Commonly in bioethics, the purpose of the case study or hypothetical narratives is to provide an illustration, or a platform on which the relative merits of predetermined philosophical positions are argued. In contrast, the personal life narratives of health-care practitioners and patients that we refer to do not set out to serve as a base for a particular ethical standpoint, or a test case for conflicting theoretical positions. However, we argue that ethical work invariably occurs through telling and engaging with these personal life narratives; through this engagement we come to understand who we are and how to live our lives. The emphasis here is not on solving an ethical dilemma, or on undertaking ethical decision making per se, but rather on enacting our lives through the telling of and engaging with stories (Frank, 1997). We emphasise our lives as being embedded in stories, within which ethical engagement occurs.

Schafer (1981) discusses the notion of self-stories and their importance as a way of forming the self. Frank (1995, p. 56) takes this up when he states:

> The self-story is told both to others and to one's self; each telling is enfolded within the other. The act of telling is a dual affirmation. Relationships with others are reaffirmed, and the self is reaffirmed. Serious illness requires both reaffirmations ....

Frank's point here is in relation to serious illness. However, we would suggest that self-stories told by practitioners in health care are similarly about forming and reaffirming the self and relationships with others, and working to give meaning to experiences. One function of narrative ethics is as a site of ethical reflection by the storyteller. It offers storytellers the opportunity to rethink and recreate themselves ethically.[8] In this process, the emphasis of the self-story is on the storyteller. However, we suggest that self-stories, or personal life narratives, fulfil another moral purpose for those who listen to and engage with the stories. As we go on to explain, actively attending and engaging with the story can be ethically enlightening and equally meaningful for the listener/s as well as the storyteller. In this paper, we focus primarily on the listener's engagement with narratives.

STORY AS PROCESS

We have argued for the importance of acknowledging everyday ethics in health care and have stressed the significance of narratives of health-care practitioners and patients in understanding the everyday ethics of health-care practice. We suggest that the *process* of storytelling and engaging with the narrative is as significant as the story itself; both the 'story as product' and the 'story as process' are important. In this paper, we pay particular attention to the 'story as process'. We suggest that through this process of engaging with stories, we become *ethically* engaged. By that, we do not mean that from stories we distil some kind of ethical essence, which will produce a solution or provide some sort of moral lesson. Rather, we are referring to a complex intellectual and emotional response to, and engagement with, the stories, which yields ethical meaning in a variety of more open-ended ways.

There is an assumption in much of bioethics that the aim of ethical discussion of health-care practice is ethical evaluation and decision making. The purpose of considering a given situation in bioethics is to identify the key ethical elements at stake, ethically evaluate these key principles and use this to come to a conclusion about what would be the ethical or most justifiable way to proceed. It is intended from this that the health practitioner gains a better understanding of how to make ethical decisions, and by implication, will make more ethically sound or justifiable health-care decisions. Whilst we take decision making to be an important part of ethical practice in health care, we argue that the bioethical focus on decision making is too narrow. An obvious limitation to this approach is that ethical practice cannot occur unless practitioners can recognise when a situation is ethically significant and an ethical decision is called for, can make the decision in the 'heat of the moment' and can actually implement it in practice.

We argue that a narrative approach broadens the range of ethical considerations beyond those that bioethics usually takes into account. The aim of our approach is not to arrive at the best ethical decision or to necessarily produce more justifiable health-care decisions. Our aim is a more modest one. We suggest that the process of engagement with stories can lead to what we term 'ethical mindfulness'. As we go on to discuss, being ethically mindful offers the opportunity to recognise and understand the ethically important moments in health care.

ETHICAL MINDFULNESS

Ethical mindfulness, as we define it, refers to a cluster of pre-dispositions and processes, rather than any single characteristic. We identify the following features of ethical mindfulness (although we are not claiming that this list is exhaustive). First, ethical mindfulness requires recognition of the ethically important moments of everyday health-care practice. The big-ticket ethical dilemmas or the major 'life and death' issues of bioethics are relatively easy to recognise. However, the ethically important moments may go unnoticed in the hustle and bustle of health-care settings. Ethical mindfulness requires the ethical sensitivity to notice and appreciate these moments for what they are.

Second, being ethically mindful means being prepared to take notice of feeling troubled when something does not feel quite right. It can be easy to disregard these sorts of feelings as unimportant, particularly when nobody else seems to have noticed anything amiss. In addition, it is often difficult to separate out the ethical concerns from clinical ones. As a health-care practitioner has noted to us: 'Knowing where a line is crossed is harder to distinguish, and separating ethical dimensions from clinical ones is murky' (Guillemin & Gillam, 2006, p. 62). Being ethically mindful is about taking notice of when lines are crossed and being attentive to the murkiness of clinical and ethical boundaries. Feeling troubled may indicate something of ethical importance (though it also may not) and deserves to be thoughtfully considered rather than just dismissed.

Third, to be ethically mindful necessitates being able to articulate what is going on, ethically speaking. We require a language with which we can think about and communicate what is ethically at stake. Bioethical principles provide an obvious and valuable set of linguistic and conceptual tools with which to do this. However, they are not the only useful set of tools available to us. We suggest that sociological concepts (together with other conceptual frameworks) may be equally beneficial in being able to understand and articulate what is ethically at stake. Just as ethical concerns are often entangled in clinical ones, they are similarly often entwined with issues of power relations, professional dominance or organisational structure. The language and concepts of sociology have much to contribute in articulating and communicating not just the sociological factors, but also the ethical factors at play in health care.

Fourth, being ethically mindful means being reflexive. This is a well-known concept in sociology, often used in research contexts. We suggest it also has a place in the process of ethical engagement where it is crucial to be aware of one's own role, views and standpoint, and to acknowledge that these can only provide a partial perspective. To be ethically mindful requires an openness to other possible interpretations. Finally, being ethically mindful requires courage. To be courageous in this context means being able to acknowledge feeling troubled, to challenge accepted practice, to expose oneself to criticism from others or, more confrontingly, to doubt oneself. Courage is often needed to question and challenge, particularly in settings where this is not the norm. The notion of ethical mindfulness is significant for us; we suggest it is what we should be aiming for in relation to ethical engagement in health-care practice. We do not suggest that engaging

with narratives will necessarily or immediately result in ethical mindfulness. However, we do believe it offers an useful pathway towards ethical
mindfulness.

ENGAGING WITH NARRATIVES

Drawing on the useful contributions of Jones (1999), Zoloth and Charon
(2002), Nelson (2002) and Frank (2005), we have formulated an approach for
engaging with narratives. This provides a structure for systematic exploration
and reflection, but also retains sufficient flexibility to allow each narrative to
be considered in its own right. Our approach uses a series of trigger questions,
which direct attention to various aspects of the story that may have ethical
significance. More importantly, these questions include direct reference to
ethical principles as they are conventionally used in bioethics. Our model of
narrative ethics is not intended to be in opposition to a principlist or
philosophical-analytic approach to bioethics. Rather, it seeks to draw on
what is useful in that approach, whilst also expanding the horizons of ethical
enquiry and reflection in ways that principlist bioethics cannot achieve.

Adapting Nelson's (1999) terminology, our set of trigger questions
includes naming, sideways-looking and forward-looking questions. As we
will explain, each type of category of question serves a particular function.
The trigger questions are as follows:

Naming questions
- What are the key ethical elements?
- How do they relate to one another?

Sideways-looking questions
- How has the story been cast? What is the narrative frame, time, plot, and
  desire? How has the narrator cast himself and the other characters?
- What are the key 'ethically important moments' in the story?
- Who is telling the story? Why is the narrator telling the story in this
  particular way?
- What has been left out of the narrative? Whose voice is not being heard?
  What other stories does this story resist?
- What is ethically at stake here, and for whom?

Forward-looking questions
- What does this story tell us (that would not otherwise be heard)?
- How can engaging with this story lead to ethical mindfulness in health-
  care practice?

These questions serve as interpretative triggers. They do not necessarily have to be considered in any particular order since they are interlinked and likely to spark off one another. Similarly, it may be that not all questions are useful for all narratives. What is important here is being open to what is prompted by these questions.

The aim of the first set of questions, the 'naming questions', is to provide an avenue into the rawness of the story. We suggest that stories do not have built-in meanings that are self-evident to anyone who reads or hears them. They need to be interpreted to yield meaning. The naming questions are invariably reductionist; indeed, we suggest that it is not possible to interpret and create meaning without reduction in some form. The key issue is whether the reduction serves some useful purpose and is done with reflexive awareness of its limitations. The purpose of the naming questions is to enable us to articulate the key ethical elements and to communicate these to others using a shared language. Ethical principles in the form introduced by Beauchamp and Childress are a helpful tool for this purpose, and we make use of them. However, whereas the conventional bioethics approach would then use this to undertake an analysis of the meaning, application and relative weight of the relevant principles and would come to a judgement about what is the right thing to do in this situation, we do not proceed in this way. At this stage our purpose is simply to articulate ethical issues using a shared language, not to make an ethical judgement. In this task of articulating ethical issues, ethical principles are, in fact, not the only useful conceptual and linguistic tool. We also draw on other conceptual approaches, especially those from sociology, that help us to identify and name the ethical elements at stake.

The next set of questions are 'sideways-looking questions'. Having used relevant conceptual tools to reduce complexity and identify what makes the story an ethical one, we pose a series of questions that serve to re-contextualise the narrative, and re-introduce complexity, albeit in an organised fashion. The idea of sideways questions is derived from Nelson (1999), who advocates the telling of 'sideways stories'. A 'sideways story' is the story as it would be told by one of the characters in the original story, other than the narrator. These sideways stories enable the fleshing out of the story and of the context and the identities of the people involved, and draw attention to the constructed nature of the narrative by showing how different players would tell the story of the same event in quite different ways. Whilst we do not attempt literally to tell these sideways stories, we propose a number of questions that serve this same function, namely of highlighting the ways in which the narrative has been deliberately put together by the narrator, rather than being some sort of natural recounting. These questions, drawn largely from narrative analysis, ask about the casting of the story, in terms of characterisation, emplotment, temporal sequence and narrative frame.

These questions are revealing *ethically* in that they encourage us to reflect on and consider the standpoint, interpretations and values implicit in the way that the narrator has constructed the story. The questions *Who is telling the story? Why is the narrator telling the story in this particular way?* focus attention on the narrator and their worldview. Rather than taking for granted the interpretation that the narrator has written into the story, we are encouraged to broaden our view and consider other possible readings of who the narrator is and how and why they have come to tell the story in this particular way. The questions *What has been left out of the narrative? Whose voice is not being heard? What other stories does this story resist?* further open up the narrator's version to contestation. They emphasise that the narrator's version is not the only possible one and that the narrator does not have ultimate authority over its interpretation. This is an ethically vital point; decisions and practice in health care are deeply influenced by whose version of a story is accepted as authoritative. Hence it is of considerable ethical importance not to accept a narrator's interpretation unquestioningly.

Asking *What are the key 'ethically important moments'?* has a somewhat different purpose. It asks us to consider the plot as it is presented by the narrator and look for places where there is an unexpected turn in the story, or where it could have unfolded differently. In these places are likely to be found the ethically laden moments that may otherwise go unnoticed. These moments may consist of an opportunity that is taken up or missed, an unrecognised assumption that leads events off in a particular direction, a crisis that is avoided, a conflict that is ameliorated or inflamed, and so on. None of these will appear as dilemmas as such and may go unnoticed if not explicitly sought out.

The question *What is ethically at stake here, and for whom?* gathers together insights from all the previous questions, asking us to consider what is of particular ethical significance. It leads to a final set of questions, which are 'forward-looking' in that they ask us to consider the implications of the insights gained from reflecting on the story. The questions *What does this story tell us (that would not otherwise be heard)?* and *How can engaging with this story lead to ethical mindfulness in health-care practice?* are adapted from Nelson. Nelson (1999, p. 45) stresses the importance of 'tell[ing] the story forward', to consider where we could go from here. Although Frank (2004a, 2004b) sees the process of narration as ongoing and perpetual, Nelson proposes the forward-looking story as a closing story. Although we think that this forward-looking step is crucial, our view differs from that of both Frank and Nelson. We are conscious that in health-care settings there is an imperative to act. For most health-care practitioners, it is not enough to remain at the level of the story for its own sake; we still need to address the practical issues of what to do. Despite this necessity to act, we do not believe that there is a single 'closing story' available that will produce a solution to the problem or a guide for what to do next time a similar situation arises. Instead, we see the naming and sideways questions asked of each particular story as producing insights which feed into ethical mindfulness. One way to bring this about is by reflecting on what the telling of a story and the process of engaging with it has revealed that would otherwise not have been heard and understood.

HANNAH'S STORY

So far we have been writing *about* narratives. It is appropriate and important to also *engage with* narratives. For this reason, we present Hannah's story. This story is written by Hannah, one of our graduate students. At the time of the experience, Hannah was a newly qualified radiotherapist. The story relates to events that took place six years previously, but as will become obvious, they continue to trouble Hannah. We first present the story and then proceed to engage with it using our narrative approach.

One of the paediatric patients that I was responsible for treating when first qualified was a two year-old boy called Charlie. He was the stereotypical gorgeous little blonde-haired, blue-eyed toddler who would have been perfect for any television advertising campaign. I can't remember now the exact details of his original diagnosis but at 2 years of age, when we first met Charlie, we were treating a cancer that was eating away at his jaw. It isn't very often in radiotherapy that we are able to see the tumour that we are treating as they are usually internal. In Charlie's case the tumour was enlarging one side of his face, and on opening his mouth we could see both the tumour and the bone that it was eating away at.

Charlie was having daily radiotherapy treatment that involved having a perspex mask placed over his face. This was then clipped into the treatment bed. After getting Charlie in the right position we would line up the machine with the marks on the shell and would leave the room to deliver his treatment. This would usually take about ten minutes. As Charlie was so young he needed to be anesthetised each day, which in itself is a procedure that carries significant risk for any person. This meant that he would be unconscious for the time that he was in the treatment room.

Every morning Charlie would come in with his mum. Between the radiotherapists, the team of paediatric nurses and his anaesthetists we could coax him into having the anaesthetic. Charlie knew what the trolley holding the anaesthetics meant and I remember one morning he looked at us and shook his head, turned on his heels and toddled down the 25 m corridor to the door leading outside.

As with any patient undergoing radiotherapy for an extended period of time you learn to relate to them on one level or another. In Charlie's case his relationship with me was based on Hi-5, a young children's pop band. His mum taught me the words (three lines that I will never be able to forget) and Charlie would make me sing so he could do his dance. In return I taught him how to do a "high five". His mum once told me that she was sick of him running round the house and sticking his hand up for her to give him a high five, although she obviously loved it. I told her she had already had her payback as I couldn't get their hit song out of my head.

Treating Charlie was always going to be emotionally difficult, but this was made harder as I found out beforehand from my colleagues that he could have undergone surgery to remove the tumour. However, as Charlie's parents were Jehovah's Witnesses and would not consent to a blood transfusion, no surgeon would operate on him. I couldn't understand, and thought it selfish that his parents would make a decision on the life of their child based on their religion. Surely their child's welfare and chance at a life (when the flipside was death) was more important than what was dictated to them by their religion. I met Charlie's 14-year-old brother and wondered what his view was on his parent's decision and his thoughts about Charlie's impending death (which at this stage was a reality).

One day, a few weeks into the treatment, the tumour had started breaking down and Charlie's mother was in the treatment room as usual. Due to the effects of the treatment Charlie would constantly have saliva (sometimes blood-stained) coming from the left side of his mouth and the smell when cleaning it was of rotting tissue. However disgusting this may sound, he still had his angel face and loveable persona and of course, it was out of his control. Charlie's mother couldn't cope with these bodily fluids and was visibly embarrassed by them. I had to reassure her that it was fine and that it didn't bother us, that he had no control over it and that it was not her fault that this discharge was happening, (although we did think it was her fault that Charlie was in this situation).

Charlie died a couple of weeks after his treatment finished and I soon received from his parents, a beautiful letter with photos that his mother had taken of us during treatment. I don't know what happened to that letter and I wish I could find it now.

Reflecting on my experience of treating Charlie I would not have changed my professional practice of how I dealt with the patient or his family if I had the opportunity. Looking back now, six years later, it wouldn't be my actions that I would have changed but how I thought about Charlie's parents and the decisions that they made.

I feel guilty that I made my judgement of his parents by mimicking that of the more experienced radiotherapists that I had only just started to work with. I feel bad that I had such a strong emotional response to his parent's decision being the wrong one without knowing the full extent of the decision they actually had to make. I based my thoughts of their religion on the one piece of information that I got from the other therapists. I was very narrow-minded. Without realising, over the following years I had blamed Charlie's death on the decisions made by his parents, when in reality there may have been no difference in the outcome if he had the surgery or not. I felt that the parents were "harming" Charlie by not choosing the best treatment (although I never found out what that was).

I have often thought about Charlie and his family. I believed that the ethical dilemma that I had with their story was related to their religious beliefs. My belief was based on the gossip I had heard in the staffroom. At that time, I felt insincere when dealing with the parents. Now, on reflection, I realise that there were many more issues involved. I realise that their decision may not have been unethical at all. I am glad, now, that my professionalism had overridden my urge to tell them what I thought of their choice.

What troubles me most about this situation now is not so much the ethics surrounding the family's decision but the way that I had allowed other therapists to influence my opinions. The power relationships within the radiotherapy department between newly qualified therapists and the more experienced staff was the main reason that I felt corrupted. The culture in the department of the more experienced staff teaching the less experienced by their actions extended from the clinical practices to the bases for forming attitudes and opinions. This is the first time that I realised that this "gossip culture" had affected my thoughts and views. I think the difference with my practice now is that because I have had more exposure to different cultures and religions I am more aware and respectful of different ideas. I cringe when I think that I just took on board the ideas of other more "experienced" radiotherapists without analysing them for myself. I was so used to learning their practical skills by imitation that I wasn't strong enough to distinguish between the practical skills and forming an opinion.

ENGAGING WITH HANNAH'S STORY: A NARRATIVE ETHICS APPROACH

We have presented Hannah's story as a product. In doing so, what may go unnoticed is the process and the work of Hannah as a storyteller. Hannah has selected which events to include and exclude and has organised the events into a narrative form with both a plot and a time sequence. She has characterised the players in the story including, notably, herself. Hannah has written the story in the first person, a task which many health professionals find difficult to do, since it goes against years of clinical training in being objective and presenting cases in the approved de-personalised fashion. Hannah's reflection on her narrative shows some of the insights that she gained from this process. This is clearly not just a straightforward story recounting events associated with a memorable patient. There are clear indications that for Hannah, telling the story has been a process of meaning making and re-creation of herself. The real issue for Hannah was how she thought, rather than how she acted, and this is a notable example of the sort of ethical work that can be done in the process of storytelling. The gain in ethical mindfulness is very apparent. However, rather than focusing on this aspect, we want to describe and demonstrate the next stage of the process, namely our engagement with the story using the trigger questions described above, and show how this can lead to ethical mindfulness. Although we cannot present a comprehensive interpretation here, we aim to provide an indication of what can be achieved through this process of engagement.

HANNAH'S STORY: NAMING QUESTIONS

The naming questions aim to identify and articulate what makes this story an ethical one. Here the bioethical principles of most obvious importance are respect for parental autonomy and the best interests of the child. Generally in bioethics, parents are regarded as having both the ethical and the legal right to be decision makers for their children in relation to medical treatment. However, this right is recognised as a limited one, which can be overridden when the parents' decisions are patently not in the child's best interests. Charlie's parents have decided against surgery and for radio-therapy. However, both of these decisions are ethically open to question, as it is not clear that either of them serve Charlie's best interests. Surgery may have substantially improved Charlie's chance of long-term survival, but without it, radiotherapy may be futile, or perhaps may even exacerbate Charlie's suffering, with no hope of any improvement in his condition.

Trying to resolve this question is not straightforward, since it all hinges on the question of what counts as being in Charlie's best interests and who is best placed to decide this. We need a closer scrutiny of the notion of 'best interests' to sort this out. A child, or any person, has an interest in many things, and these include not just physical health, freedom from suffering and continued life, but also emotional and psychological matters such as personal relationships, love and nurturing, happy and rewarding experiences, hope for the future, and so on. The problem is that none of these things is easy to assess or weigh up; hence these sorts of issues remain contentious, even intractable, in bioethics.

Another ethically important principle at stake in this story is personal and professional integrity. Hannah has her own views about the ethics of treating Charlie's tumour, even though she is not the clinician who made the decisions. Ethically speaking, it is entirely appropriate for her to have such views, and to have them considered, since Hannah, like all health professionals, is an independent moral agent, not just an automaton following orders. Acting according to one's conscience is tricky, since health professionals are also ethically required to respect the autonomy of their patients. But in a situation like this, it would be widely accepted that if Hannah felt strongly that radiotherapy treatment for Charlie was wrong, then she would have a right to conscientious objection and could withdraw from the treating team.

These are the key ethical issues in terms of ethical *decision making*, but they are not the only ethically relevant features of the situation. There are also important social, cultural and professional factors at work which have a significant bearing on ethical *practice*. A sociological lens brings into view a number of these issues: the power dynamics between Hannah, the junior radiotherapist, and her more experienced colleagues; the influence of professional and organisational cultures on individuals; the processes whereby novice health-care practitioners gain entry into a professional system; as well as the tensions between personal, professional and clinical values. All these points are played out in Hannah's story. Each has important sociological theoretical bases that shape and inform our understanding of health-care practice and the individuals involved. Although these sociological concepts may not be readily labelled or identified as 'ethical principles', they have much to offer in terms of ethical analyses. Identifying and naming these allows us to take better account of the way ethical issues are perceived, what options for action are seen as possible in the situation, and what forces are operating to influence the way people think and act. Having identified and named these ethical elements, we go on to pose the 'sideways-looking questions', which re-contextualise the story, and draw explicit attention to how the story has been framed and constructed. The sideways-looking questions will bring us back to some of these ethical elements, but in different ways.

HANNAH'S STORY: SIDEWAYS LOOKING QUESTIONS

The sideways-looking questions are a window into the implicit ethical dimensions of the story. In asking how this story has been cast, on one level we can say that this is a rather stereotypical story of a young child dying a premature and tragic death. However, closer consideration reveals otherwise. Charlie's death takes place 'off-stage'; Charlie's death is not a focus of interest and it is not what engages the reader's imagination and emotions. Focusing on the characterisation, emplotment and temporal sequence shows that the story is more centrally one of relationships. Of interest to us are the ethical dimensions of these relationships.

In examining how the story is constructed, we find it comprises a series of vivid snapshots or moments, rather than having a strongly linear plot. Each moment tells us something about the relationships between the story's various characters. In these snapshots, Hannah is a central, active character, but between the different takes, her characterisation changes. Hannah moves in and out, from her active practitioner role to distancing herself as she questions and makes judgements about the situation. In this interplay, we get a feel for the ethical importance that she places on relationships. In effect, her ethical thinking happens through and is reflected in her portrayal of these relationships – between Hannah and Charlie, Hannah and Charlie's mother, and Hannah and the other radiotherapists.

The characterisation of Charlie's mother is interesting and significant. At the beginning of the story, she is presented in a warm and intimate way; Charlie's mother is presented to us as 'Mum' and seems to be Charlie's loving protector. She is actively and intimately involved in helping Charlie deal with the radiotherapy; by teaching Hannah the Hi-5 song, she is trying to help the staff to help Charlie. However, as the story unfolds, she is portrayed very differently. When Charlie's tumour is breaking down, she changes from being Charlie's 'Mum' to Charlie's 'mother'; she is presented as disgusted and embarrassed by Charlie's rotting tissue and accompanying smell. She is distanced from Charlie, no longer on his side, and no longer able to cope. This is a very negative picture. Why the change in characterisation? Perhaps it signals Hannah's deep ambivalence or change of attitude towards Charlie's mother. At first, Hannah thought of Charlie's mother as a model 'good mother'. However, after finding out about Charlie's parents' religious beliefs and refusal of surgery, Hannah presents Charlie's mother as an impediment to caring for Charlie, rather than as an ally. Charlie's mother becomes an obstacle because she has not allowed Charlie to have surgery and also because she ends up needing to be cared for herself, requiring reassurance and comfort when Charlie's tumour deteriorates.

By the end of the story, the letter sent by Charlie's parents seems to redeem Charlie's mother; she is again the loving and caring parent, and the photograph she sends also acknowledges Hannah's relationship with Charlie. This incident highlights a very important voice that is missing from the story, namely that of Charlie's mother. Charlie's mother has her own story, and we imagine that she would tell it very differently from Hannah's version. The letter and photograph hint poignantly at this; they speak of a whole world of meaning that Charlie's parents attach to Charlie's life and death, which we, as the audience, have no access to.

This complex characterisation of Charlie's mother carries ethical significance. It has resonance with one of the major issues that the naming questions drew out, namely whether Charlie's parents are acting in Charlie's best interests or not. But it deepens and personalises this rather abstract concern of 'best interests of the child'. In the story, this question of whether Charlie's parents have made the right choice in deciding against surgery is played out in the portrayal of the relationships between Charlie's mother and Charlie, and between Charlie's mother and Hannah. We see Hannah trying to sort out whether Charlie's mother is 'on his side' or not, and we also see very clearly Hannah's feelings of guilt that she had judged his parents on the basis of very little information.

The relationship between Charlie and Hannah is also interesting. Charlie is a totally engaging and winning character from the moment he is first introduced, and we feel the strong sense of the attachment Hannah has for him. Hannah displays a strong loyalty towards Charlie, to the extent of wanting to defend his image and ensure that the reader still sees him as cute and lovable, even when his tumour is foul and repugnant (indeed, Hannah's separation of Charlie and his tumour is striking: They are almost two different characters). Again, this relationship between Charlie and Hannah is ethically significant. It is not by accident that Hannah characterises herself and Charlie in this way. Hannah casts herself as the advocate and defender of Charlie, roles that are ethically laden.

Considering the relationship between Hannah and Charlie's mother highlights a notable ethically important moment and a potential turning point in the story. This occurs during the moment of treating Charlie when his tumour is breaking down. His mother 'cannot cope' and is 'visibly embarrassed', and as Hannah says, 'I had to reassure her that it was not her fault'. This is a crucial point where Hannah could have revealed to Charlie's mother what she actually thought, namely that this really was her fault. Things could have gone very differently at this point, but interestingly, they do not. We find out later that Hannah was tempted to speak her mind, but as she says, she is glad that her professionalism had overridden this urge. The impression that comes through about this moment is Hannah's sense of professional obligation to Charlie's mother. Hannah felt she was required to try to help Charlie's mother and to reassure her. However, there is also a feeling of reluctance, even irritation in Hannah's words, as she adds that they nonetheless thought it was the fault of Charlie's mother that Charlie was in this situation. It is perhaps revealing that Hannah focuses on reassuring Charlie's mother that she was not at fault, since this is clearly the issue that was really bothering Hannah at the time of the event. We do not know what Charlie's mother was actually distressed about; feeling guilty may have had nothing to do with it. Hannah does attempt to explain this apparent contradiction between what she said and what she felt, but in such an unconvincing way that it actually says more about the strength of her professional obligation towards Charlie and his mother than her genuine feelings at the time.

Posing the sideways questions also draws our attention to the voices that are not heard in this story, namely Charlie's mother, and indeed all other members of Charlie's family including, significantly, Charlie's father. Of equal importance are the absent voices of Hannah's radiotherapy colleagues. This is significant as Hannah clearly feels angry with her colleagues; she speaks of the 'gossip culture' in the department and of feeling 'corrupted' by their views. Hannah tells of the power relationships between the experienced and novice radiotherapists and of her taking for granted that what her experienced colleagues said must necessarily be right because of their status in the department. We are given the impression that this is an established culture that is not open to questioning, and certainly not by a junior staff member. We can only speculate on the versions of the story that could be told by Hannah's colleagues: versions that centre on Hannah as the novice radiotherapist undergoing her 'initiation' into organisational culture, past professional experiences with difficult Jehovah's witness parents, or more likely, this was another 'case' in their busy schedule that was not particularly memorable.

Taking into account whose voices are left out of this story leads us to consider what is ethically at stake, and for whom. We have explored what is ethically at stake in terms of Charlie and the decisions about his treatment, but there is much more at stake than this. There is also Hannah's standing as an ethical health-care professional and her professional relationships with her colleagues. Hannah is striving to become a clinically competent practitioner and she is dependent on her colleagues to achieve this. However, it is clear that she also yearns to be professional and ethical, and it is here where the tensions arise. Hannah was swayed by the opinions and attitudes of her senior colleagues and is now disillusioned that these had shaped her professional attitudes, when they were quite contrary to her own set of values. Hannah feels that her moral agency and integrity are in jeopardy, though not in the way envisaged in the earlier discussion of the naming questions. Hannah feels that her integrity is threatened not by her actions, but by her thoughts, or more specifically by the way in which she has been influenced by others in her thinking. This is a much less obvious but probably more pervasive and powerful type of pressure on integrity.

HANNAH'S STORY: FORWARD-LOOKING QUESTIONS

As we have shown, there are many possible interpretations of this story, each highlighting the significance of everyday ethics. In posing forward-looking questions we look to how this story could have been otherwise, and it is here that we can suggest some implications for practice. Hannah's story is about a network of relationships: certainly between patients and practitioners, but of particular interest to us, relationships between practitioners. Hannah's story allows us to hear a number of issues that would otherwise not be heard. We are given a glimpse into what it is like to be a novice learning the ropes of being a professional health-care practitioner. This offers us a reflection on how professional attitudes and ethical integrity are developed in health-care practice. Much effort is spent within clinical practice on teaching and learning clinical skills and knowledge, and role modelling plays an important part. However, modelling extends beyond practical skills into the more tricky realm of values and attitudes. This is of vital importance in terms of ethical practice, since it highlights the way in which individual practitioners work within a web of influences and relationships; ethical values are not formed in a vacuum. Developing ethical mindfulness very much depends on being aware of, and being reflexively critical about, these influences.

CONCLUSION

Engaging with Hannah's story and using the interpretive trigger questions demonstrates, by example, what a narrative approach has to contribute to bioethics. We argue that in this process of engagement we become ethically mindful. Hannah's story does not involve ethical dilemmas that require difficult ethical decisions. It is a series of snapshots or moments that, on their own, may go unnoticed; they are everyday events common in many radiotherapy departments. However, despite their everydayness we argue that they are ethically significant. Being sensitised to this is important as it enables us to begin to seriously engage with the story on ethical terms. This engagement is complex. We need to be able to identify what it is that makes the story an ethical matter and a set of diverse conceptual and linguistic tools is required to articulate and communicate this. Furthermore, to be ethically mindful requires reflexivity; this means being open to the different possible versions and interpretations of the story. This is where the use of the sideways trigger questions is particularly useful. We are made to consider how the story is cast, who the storyteller is, how the characters have been framed, and significantly, how the story could have unfolded differently. As people who both tell and engage with stories, we emphasise that this is not easy work. It requires courage and willingness to open yourself up for questioning. In Hannah's reflection, we sense her feelings of doubt and uncertainty and self-questioning in facing up to her 'prejudices'. In engaging with Hannah's story we share these emotions and invariably consider how we make sense of the situation, what we would have felt and how we would have acted in the same situation. Storytelling is not an easy way out of ethical reflection. It is personally challenging, but this is the very reason for its value.

In our approach, we take seriously the work of storytelling and engaging with stories. We argue that through this comes a process of ethical engagement and ethical mindfulness. This approach brings together bioethics and sociological approaches. We suggest that narratives bridge the gap between abstract ethical principles and the particularities of real-life ethics, and from this interplay arises the potential for sustained attention to the ethically important moments in health-care practice.

NOTES

1. In this paper, we do not distinguish between 'narrative' and 'story'. Although we are aware of, and acknowledge, the linguistic and etymologic distinctions between the terms, we, like many other authors, use the two terms interchangeably. We agree with Hunter (1996), when she states that 'In using the word 'narrative' somewhat interchangeably with 'story' I mean to designate a more or less coherent written, spoken, or (by extension) enacted account of occurrences, whether historical or fictional' (p. 306).
2. Pseudonyms are used throughout the paper.
3. For a historical overview of narratives and narratology see Onega and Landa (1996).
4. See Ellos (1994) for a discussion of the linguistic foundations of narrative ethics.
5. The key text of this period was Beauchamp and Childress (1979). After numerous editions, this text continues to be influential.
6. These critiques arose from both within and outside moral philosophy. Feminist philosophers such as Baier (1998), as well as religious scholars such as Burrell and Hauerwas (1977) were prominent in the late 1970s in mounting these critiques of principlism and advocating for narratives as a response.
7. For a discussion on different categories of uses of narratives in ethics, see Nelson (2001) and Chapter 2 of Guillemin and Gillam (2006).
8. See Rorty (1989) for a discussion on the effects of literary texts and their potential for self re-creation.

ACKNOWLEDGMENTS

We wish to thank Genevieve Gaffney for her considered and thoughtful contributions to this paper.

REFERENCES

Baier, A. C. (1998). Ethics in many different voices. In: J. Adamson, R. Freadman & D. Parker (Eds), *Renegotiating Ethics in literature, philosophy and theory* (pp. 247–268). Cambridge: Cambridge University Press.
Beauchamp, T., & Childress, J. F. (2001). *Principles of biomedical ethics*. New York: Oxford University Press.

178   MARILYS GUILLEMIN AND LYNN GILLAM

Beauchamp, T. L., & Childress, J. F. (1979). *Principles of biomedical ethics*. New York: Oxford University Press.
Burrell, D., & Hauerwas, S. (1977). From system to story: An alternative pattern for rationality in ethics. In: H. T. Engelhardt & D. Callahan (Eds), *The foundations of ethics and its relationship to science: Knowledge, value and belief* (Vol. 2, pp. 111–152). Hastings-on-Hudson, NY: Hastings Center.
Ellos, W. J. (1994). *Narrative Ethics*. Aldershot: Avebury.
Frank, A. W. (1995). *The wounded storyteller: Body, illness and ethics*. Chicago: University of Chicago Press.
Frank, A. W. (1997). Enacting illness stories: When, what, and why. In: H. L. Nelson (Ed.), *Stories and their limits: Narrative approaches to bioethics* (pp. 31–49). New York: Routledge.
Frank, A. W. (2004a). Asking the right question about pain: Narrative and *phronesis*. *Literature and Medicine, 23*(2), 209–225.
Frank, A. W. (2004b). Ethics as process and practice. *Internal Medicine Journal, 34*, 355–357.
Frank, A. W. (2005). *Narrative theory and method in the ethics and practice of social research*, Workshop, University of Melbourne, Melbourne.
Guillemin, M., & Gillam, L. (2006). *Telling moments: Everyday ethics in health care*. Melbourne: IP Communications.
Hunter, K. M. (1996). Narrative, literature, and the clinical exercise of practical reason. *Journal of Medicine and Philosophy, 21*(3), 303–320.
Jones, A. H. (1999). Narrative in medical ethics. *British Medical Journal, 318*(7178), 253–256.
Montello, M. (1995). Medical stories: Narrative and phenomenological approaches. In: M. Grodin (Ed.), *Meta medical ethics* (pp. 109–123). Dordrecht: Kluwer.
Nelson, H. L. (1999). Context: Backward, sideways, and forward. *HEC Forum, 11*(1), 16.
Nelson, H. L. (2001). *Damaged identities: Narrative repair*. Ithaca: Cornell University Press.
Nelson, H. L. (2002). Context: Backward, sideways, and forward. In: R. Charon & M. Montello (Eds), *Stories matter: The role of narrative in medical ethics* (pp. 39–47). New York: Routledge.
Onega, S., & Landa, J. A. G. (Eds). (1996). *Narratology: An introduction*. New York: Longman.
Rorty, R. (1989). *Contingency, irony and solidarity*. Cambridge: Cambridge University Press.
Schafer, R. (1981). Narration in the psychoanalytic dialogue. In: W. J. T. Mitchell (Ed.), *On narrative*. Chicago: University of Chicago Press.
Zoloth, L., & Charon, R. (2002). Like an open book: Reliability, intersubjectivity, and textuality in bioethics. In: R. Charon & M. Montello (Eds), *Stories matter: The role of narrative in medical ethics* (pp. 21–36). New York: Routledge.

MAKING THE AUTONOMOUS CLIENT: HOW GENETIC COUNSELORS CONSTRUCT AUTONOMOUS SUBJECTS

Daniel R. Morrison

Although philosophers, lawyers, physicians, and others have produced a large corpus of literature on decision making in health care that is often labeled "bioethics," sociologists are relatively new to the field. While sociology may be late in theorizing the new profession of bioethics, and its practices, academics with an interest in bioethics are hardly alone. There is much to study. Conrad and DeVries (1998) note how active the field is, as evidenced by the avalanche of announcements they receive for conferences, journals, and symposia. How can medical sociologists bring their specialized knowledge to the field? How can sociologists be both critical (sociology "of") and helpful to (sociology "in") the practice of bioethics (DeVries, 2004)?

In this chapter, I argue that sociologists should go to the field, in order to gain an empirical understanding of how bioethics is practiced within diverse medical settings. This call is not new, as many scholars have discussed the merits of ethnography in understanding how bioethics is practiced (see DeVries & Subedi, 1998). Sociologists should also think critically about the boundaries of bioethics as a discipline, questioning what counts as a problem for bioethics. While philosophers and lawyers may examine the ethics or legality, respectively, of certain medical interventions, researches,

Bioethical Issues, Sociological Perspectives
Advances in Medical Sociology, Volume 9, 179–198
Copyright © 2008 by Elsevier Ltd.
All rights of reproduction in any form reserved
ISSN: 1057-6290/doi:10.1016/S1057-6290(07)09007-9

and routine practices in the abstract, I argue that one of sociology's strengths is in determining the discursive work of bioethics. Sociologists of medicine, bioethics, and organizations can benefit from the study of bioethics in practice.

My case study is genetic counseling. The origins of modern genetic counseling can be traced to 1969, and to the development of a new master's-level science degree in genetic counseling (Rapp, 1988). Established at Sarah Lawrence College, the program primarily catered to female students, who "... seemed especially suited to a field that was designed to counsel pregnant women. And 'counseling' was a field in which 'female qualities' seemed particularly appropriate" (Rapp, 1988, p. 144). The cultural conception of women as caring, compassionate listeners seemed to make women the "natural" choice for this new, lower-status profession, instead of the more technically proficient geneticists, who were more likely to be male.

Technical advances were not the only impetus for ethical guidance in medical professions. According to Rapp, "'Genetic counseling,' a label coined in 1947, initially stood for a position of ethical neutrality, favoring personal choice in the century-old eugenics debate ..." (1988, p. 144). The eugenics debate, which raged throughout early 1900s in America, is analyzed elsewhere (see Kevles, 1985). Although the new genetic counseling was not established until 1969, medical genetics, often practiced by male physicians, was alive and well. By 1963, at least 28 genetics centers were in operation. Most of these centers were housed at major medical centers affiliated with research universities, including Johns Hopkins, Boston University, and the Universities of Wisconsin, Washington, Texas, Oklahoma, and Virginia (Reed, 1963). These universities were at the vanguard of research and technologies that have provided much food for thought among contemporary bioethicists. They counseled patients and conducted surgery and research in the hope of bettering the "germ plasm" in America.[1]

Here, I argue that genetic counselors take the dominant discourse of bioethics, whose focus is on patient autonomy, and translate this concept using "nondirective" methods. Indeed, the preservation of client/patient autonomy is a dominant feature of the genetic counseling literature, and a key feature of graduate training in genetic counseling. The research is motivated by a desire to understand the ways in which genetic counseling practice does or does not create autonomous clients. What does "nondirective" counseling allow these professionals to do, or not do? What practices does it include or exclude, and what are the consequences? In other words, what technologies do genetic counselors use in order to create the type of client that they understand is to benefit from their practice? In the pages to follow, I will briefly review the sociological literature on genetic counseling and discuss the tradition of principlism in bioethics. Next, I offer selections from in-depth interviews I conducted with 10 genetic counselors from multiple locations within the United States. These interviews provide another glimpse into the work and practices of this unique profession. In my analysis, I focus on the ways in which genetic counselors understand their roles in protecting client autonomy, and I argue that autonomy is created processually through the genetic counseling session. Understanding autonomy as a fluid, ongoing construction can help sociologists more clearly theorize the bioethical enterprise. Finally, I gesture toward a more relational understanding of autonomy (see Donchin, 2001), which may be useful for the practice of genetic counseling and bioethics.

LITERATURE REVIEW

The issues raised by bioethics have been discussed broadly within medical sociology. Scholars such as Bosk (2002), Rothman (1986), DeVries (2004), DeVries and Subedi (1998), and others have discussed the social origins, organization, and consequences of various aspects of bioethics, while many authors have discussed the ways in which bioethics may be blind to social context. Fox and DeVries note that all contributors to the DeVries and Subedi (1998) text fault bioethicists for their failure to recognize the multiple social, cultural, and historical influences on their ethical thinking and the failure to recognize the broader implications of their work for society. The collection of essays in DeVries and Subedi is an exceptionally rich source of sociological reflection about bioethics, its origin, social organization, and implications. This text stands in contrast to previous work by sociologists who served within bioethics as consultants or advisors to bioethics committees. Since its publication, relatively fewer works have sought to understand the world of bioethics through a sociological lens, although the number of books and journals on bioethics has proliferated.

The sociological literature on genetic counseling is somewhat less developed. Bosk's (1992) shop-floor ethnography of genetic counseling provided an early account of genetic counseling in the late 1970s and early 1980s. This text focused primarily on the relationships that genetic counselors have with other medical professionals and the ways in which genetic counseling serves as a "mop-up" service for physicians and "shock absorbers" for the organization.

Rapp (1988, 1999) has published a series of articles and a book on the social impact of amniocentesis in her long-running study of the communication process between genetic counselors and their diverse clientele. Through fieldwork and in-depth interviewing in New York City, Rapp describes the ways in which scientific discourse fits, or does not fit, the linguistic and cultural skills of clients. Rapp pays particular attention to women as clients and genetic counselors in her work, resulting in a particularly strong addition to the feminist literature on science and technology.

Perhaps the most cited study of motherhood that includes genetic counseling is Rothman's (1986) *The Tentative Pregnancy: Prenatal Diagnosis and the Future of Motherhood*. Rothman interviewed women who were faced with the decision of whether or not to undergo amniocentesis after speaking with a genetic counselor. Here, Rothman explores not only the reasons that women give for the choices they made, but also the consequences, focusing on what she calls "the tentative" pregnancy, the period of time between an amniocentesis and its results. During this time, the mother and baby are in limbo. Rothman argues that by changing the way mothers think about their fetuses, the technology and information now available changes the experience of motherhood, and the attachment that a woman feels toward the baby she carries. Rothman also discusses future developments, including "simple" blood tests for disorders that are now only "caught" via amniocentesis. She wonders whether women will be able to refuse this "simple" blood test and whether or not people who are disabled or "defective" will be allowed to exist in the future. She also wonders whether or not sophisticated technologies will raise our standards for what counts as a child worth keeping. This focus on individual decisions, Rothman notes, makes the job of mothering a fetus even more difficult, and isolates women during a very important time for connection-building with the child and with her support system, both of which are important to the health of future children. These individualistic interventions and surveillance are contrasted with the lack of support for environments in which it is safe to raise children, especially in light of chronic air and water pollution.

While most of the literature on nondirectiveness in genetic counseling has focused on its presence or absence, treating directiveness and nondirectiveness as binary, Oduncu (2002, p. 58) notes that the two concepts are not mutually exclusive. In reality, he argues, "... there is a vast grey zone between the two, and most of what happens in genetic counseling falls into this grey area." In the past 15 years, there has been considerable debate about the ability of genetic counselors to be nondirective in their work (see Clark, 1991; Michie, Bron, Bobrow, & Marteau, 1997; Kessler, 1997, as cited in Oduncu, 2002). Taken together, this literature primarily deals with the psychodynamics of the relationship between the genetic counselor and his/her client (e.g., Oduncu, 2002). Clark (1991), for example, worries that the offer of prenatal genetic diagnosis entails a tacit recommendation for abortion if any abnormality is found. He argues that this chain of reasoning is "built in" to the structure of the genetic counseling encounter. Below, I will present some evidence in support of this statement. Hodgson and Spriggs (2005) disagree, arguing that the primary aim of genetic counseling is the facilitation of autonomous decision making. They also argue for a practical descriptive account of autonomy, using a fictional case study as an illustration of their approach. Although they describe the choices that a fictitious couple would have when faced with a prenatal diagnosis of Down's Syndrome, the authors focus on the facts that the couple need to know. They also recognize that critical reflection on these options is also necessary. These authors do not address the ways in which these options are presented, or the support that genetic counselors can provide in helping a couple reflect on their most important values when making a decision about the future of the pregnancy. Further, Hodgson and Spriggs continue to focus on the psychology of the encounter between client(s) and counselor, understanding the social context within which this encounter lies. In this chapter, I argue for an important sociological angle on this relationship and the importance of the cultural and organizational context in which it takes place. Other scholars within genetic counseling called for studies that peer into the "black box" of counseling (Biesecker & Peters, 2001).

Previous studies have also noted that the term "nondirective" was borrowed from the psychotherapy of Carl Rogers (1942; as cited in Oduncu, 2002). Grounding genetic counseling in the context of developments in psychotherapy not only is an interesting object of study for the sociology of organizations, but also foregrounds a particular aspect of the idea of nondirectiveness that has not been empirically observed in process studies of genetic counseling.

PRINCIPLISM IN BIOETHICS

Philosophical grounding for nondirective counseling can be found in Beauchamp and Childress' (2001) text *Principles of Biomedical Ethics*. Now in its fifth edition, this text offers four principles that Beauchamp and Childress claim should be used as guides to ethical decision making within health-care settings. While not specific to genetic counseling, Beauchamp and Childress' work is helpful in understanding the practice of biomedical ethics throughout the health-care industry. The principles are respect for autonomy, nonmaleficence, beneficence, and justice. Before focusing on genetic counselors' respect for client autonomy through nondirective methods, I will briefly define each principle.

Beauchamp and Childress caution readers not to understand autonomy as the principle that overrides the other three. Although it has been suggested that this is the case in the practice of biomedical ethics (Evans, 2002), these authors deny that autonomy should be seen as the preeminent principle. Specifically arguing against a definition of autonomy that is excessively individualistic, excessively focused on reason, or excessively legalistic, they write, "Personal autonomy is, at a minimum, self-rule that is free from both controlling interference by others and from limitations, such as inadequate understanding, that prevent meaningful choice" (Beauchamp & Childress, 2001, p. 58). This definition of autonomy clearly fits with genetic counseling's focus on nondirective methods for helping clients understand the information that genetic tests do and do not provide. Reed (1963) advocates nondirective genetic counseling. More recently, Weil (2000, p. 121–122) has defined nondirective counseling:

> ... nondirective genetic counseling is defined as noncoercive or nonprescriptive, in which the genetic counselor refrains from giving advice, telling counselees what to do, or making therapeutic recommendations ... Another aspect involves whether the counselee's questions are answered in a manner that addresses the underlying emotions and concerns, which is empowering, or in a directive or dismissive manner, which implies that the genetic counselor's agenda and perspective are the only valid basis for discussion.

Professional judgment is often critical to a counselor's success. Counselors provide much more than mere information when being nondirective. As one genetic counselor put it, to be completely nondirective would mean giving clients information in a sequence that is random, unstructured, ungrounded, and probably unclear. Professional practice (and practical necessity) dictates that genetic counselors use their best judgment when determining the types of questions and information that clients need in order to make their best decisions. Some of the tools they use to accomplish this will be discussed below.

Nonmaleficence is the principle that asserts an obligation not to inflict harm on others (Beauchamp & Childress, 2001). This principle has been commonly associated with the Hippocratic tradition of medical writings, although the origin of Hippocrates' writings has been subject to some question (Edelstein, 1967; cited in Veach, 2000). This principle clearly applies to the work of genetic counselors in that there are cases one could imagine in which genetic counselors inflict harm upon their clients by revealing confidential information to outside parties.

Morality, for Beauchamp and Childress (2001, p. 165), requires that we treat persons autonomously, refrain from harming them, and contribute to their welfare. Actions that benefit others fall under the category of beneficence. The authors distinguish between two principles of beneficence: positive beneficence and utility beneficence. "Positive beneficence requires agents to provide benefits ... utility requires that agents balance benefits and drawbacks to produce the best overall results" (p. 165). In the context of genetic counseling, the principle of beneficence surely applies. Here, counselors provide information to clients (a benefit, although not necessarily a positive one) that they can then use in order to make decisions.

The final principle, justice, is especially difficult to codify. Beauchamp and Childress (2001, p. 226) resolve this dilemma by analyzing the terms "justice" and "distributive justice". Justice is interpreted as what is fair, equitable, and appropriate in light of what is owed to a person or persons. By contrast, distributive justice refers to "... fair, equitable, and appropriate distribution determined by justified norms that structure the terms of social cooperation" (p. 226). Justice is always the relation of one to another, or one to an institution. It is here that one could locate many questions about the practice of genetic counseling within the United States. Questions that turn on social inequalities such as racial, gender, and class status can all be asked under the principle of justice. These inquiries are surely important, yet are not my focus here.

Of course, there are other schools of thought within the larger bioethics discourse. Examples include casuistry, narrative, feminist, and utilitarian, among others (see Nelson, 1997). These approaches focus to varying degrees on the divide between abstract, conceptual principles and arguments that, some say, are disconnected from how people understand and make meaning from their experiences of illness and suffering within medical settings. Other approaches take a more ethnographic or case-based (as in casuistry) approach to ethics, seeking to understand how an ethical life can be led among the various contingencies and competing values that make life more complicated than abstract principles would lead one to believe. For our purposes in thinking about genetic counseling as a practical case of bioethics, Beauchamp and Childress (2001) provide a useful frame. By focusing on the use of client autonomy, we can come to understand something about how genetic counselors understand their work, and what this practice can tell us about the ways in which autonomy is employed in bioethics.

Sociologists who study the social context of bioethics have, for some time, been concerned about the use of abstract principles in deciding real cases. Work by DeVries and Subedi (1998) brings together sociologists who are concerned about bioethics' seemingly tin ear to social and political contexts and the consequences of their work. For example, Light and McGee (1998, p. 5) write, "Sociology insists that individual behaviors and choices emanate from the norms and customs of their setting and form institutional structures". They argue that bioethicists strip people of their sociocultural contexts in ways that are unreflective and unnecessarily narrow. This unhealthy reductionism denies the sociological fact that persons are necessarily embedded in reciprocal and enduring relationships with others. DeVries and Conrad (1998, pp. 233–234) put it this way:

> ...sociologists can show bioethicists how social structures, cultural settings, and social interaction influence their work. A bioethicists who adopts a sociological imagination (see Mills, 1959) can reflect on the practice of bioethics, to understand how the task of bioethics is constrained by disciplinary habits, professional relationships, cultural 'ways of seeing,' institutional needs, economic demands, and arrangements of power and prestige.

In the same way that DeVries and Conrad seek to put bioethics into its appropriate social and historical context, I seek to provide a critical, interpretive account of genetic counseling as one site where bioethics is practiced, a place where autonomous selves are constructed. For this to be true, genetic counselors must indicate that they believe their practice to enhance client autonomy. Before we get to the evidence, a brief note about methodology.

METHODS

I conducted a series of interviews with genetic counselors from September 2005 until late 2006. The work is exploratory. The genetic counselors were identified using snowball sampling, starting with one key informant. Because of this convenience sample, the analysis here is not generalizable to genetic counseling within the United States. The 10 genetic counselors I interviewed were all women between the ages of 25 and 55. Like most genetic counselors, they practice within major medical centers. Eight of the 10 counselors I interviewed were Caucasian, one African American, and another Asian American. All counselors I interviewed specialized in either prenatal or pediatric counseling, or were generalists. Although a considerable number of genetic counselors work with adult clients in cancer genetics, I did not interview any genetic counselors who specialized in this area. Although all counselors had experience counseling one-on-one, one counselor had spent some time working in a research setting. Counselors had between four months and 20 years of experience. Four practiced in the eastern United States, two in the mid-west, and four in the mid-south. I interviewed eight participants face-to-face, and two over the phone. Interviews lasted between 45 min and nearly 2 h. I used a semi-structured interview protocol, which asked respondents to describe their work processes, the type of counseling they practice, and their thoughts on nondirective counseling methods. All interviews were transcribed. The complete set of transcripts run to 93 single-spaced pages.

GENETIC COUNSELORS AND NONDIRECTIVE COUNSELING

So, how do genetic counselors go about their work? What sorts of technologies do they use in their daily interactions with their clients, both pediatric and prenatal? Most importantly, how does their practice help construct autonomous clients? Previous studies have provided a glimpse into the history and development of genetic counseling as a field (Rapp, 1988; Rothman, 1986; Resta, 1997; Heimler, 1997; Reed, 1979), although limited space prevents a comprehensive review.

Genetic counselors help construct autonomous clients (that is, they practice nondirective counseling) by contracting, "providing information," "giving options," "translating," "reflecting," and providing empathy and support. Of course, not all counseling sessions provide each, and no single counselor provides each equally well. These practices are connected, with one often leading to another. Nevertheless, the distinctions may be analytically useful for sociologists and bioethicists who seek to gain purchase on the ways in which autonomy is fostered within medical settings. Each counselor whom I spoke to discussed some version of each of these concepts, and together, they seem to define what they believe to be nondirective counseling. Although the definition of nondirective counseling is not without controversy, the counselors I spoke with seem to agree that it is defined by what it excludes: telling clients what to do, or recommending, even to the slightest degree, one course of action over another. This is especially true for prenatal genetic counseling, where termination is often discussed as a possibility. Consistent with the findings of a large-scale survey of genetic counselors (Bartels, LeRoy, McCarthy, & Caplan, 1997), each counselor I interviewed expressed strong support for the use of nondirective methods in their counseling.

CONTRACTING

Contracting, or providing a set of goals for the counseling session, was frequently mentioned as a way that counselors establish rapport with their clients. Often, but especially in prenatal settings, genetic counselors may only see their clients once, for about an hour. Contracting helps counselors narrow down the focus of the counseling session, bringing into line the expectations of the client with the work that the counselor must do. Counselors of prenatal women indicated that many times their clients were unsure as to why they were referred to the genetics clinic for counseling. For example, one counselor said, "I've had women come in who have absolutely no idea why they're there. No clue." Even if their clients do have some understanding of why they might be referred to a genetics clinic, they still may have the wrong impression. One counselor indicated that clients may have the impression that they were referred because of past drug or alcohol abuse, which may impact fetal development but are not the main reason for prenatal genetic counseling. "Advanced maternal age" is a very common "condition" that, as part of the standard of care, calls for genetic counseling. Rapp (1988) and Rothman (1986) discuss some features of its impact.

Once clients enter the counseling room, genetic counselors begin focusing the session. Oftentimes, they solicit information about their client's understanding of the purpose of the visit. One genetic counselor said, "... initially what I do is just say, 'Well, tell me why you're here'. 'What do you know about your session today?'... [A]nother question is, 'What do you want to get out of today's session?'" This line of questioning was echoed by an experienced counselor, who said, "... you'll have a family come in, and you ask them, 'I've read your chart, so I have some idea of why you're here, but what is your impression of why you're here?' or 'What are you looking for today?'" Other counselors indicated that contracting helps "set the tone" and provides "[a] sort of set parameters on what's going to happen." Sometimes, counselors will provide a brief session on how, through the systems and standards of practice common to contemporary medicine, they were referred for counseling. Another counselor said, "... one of the things I start of my counseling is asking them what their main concerns are, because a lot of times, what they're coming into this with ideas about is different from what their doctor referred them for." These types of questions position the client as the source of some knowledge about the encounter, and may provide some opportunity for the client to direct the session. As Rapp (1988) has noted, however, the discussion quickly focuses on the medically relevant, scientific information that the counselors need to collect and disseminate.

Many of the counselors I spoke with felt that contracting may help build rapport and put clients at ease with the unfamiliar environment and interaction. One spoke strongly about the negative connotations that the phrase "genetics clinic" has for some patients. This, the counselor recognized, can cause anxiety. One way in which genetic counselors deal with this, as a part of contracting, is laying out the goals for the session. Here is how one counselor described her approach for a pediatric session:

> ... I try to put them at ease with that, and just say, 'Sometimes people can be a little nervous when they are referred to the genetics clinic and wonder what's going to happen. So here's what's going to happen. I'm going to ask you for some information, the doctor is going to come in, take a look top to toe ... look for unusual things, things that most people wouldn't even look at, how widely spaced the eyes are, take a look at everything .... There's nothing hidden on our part. What we're suspecting, we'll tell you what we're suspecting, and then try to figure it out and then give you that information. We'll tell you what that information means, what that test means...'

By providing their clients with a set of goals for the counseling session, genetic counselors steer the conversation toward the "real" reason that the client(s) have come into contact with their services. The medical chart, the physician's recommendations, and the public health surveillance system all contribute to the counselor's understanding of the reason for the visit. The extent to which many, or most, clients are informed of these facts is unclear, although several counselors mentioned confusion about what genetic counseling means for them. Sometimes, genetic counselors identify unusual features before parents notice any problem, though this is rare. More common is the case in which a family has contacted a number of specialists without a confirmed diagnosis. Families then see genetic counselors in order to find out what genetic testing may be available.

PROVIDING INFORMATION

Once the counselor and client have finished "contracting" their session, the counselor often begins to provide her client with various types of information. In a pediatrics setting, this often involves discussing the symptoms and morphology of a child, as seen in the quote above. Here, counselors seek to inform their clients of the availability of various types of genetic testing. Of course, in prenatal cases, many screening tests are available through a "simple" blood test, while amniocentesis is a more invasive, more risky procedure. If a woman has one child with a genetic condition already, counselors reported that they discuss recurrence risks, i.e., the risk of conceiving a baby with the same genetic condition.

The counselors whom I spoke to seemed to see providing information as one of the most important aspects of their work, and a key to creating a nondirective environment. One counselor said, "… in my experience, I was mostly just giving information." Despite this statement, many counselors linked the notions of providing information and allowing free choice. All 10 counselors I interviewed discussed the way in which providing information *was* respecting a client's autonomous decision-making capacity. Perhaps, this view results from genetic counseling's roots in the client-centered psychotherapy of Rogers (1948; as cited in Oduncu, 2002). One counselor put it this way: "… I tell them [clients] that this information is important, that they'll be able to make decisions for their family." Another said, "… information, when you're looking at the ethics of patient autonomy, information helps the patient become autonomous." A 20-year-veteran counselor said, "… I'm trying to … give them the factual information they'll need to make decisions." These statements strongly link the idea of providing more information to clients with maximizing client autonomy. The idea is that if a client has more information, she will be more empowered to make a decision about whether or not to undergo screening or genetic testing for various conditions. One counselor said precisely this when she indicated that she has told clients, "… it's your decision to make, and you can be empowered by the feeling like you're making the right decision for you." Another, speaking of a prenatal counseling session, said:

> … [I] approach it as an informational sort of thing first, and then, once you give them all the information, try and help them go through their own thought processes, their own personal experiences. Have them sort of look in and see what they might want to do and why they might want to do that. So, a lot of it is really informational. And then, once they make a decision, it's giving them more information and once they get … [the test results] …

Thus, information is linked to autonomy, empowerment, and responsibility. These features, so central to the notion of freedom, undergird a substantial portion of genetic counseling practice. By establishing the goals of the session and "providing information," genetic counselors may distance themselves from the outcomes of decisions that clients make. Clark (1991) makes this point when he indicates that prenatal genetic counselors rarely follow up with their clients, and do not often participate in support groups for children with genetic conditions such as Down's Syndrome.

GIVING OPTIONS

Genetic counselors report that their clients have a wide variety of reactions to the information that they provide. In some cases, clients almost immediately decide whether or not to undergo amniocentesis or other screening. One counselor who had experience with working in the north and upper mid-west, as well as the south, indicated that, in general, there is some regional variation in willingness to receive information prenatally through amniocentesis. Of course, clients varied widely in the level of education and general understanding of science, and genetic counselors reported that they try to keep "science talk" as simple as possible. One counselor said, in order to make sure her clients understand the information she presents, "... I try to keep things fairly simple ... very concrete and very simple to present, and I try to do it with multiple methods of hearing and seeing the information." Because many clients graduated high school (or not) a decade or more ago, counselors often provide only the most basic scientific information, although, as Rapp (1988) points out, even this information is difficult for some clients to grasp.

Even though counselors seek to provide information in a way that is most helpful and easily understood by their clients, the best information may not help clients make a decision. When clients have difficulty making a decision, counselors report that they often provide options or scenarios for them to consider. These options may come from past clinical experience, training during graduate school, or publications. The counselors whom I spoke to were careful to say that they include "both sides" when describing options to their clients. One counselor, while discussing a prenatal counseling session, reported:

> ... [I say that] these are some of the reasons why we offer this testing: For people who want to know ahead of time for reassurance, for people who might make decisions that are different based on some information that they get, to help plan for the rest of the pregnancy, delivery options, you know, how the rest of the pregnancy is going to be handled, and to plan for care of the child after the child is born.

Another counselor reported that she says, " 'Well, other people in your shoes ... or other people have ...' and usually suggest what other people have done, but give them both sides of the coin." The options that counselors provide their clients may change client perceptions of the genetic condition. This is a major goal of counseling. One counselor said:

> ... I definitely believe that people should make their own decisions, and that they need, in order to do that, in order to make an educated decision, they need to have all of the facts that are available, all of the potential outcomes, and kind of be able to explore each one in order to make an informed decision.

Although the choices are often cast in an either/or fashion, some counselors provide a third option. For example, one counselor, discussing a prenatal session, indicated that she provides women with the option of enhanced monitoring, "... I talk to them about the alternatives of monitoring their pregnancy through detailed ultrasound, and what the sonographer can look for to see if the baby has an increased chance of having a chromosomal abnormality ...." This "third way" could come as welcome relief for women and their partners who do not choose amniocentesis for fear of its risks, but still prefer vigorous monitoring for genetic conditions.

Some counselors indicated that they often advise their clients that a decision is not necessary during the counseling session, but that the woman, couple, or family, should consider their options carefully prior to making a decision. Often, counselors will provide printed materials, visual aids, and other, client-friendly publications that explain the condition that was diagnosed or is suspected.

TRANSLATING

Since genetic counselors often work as part of a clinical genetics team, they often interact with clinical and research geneticists, family physicians, and other medical professionals. In many types of genetic counseling, but especially in pediatrics and adult-onset disorders, families and affected individuals see both a genetic counselor and a geneticist in order to discuss testing and receive physical examinations. It is in this context that the genetic counselor helps clients become autonomous decision makers by translating medical jargon into lay language. We have already seen a bit of this in action when counselors describe the ways in which they discuss genetic information such as chromosomes, genetic tests, recurrence risks, and the like. When they meet with other health professionals, however, clients may not be provided with information that is as easy to understand.

The genetic counselors I spoke with discussed the ways in which their style of giving information was different, more culturally appropriate, and more tactful than other health professionals. Their statements resonate with those captured by Bosk (1992). One counselor identified translation as one of the key tasks in her work. She said, "Translating medical information into lay language is a huge part of [what I do]." Another genetic counselor indicated that she is attuned to the ways in which clients can misunderstand medical information, even though the clinician is communicating in the best way that she knows. She said:

> ... being more attuned to the non-medical speak, you know, and sort of translate. Something that would make sense to me in the medical sense, but then I would also be aware [that] for someone from a different background, it would, they might hear it a different way. They might misinterpret what was said because of their own background.

There is, of course, some risk that the counselor will translate in ways that are not helpful to her clients, further confusing or obscuring the geneticist's message. The counselors that I spoke with seem to think that this does not happen often.

REFLECTING

Consistent with genetic counseling's intellectual heritage in the psychotherapeutic theories of Carl Rogers, the genetic counselors I spoke to indicated that one way in which they help clients decide whether or not to have genetic testing is to reflect what clients say back to them. One genetic counselor explained Rogers' client-centered therapy in this way:

> ... it's basically where you're viewing the individual as an autonomous individual. And you're assuming that they have the tools necessary [to make a decision], and communicating with them in a way so that they have the tools necessary to get the answer ... [that] they need.

This definition requires that clients be empowered to make their own decisions about genetic testing and interventions while simultaneously making them directly responsible for all outcomes, both positive and negative. This could be one of the most striking aspects of genetic counseling: By creating autonomous subjects, the counseling session also creates a great sense of responsibility.

Counselors indicated that, in order to help clients come to a decision, they try to ensure that clients consider their deepest values and beliefs. Instead of directly confronting their clients with questions about ultimate meanings and values, genetic counselors listen to the expressed thoughts and feelings of their clients and then re-present them. One counselor described her process:

> ... people come in with different expectations, they come in with different life experiences, they come in with different points of relation to whatever the decision is that they're going to make. ... I think that part of counseling needs to be understanding what somebody else is thinking or feeling ... because they've given you the information in a setting where you're sitting down and talking ... and then being able to form a relationship enough with them that you can give back to them what it is that they've been telling you, and sort of see whether you can clarify something or help them see something in a different way that may move them towards a decision.

The quote above captures several important aspects of the "reflecting" process that genetic counselors understand is operative in providing autonomy to their clients. Because clients already possess unique points of view, values, and life goals, the counselor must identify these deep feelings and then express them back to the client. Another counselor said that she often provides couples with an opportunity to discuss testing options or test results, trying to:

> ... just [give] them a few minutes to talk, and then listen, and then ... [I] reframe what they're saying back at them and lay it before them and say, 'So, this is what I've been hearing. You kind of feel this way', and you wait for the nod of affirmation or the no, you misunderstood them. 'And you kind of feel this way'.

By reflecting clients' statements, the counselor may help them clarify their understanding of the meaning of the options that they have been given. This clarified understanding can go beyond just providing information to reveal a client's core beliefs and life goals. If genetic counselors are able to help clients clarify their core values and beliefs with respect to genetic testing, then more autonomous choices may be available to them. Some authors (see Donchin, 2001) have critiqued this understanding of autonomy from a feminist standpoint, arguing that it does not take into account the social relations that help shape personal identity.

EMPATHY AND SUPPORT

Genetic counselors also report providing psychosocial support to their clients. As one counselor put it, "it's not just giving information and walking away. This is heavy information, it has implications for you, for your other family members, and so we need to be there to make sure that the client ... understands that information ...." Counselors report that they often verbally acknowledge the difficulty of making decisions that can have far-reaching consequences. With women of "advanced maternal age," counselors often report providing reassuring information to women, who, having chosen amniocentesis, receive a negative (that is, no genetic abnormalities) result.

Other counselors report that they refer clients to support groups and other external agencies. These external groups provide the ongoing psychosocial support that clients may need when parenting a child with a disability, or living with a genetic condition such as sickle cell disease. As such, these counselors become resource officials, collecting information on meeting times, locations, and government and other social support groups that can help clients manage the day-to-day challenges of living with a condition or parenting a child with a genetic condition. Of course, there is a wide range of interventions and management techniques for each condition. Two genetic counselors likened this to social work.

AUTONOMY WITHIN GENETIC COUNSELING AND BIOETHICS

Although Beauchamp and Childress (2001) are clear that client autonomy should not be seen as more important than the other three principles of nonmaleficence, justice, and beneficence, this is not always the case in practice (Evans, 2002). Evans found that when there is conflict between the four principles, health professionals, with the aid of bioethicists, often defer to a patient's request, regardless of the consequences for a patient's quality of life. Genetic counselors, through contracting, providing information, giving options, translating, reflecting, and providing empathy and support seek to help clients become their most autonomous selves. Their work involves understanding clients as always already autonomous and fully capable of examining their core values, beliefs, and philosophies of life. The extent to which this is true varies widely due to differences in counselors, settings, geography, and a client's race, class, and gender.

Some authors have argued that bioethicists advocate for a form of patient autonomy that is too strong. One example is Schneider (1998) who notes that, contrary to bioethics' fascination with patient autonomy, few clients actually want the responsibility that they have been given. Far from welcoming the additional burden of understanding, synthesizing, and reflecting on the options now available to them, some may prefer more guidance. As an aside, Schneider points to genetic counseling as an area where mandatory autonomy is operative. The tools genetic counselors use to construct client autonomy could provide clients with a sense of responsibility that is unwelcome.

Yet genetic counselors often face significant constraints when providing this autonomy. Most of the counselors I interviewed reported seeing from four to eight clients each day and spending between 2 and 4 h preparing to see each client. These professionals coordinate testing, report results, schedule exams and client consultations, keep up with advances in genetic testing, and provide a space where critical reflection can take place. More process studies of genetic counseling should be conducted so that scholars can determine the extent to which counseling sessions include significant space for the critical reflection required of more autonomous decisions. Perhaps, counseling should provide less, not more, information, so that clients can have the time to reflect on their options and determine which values are most operative in a given situation.

CONCLUSIONS: AUTONOMY AND RELATIONSHIP

The goal of this chapter has been to provide an account of the ways in which genetic counselors seek to create autonomous clients. Taking a closer look at the tools genetic counselors use to create autonomous clients (who, in turn, make more autonomous choices), focuses our attention on the process at work, both in the relationship between the counselor and the degree of autonomy that it provides. Perhaps this view of how autonomous selves are constructed in practice can help sociologists of bioethics understand the many ways in which bioethical principles are used. Bioethicists may find ways to refine theories of autonomy to focus on its processual and relational aspects. As Donchin (2001) argues, autonomy should be understood as relational, not overly individualistic.

One of sociology's central themes is that social structures, culture, and social interaction impact individual lives in ways that individuals themselves cannot control. This seems especially relevant to the study of the role autonomy plays within bioethics and genetic counseling. Many sociologists have argued that bioethics and bioethicists often fail to take into account social context, historical forces, and changing social relations when formulating bioethical theory. Individuals are always already embedded in social relationships, and these relations help constitute personal identity. Although several genetic counselors spoke of the importance of recognizing a client's background and life experiences, few spoke of the extensive social relationships in which clients are embedded. Heterosexual couples were the most frequently, if rarely, mentioned type of social relationship that the genetic counselors I interviewed saw as relevant to the counseling session. This was particularly true of counselors who worked with women who were pregnant or may become pregnant.

With the collective construction of identity in mind, it may be helpful for genetic counselors and bioethicists to consider the broad social networks within which their clients are embedded. Because individuals receive their moral and ethical sense from their social relationships, counselors may ask their clients to reveal more about the types of ethical and moral instruction that their clients bring with them into the counseling room. Doubtless, many counselors are aware of these issues. Yet because counselors seek to create autonomous clients, who make choices as individuals (or couples) alone, they may miss an important source for the values that a client expresses. If genetic counselors were more aware of the different moral, religious, and ethical perspectives common to the contemporary United States, then they might counsel their clients in a more culturally appropriate manner.

NOTE

1. Kevles (1985), Rothman (1986), and others discuss the eugenics movement in the United States and Europe.

REFERENCES

Bartels, D. M., LeRoy, B. S., McCarthy, P., & Caplan, A. L. (1997). Nondirectiveness in genetic counseling: A survey of practitioners. *American Journal of Medical Genetics, 72*, 172–179.

Beauchamp, T. L., & Childress, J. F. (2001). *Principles of biomedical ethics* (5th edn.). New York: Oxford University Press.

Biesecker, B. B., & Peters, K. F. (2001). Process studies in genetic counseling: Peering into the black box. *American Journal of Medical Genetics (Seminar in Medical Genetics), 106*, 191–198.

Bosk, C. L. (1992). *All god's mistakes*. Chicago: University of Chicago Press.

Bosk, C. L. (2002). Now that we have the data, what was the question? *American Journal of Bioethics, 2*, 21–23.

Clark, A. (1991). Is non-directive genetic counselling possible? *The Lancet*, *338*, 998–1001.
De Vries, R. (2004). How can we help? From sociology in to sociology of bioethics. *Journal of Law, Medicine, & Ethics*, *32*, 279–292.
DeVries, R., & Conrad, P. (1998). Why bioethics needs sociology. In: R. DeVries & J. Subedi (Eds), *Bioethics and society: Constructing the ethical enterprise* (pp. 233–257). Upper Saddle River, NJ: Prentice Hall.
DeVries, R., & Subedi, J. (Eds). (1998). *Bioethics and society: Constructing the ethical enterprise*. Upper Saddle River, NJ: Prentice Hall.
Donchin, A. (2001). Understanding autonomy relationally: Toward a reconfiguration of bioethical principles. *Journal of Medicine and Philosophy*, *26*, 365–386.
Evans, J. H. (2002). *Playing god?: Human genetic engineering and the rationalization of public bioethical debate*. Chicago: University of Chicago Press.
Heimler, A. (1997). An oral history of the National Society of Genetic Counselors. *Journal of Genetic Counseling*, *6*, 315–336.
Hodgson, J., & Spriggs, M. (2005). A practical account of autonomy: Why genetic counseling is especially well suited to the facilitation of informed autonomous decision making. *Journal of Genetic Counseling*, *14*, 89–97.
Kevles, D. J. (1985). *In the name of eugenics: Genetics and the uses of human heredity*. New York: Knopf.
Light, D. W., & McGee, G. (1998). On the social embeddedness of bioethics. In: R. DeVries & J. Subedi (Eds), *Bioethics and society: Constructing the ethical enterprise* (pp. 1–15). Upper Saddle River, NJ: Prentice Hall.
Michie, S., Bron, F., Bobrow, M., & Marteau, T. (1997). Nondirectiveness in genetic counseling: An empirical study. *American Journal of Human Genetics*, *60*, 40–47.
Nelson, H. L. (Ed.) (1997). *Stories and their limits: Narrative approaches to bioethics*. New York: Routledge.
Oduncu, F. S. (2002). The role of non-directiveness in genetic counseling. *Medicine, Health Care and Philosophy*, *5*, 53–63.
Rapp, R. (1988). Chromosomes and communications: The discourse of genetic counseling. *Medical Anthropology Quarterly*, *2*, 143–157.
Rapp, R. (1999). *Testing women, testing the fetus: The social impact of amniocentesis in America*. New York: Routledge.
Reed, S. C. (1963). *Counseling in medical genetics* (2nd edn.). Philadelphia: W.B. Saunders Company.
Reed, S. C. (1979). A short history of human genetics in the USA. *American Journal of Medical Genetics*, *3*, 282–295.
Resta, R. G. (1997). The historical perspective: Sheldon Reed and 50 years of genetic counseling. *Journal of Genetic Counseling*, *6*, 375–377.
Rothman, B. K. (1986). *The tentative pregnancy: Prenatal diagnosis and the future of motherhood*. New York: Viking.
Schneider, C. E. (1998). *The practice of autonomy: Patients, doctors, and medical decisions*. New York: Oxford University Press.
Veach, R. M. (2000). *The basics of bioethics*. Upper Saddle River, New Jersey: Prentice.
Weil, J. (2000). *Psychosocial genetic counseling*. Oxford monographs on medical genetics, no. 41. New York: Oxford University Press.

PART III: MACROSOCIOLOGICAL PERSPECTIVES: BIOETHICS IN THE POLICY ARENA

Because discussions of bioethical decision making often take place around specific cases that highlight the individual, the ethical issues these instances bring to the fore are often framed as problems of a deeply personal – and hence *individual* – nature. While the decisions of ethical bodies located at the intersection of the individual and the biomedical establishment have ramifications at the level of the individual, often constructed as a patient, discussions of bioethics directly inform policy in ways that affect large numbers of people – both as participants in the discussions around issues defined as bioethical in nature and as recipients of policies meant to reflect prevailing bioethical norms.

The three papers in this section directly address what happens when bioethics meets the world of public policy by focusing on three key aspects of this process. First, these authors offer theoretical ways to understand how public "debates" around scientific understandings of bioethical issues produce seeming consensus on appropriate courses of action. Second, they show how an array of institutions then become participants in enacting, at the level of individual, policy approaches that emerge from this consensus. And third, these authors offer concrete examples to show how seemingly thorough examinations of bioethical issues – conducted by appointed "experts" in the given field – obscure important issues by framing discussions toward a particular policy outcome and away from several others possible options whose consideration remains unarticulated.

Overall, these papers, either directly or implicitly, take the terms "bioethics" or just "ethics" and subject them, and the issues considered under their purview, to necessary sociological inquiry. The authors first step back and look at how certain issues come to be constructed as "ethical problems" in the first place. Second, they show how these constructions of the problem then influence the content of public debates around, and policies designed to address, the particular issue as narrowly defined. And third, they begin to consider how inequalities, on multiple levels, influence the policy outcome that these constructions and debates engender.

Herrmann and Könninger's paper focuses directly – and most theoretically of the three – on how the discourse around ethical discussions is formed. Eschewing the term "bioethics," they use the term "ethics" precisely because they are offering a model for understanding how ethical discourse enters into public discussion that can be applied across policy arenas. Explaining that ethics discourse functions "not as mere representations but rather as interpretations of reality," they are interested in how this process takes place, focusing specifically on the functioning of ethics commissions – with their mandates to publicly disseminate their findings – in France and Germany. Arguing that there are no "ethical problems" (seen as concrete) but rather "ethical problematisations" (viewed as a process), they identify two key aspects of this process: first, how issues come to be defined as problematic in the first place and second, "the problematisation of government in relation to these issues."

Their chapter is concerned mostly with the latter – namely, how ethical issues come to be considered governable. Ethics then, for Herrmann and Könninger, serves as "a frame that delineates the politico-epistemic space within which biomedical issues are defined, made governable and are governed." It is in articulating this theory of governing that Herrmann and Könninger make their theoretical contribution and do so by drawing directly on Michel Foucault's theory of governmentality with its focus on "the conduct of conduct." Distinguishing governmentality from government, Foucault's theory eschews a state-centered conception and considers the way that individuals, in liberal societies predicated on notions of "individual freedom," are encouraged to govern themselves. Governmentality, then, considers both governing – at multiple locations – and the forms of thought and knowledge that make governing possible in the first place.

Embedded in these thoughts and knowledge, despite the emphasis on individual autonomy, are normative assumptions, heavily mediated by expertise, knowledge and experts, about how individuals should conduct themselves. To make this theory concrete, Herrmann and Könninger focus on how governmentality operates through ethics commissions in France and Germany. These commissions – required to engage in "public bioethics exercises" – lead discussions on ethical deliberations where the public is encouraged to have opinions on these issues, but ones that reflect the scientific and ethical understandings generated by experts. As Herrmann and Könninger explain, through this public "stimulation of discourse," the public is integrated "into the expert guided process of rational reflection ... integrate[d] ... into the nexus of power/knowledge" that is part of being the subject of liberal self-government. Individuals are invited to weigh in on ethical issues with policy ramifications in ways that appear to be open and public but that, in fact, form microcosms of the expert-driven problematizations that are already heavily constructed by the time the public is handed these issues to deliberate.

While not directly engaging the theory of governmentality, Mukherjea's article is a perfect case study of how key public health decisions are deliberated and made by people and organizations who stand in for, but do not always directly represent, government. By moving the frame from biomedical to public health issues, her chapter also offers an important window into how the construction of public health problems leads directly toward certain solutions and away from others in ways that reflect persistent social and global inequalities.

Mukherjea tackles directly the complexity of the issues framing the discussion of male circumcision and its purported reduction in the transmission of HIV/AIDS. She opens her article outlining the increasing support this approach has received from a range of organizations and people including non-profits, public health workers, NGOs, and former US presidents. This support has been bolstered by expert knowledge that has found positive correlations, in localized contexts, between reduced HIV transmission and male circumcision. She eschews the increasingly familiar debate around the topic – in its simplistic form, male circumcision can save lives versus circumcision is a human rights abuse (a debate whose elaboration of its underlying assumptions would make a nice contribution to this volume's second edition) – instead using discussions of male circumcision's HIV-prevention potential as an opportunity to consider both what HIV-prevention alternatives are rendered invisible by the attention heaped on male circumcision and some of the reasons why these alternatives are rendered invisible.

Mukherjea focuses on the social, cultural and historical issues surrounding male circumcision as it has entered public health discourse. These issues are precisely the ones that get ignored in biomedical discussions, but Mukherjea's article reminds us that dangerous terrain can be mindlessly traversed without these considerations. Taking a critical look at the history of the public health debate around male circumcision, Mukherjea shows how "uncertain science" has informed an issue that is a "heavily racially and culturally infected one." Race, ethnicity and gender matter deeply in this article – both in explaining why male circumcision has come to receive such a privileged place among an array of HIV-prevention approaches – and in helping Mukherjea develop her thoughtful and complex stand on this complicated topic. While not wholly against male circumcision, she explains that she is "deeply uncomfortable with the cultural and ethical assumptions that underlie much of the excitement and conversation about these findings and their possible applications."

As Mukherjea points out, the discussion about male circumcision is focused on its application in the global South – precisely the region of the world where discussions of HIV usually are coupled with consideration about "cheapness." Circumcision, promoted based on empirical data as to its efficacy, is heavily weighted with cultural and economic imperialism but presented solely as a pragmatic and cost-effective approach to the problem of HIV transmission. As Mukherjea notes, discussions of HIV in the global South rarely center around HIV treatment, considered too costly, but on HIV prevention and, by focusing on such a "radical intervention" as male circumcision, the discussion of circumcision "... contains within it an underlying despair at the potential efficacy of educational programs" – programs that flounder under the assumption, despite evidence to the contrary, that "men and women cannot be adequately counseled to make informed decisions regarding their own health."

But, as Mukherjea points out, women, especially, are not being given the option to take their own health into their hands. Because the public health problem has become narrowly defined as the prevention of HIV transmission and this problem is viewed as the transmission of HIV by men, circumcision is promoted while other options for women – such as microbicides – receive far less attention and resources. As Mukherjea explains, the emphasis on male circumcision constructs a form of masculinity in the face of "political scarcity and political marginalization" while ignoring gender as relational and the ways in which women, in the global South, must also navigate complex and "circumscribed" relations.

By linking bioethical issues to the public health arena – where they directly become a matter of policy – and by showing us the range of actors concerned in public health debates, Mukherjea broadens this volume's frame globally and institutionally. She concludes her article suggesting that we consider, with respect to public health policy, the following three issues: first, how we choose to prioritize certain populations over others; second, the ethno-political and racial implications of these policies; and third, a global political economic perspective. Overall, Mukherjea reminds us to consider bioethical issues as they play out at the "world population" and "community" perspective, the ways in which public health discourse obscures as much as it reveals, and also reminds us of the reasons for why this silencing takes place.

Ettore's article takes us back to familiar locations for bioethical examinations – both geographically, in the Western, highly medicalized context, and topically, with a focus on genetic technologies and biomedical prenatal practice. Echoing Mukherjea's concern with social justice and Herrmann and Könninger's concern with knowledge and power, she examines how "genomic governmentality" – as a "social institution and moralizing regime"—focuses on women's reproductive capacities while simultaneously negating women's embodied experiences.

Ettore urges the reader to see the unintended consequences of this negation of women's embodied experiences and guides the reader by focusing less on reproductive *policy* and more so on reproductive or prenatal *politics*. She defines the latter as "the application of specific ideological beliefs, knowledge and medical procedures on developing foetuses." The central idea of Ettore's argument is that by focusing on fetuses, this politics ignores pregnant women who, in her view, "bear the brunt of damaging beliefs and painful procedures." Linking this politics to knowledge, Ettore explains that "prenatal politics operate in the discursive spaces of knowledge and practices generated by the unversalising system of reproductive genetics." As in Herrmann and Könninger's work, we see how expert knowledge around ethical issues encourages a focus on the individual while also demanding a somewhat uniform perspective on biomedical issues. The result of this reliance on expertise, according to Ettore, is that women's embodied experiences are negated. Women are required to practice "reproductive asceticism" for the sake of their fetus while simultaneously being encouraged to disregard themselves in the process.

Much as Mukherjea's work encourages a consideration of the complexity of the people upon whom circumcision is being encouraged, Ettore asks the reader to consider an "embodied ethics" through which "the corporeal experiences of moral, gendered individuals" – the women subject to genetic reproductive technologies – are brought to the forefront. Rather than excluding women from full moral agency, she encourages an approach that starts with the premise that women's experiences are reflected in the stories we tell about reproductive technologies and the research we conduct about their effects. She calls for an "empathic social science" when examining these issues and a "responsible ethics framed by and through embodied relationships" when considering the politics of genetic reproductive technologies.

Combined, these three chapters urge us to move beyond the individual while simultaneously considering how the individual figures in public narratives about policy decisions that are fraught with – or framed as – ethical issues. By focusing on how ideas about ethical issues are constructed and then how these constructions inform public debates, these four authors require us to move outside of the realm in which decisions are made and to consider the conditions under which consensus of opinions is subtly encouraged through the use of expert knowledge. By highlighting the construction of expert knowledge and its relation to policy and politics, they encourage us to consider the implications behind what factors are included in public discussions and what factors are considered outside the realm of consideration. These three chapters help us to broaden our sociological inquiries into bioethical issues institutionally and geographically, and to consider the narrow frame around which the governance of bioethical issues is constructed as an important area for critical sociological inquiry.

Rebecca Tiger
Editor

"… BUT YOU CANNOT INFLUENCE THE DIRECTION OF YOUR THINKING": GUIDING SELF-GOVERNMENT IN BIOETHICS POLICY DISCOURSE

Svea Luise Herrmann and Sabine Könninger

INTRODUCTION

Since the beginning of the 1980s, we can observe the emergence and proliferation of different processes and institutions of *ethical* debate throughout Europe and the Western world; these processes and institutions are supposed to inform and improve opinion-building and decision-making processes in the policy field of the biosciences and especially biomedicine. National boards of ethics, ethics commissions, citizen's consultations or conferences have been established throughout; they all have in common the task to debate the ethical aspects of biomedical research and practice, and inform politics as well as the public about the ways of dealing with biomedicine in 'ethically' justified ways. Conflicts in the field of biomedicine have increasingly become framed in terms of ethics, and policy makers have to explain and defend their decisions with reference to ethics. The language of ethics has become the major medium for the debate about biomedical

Bioethical Issues, Sociological Perspectives
Advances in Medical Sociology, Volume 9, 205–223
Copyright © 2008 by Elsevier Ltd.
All rights of reproduction in any form reserved
ISSN: 1057-6290/doi:10.1016/S1057-6290(07)09008-0

issues. This development is accompanied by the emergence of a new cast of professionals: the 'ethics expert', who becomes a member of a commission or an advisor to governments or organisations. Bioscientific practice and development seem to be inevitably *ethical* issues. Consequentially, controversies or conflicts appear to be solved best through *ethical* deliberations. One can justly speak of an *ethics regime*[1] that surrounds, stimulates and penetrates discourses, institutions and practices concerning conflicts and policy making in the issue area of biomedicine.

While the goal of ethical bodies or debates is the improvement of policy making and the control or limitation of biotechnological practices, empirically the success of the ethics regime in this respect is at least doubtful: Looking at the outcomes of ethical debate and advice we can observe that many, if not most, of the debates, statements or recommendations by ethics bodies or newly implemented regulation do not lead to limitations, but rather to the deregulation or re-regulation of biomedical development, at least in Europe. Empirically, the ethics regime does not provide an effective system for societal/political limitations or control of biomedical or techno-scientific development. However, on another level, which will be the focus of this paper, the ethics regime is very successful: As we will show, it has a more important function, that is the formation of a guiding frame for newly arising forms of self-government in the area of biomedicine and bioethics. Via the *activation* and *proliferation* of ethical debate, the *guidance* of participants and the formation of speaker positions, the ethics regime shapes the frame for the production and organisation of discourses on biomedical issues, rather than providing a substantial normative orientation for action, let alone the shaping of biomedical developments. On the contrary, biotechnological 'progress' remains the undoubted prerequisite for debate, and not its topic.

Committed to Foucault's understanding of discourse, we do not take the 'ethical character' of bioscientific issues for granted, but instead understand *ethics* as a historical form of problematisation that has particular consequences for the government of bioscientific development. The focuses of the paper are effects of *ethical problematisation* with regard to new forms of self-government that arise in the context of the ethics regime.

With reference to Michel Foucault's notion of *governmentality*, in this article we will particularly focus on transformations of *government*[2] related to the emergence and proliferation of the ethics regime. The empirical data suggest that we are witnessing, at the moment, a shift towards new forms of self-government accompanying the establishment of a *mentality* shaped by the ethics regime. In this paper we will focus on two types of self-government: as regards the use of one's own body and as regards the participation in bioethical debates.

The analysis is part of an ongoing research project on 'Ethical Governance?'[3] in Germany, France and Great Britain. The project analyses what we have called 'governmental ethics regimes' referring to a range of institutions, discourses and practices initiated or supported by governmental institutions and directed at linking ethical considerations to policy making especially in the field of biomedicine and biotechnology. The project studies the emergence and development as well as effects of new institutions and processes of 'ethical reflection' and their linkage to policy making since the late 1970s. In what follows, we will focus on developments in Germany and France, as two examples of the establishment of ethics regimes. Although the ethics regimes differ in the two countries as regards, for example, the number of institutions set up or the processes initiated as well as their design, scope or duration, and not the least, concerning competences and outcomes of the different instances, we find striking similarities as regards a tendency to stimulate and frame guided self-government in both countries. We analyse several instances through which individuals are invited to ethical self-reflection and self-government such as abortion policy, the writing of a living will or, on a more general level, the organisation of *Journées annuelles d'éthique*, *espaces éthiques*, *Schülerforen*, or citizen's conferences.

ETHICS AND GOVERNMENTALITY

While today, issues of biomedical developments appear as genuinely *(bio)ethical* issues, we suggest to doubt an intrinsic relation and to ask instead what 'ethics' means and does in relation to debates on biomedicine. Most, if not all, socio-political issues imply normative questions, without, however, explicitly referring to ethics. The nuclear power conflicts of the 1970s and 1980s in Europe, for instance, were also marked by conflicts of value, such as responsibility towards future generations; however, there were no ethics institutions established and controversies were not debated in terms of ethics. In the nuclear power conflicts, not 'ethics' but 'risk' was the battleground and risk discourse was the main medium in which technology conflicts could be debated (cf. Beck, 1992). The explicit reference to ethics as a frame for dealing with political conflicts came up, at least in Europe, in connection with the development of new biomedical practices and technologies, most prominently IVF and human genetic technology.[4]

In line with post-positivist theory, and committed to Michel Foucault's understanding of discourse as productive rather than descriptive, we perceive ethics discourses not as mere representations but rather as interpretations of reality. In accordance with Bacchi (1999) we suggest to speak of ethical *problematisations* rather than ethical problems. Thus, instead of understanding ethics as inherent quality of biomedical issues per se, our analysis is based on the assumption that 'ethics' is a historically particular form of problematisation that provides a frame for the interpretation of a situation or issue and determines what is problematic about it (Rein & Schön, 1993, p. 153) and that also inherently suggests ways to deal with it. Thus, the notion of problematisation embraces two interrelated meanings: The first is how issues are defined as problematic and the second is the problematisation of government in relation to these issues (cf. Foucault, 1991, p. 102ff.). Problematisation in terms of ethics, we claim, incorporates the emergence of particular forms of thinking about and exercising government as regards biomedical developments. In this analysis, however, we will focus on the second meaning, that is effects on government.

The use of the notion of problematisation in our analysis is based in studies on *governmentality* (Foucault, 1991; cf. also Dean, 2001; Gordon, 1991) referring to the question of how issues are defined as problematic, including questions as to how government works in relation to them. In this approach, we understand *ethics* as a frame that delineates the politico-epistemic space within which biomedical issues are defined, are made governable and are governed. On the one hand, problematisation in terms of ethics constructs the object of government, as well as the subjectivity and authority of those who govern or are governed. It delineates the narrative and argumentative tools for, and the format of, debate and defines the necessary skills and characteristics of those to participate in the debate. On the other hand, it excludes particular features or attributes of the issues and rules out specific arguments or forms of debate or action.

Governmentality studies are able to analyse forms of government that go beyond conventional state-centred conceptions. The theory of governmentality avoids a focus on government in the sense of formal political activity of an administration in favour of a broader view of different types of government including government of the self. Studies on governmentality particularly focus on the specific interconnectedness of divers forms of government in liberal societies that support individual self-government and individual as opposed to collective responsibility for social conditions.

Most importantly for our analysis, applying the theory of governmentality, we can analyse notions such as 'freedom', 'autonomy' or 'self' as well as 'participation' or 'inclusion' as integral elements of government in the ethics regime, rather than the reverse. As we can observe empirically, these notions play an increasingly important role in recommendations or statements by ethics bodies as well as in ethical debates more generally. In the ethics regime, these notions are, however, inseparably linked to expert-guided self-reflection and thus to the result of what Rose (1999, p. 4) has called "action upon action":

> ... to govern is to recognize that capacity for action and to adjust oneself to it. To govern is to act upon action. This entails trying to understand what mobilizes the domain of entities to be governed: to govern one must act upon these forces, instrumentalize them in order to shape action, processes and outcomes in desired directions. Hence, when it comes to governing human beings, to govern is to presuppose the freedom of the governed. To govern is not to crush their capacity to act, but to acknowledge it and utilize it for one's own objectives.

Especially as regards issues of biomedicine, or so-called bioethical issues, we can observe an emphasis on individual freedom and autonomy, as in 'patient rights' or 'reproductive freedom', that at first sight seems to contradict the notion of government. Liberal societies have always been challenged by the paradox that derives from questions as to how to govern in accordance with the freedom of the individuals in ways that lead to the preferred outcomes. The tension between freedom on the one hand and government on the other, can best be resolved in self-government that channels the use of freedom: Guided self-government, as Weir (1996) writes, is the ideal answer to this problem of liberalism.

As becomes obvious in the amalgamation of the two terms – *government* and *mentality* – governmentality studies are particularly devoted to understanding the interconnectedness of forms of government and forms of thought and knowledge. The fusing of these two concepts emphasises that modern government is inseparably linked to particular forms of thinking the reality of government as well as of subjects and objects of government. Liberal government, understood as a form of the conduct of conduct, necessarily has a normative dimension as it entails assumptions about how individuals or groups should conduct themselves. It entails the assumptions of the (relative) freedom of the individuals to act and of the possibility to direct or regulate the use of this freedom. "Government", in the governmentality sense, "is an activity that shapes the field of action and thus, in a sense, attempts to shape freedom" (Dean, 2001, p. 13) through increasing the predominance of apparatuses of conduct and the development of a complex of truth and knowledge (Foucault, 1991), that is through the establishment of a *mentality* that is collective and relatively taken for granted and that guides conduct/government including government of the self.

Expertise, knowledge and experts play important roles in the formation of norms and goals of government distant from the state. Liberalism particularly refers to experts and expertise when it comes to the identification and resolution of problems that 'need' disinterested advice – when it comes to the need to govern and to limit government at the same time. Instead of implementing the rules and norms of conduct, political authorities installed a set of expertise equipped with the authority to truth (Rose, 1996). The new ethical advisory boards, although they differ in their institutional design or scope of authority, comprise mostly experts who are supposed to provide expert advice. In this sense, ethics in the ethics regime, is a form of expertise.

Expertise, that is the "authority arising out of a claim to knowledge, to neutrality and to efficacy" (Rose, 1996, p. 39), provides government (in the sense of governmentality) with the necessary knowledge that enables the conduct of conduct. Experts, in return, are granted relative autonomy from political intervention so as to assure their disinterested judgement on the basis of expertise. In the ethics regime, it is a necessary condition of ethics bodies to be 'independent'. Still, the ethics bodies are not necessarily or even predominantly assumed to provide straightforward recommendations for policy making. Rather, expert advice often comes explicitly as an *offer*, or several offers in dissenting votes on one and the same issue, that the policy maker or the public might choose from. Expertise in the ethics regime becomes, to use the words of Rose (p. 54), a service that consumers might request in acts of choice.

While it is not (necessarily) the case that the new ethics bodies have great impact on policy making,[5] the ethics regime still does have effects at the level of government (in the Foucauldian sense) in that it establishes a *mentality*, a guiding frame for self-government as regards individual bodily existence as well as the participation in public debates on bioethics. In the next section we will analyse the empirical data with regard to the question as to how the ethics regime effects (and puts forth) these forms of self-government.

BODILY EXISTENCE AND THE CONTROL OF SPEECH

The concept of governmentality has already been applied to the analysis of forms of governing individual bodily existence or bioethics. Memmi

(2003, 2005) and Rose (2001, 2005), for example, situate 'bioethics' within the wider framework of the transformation of biopolitics (Foucault). In their perspective, biopolitics no longer operates through forms of external, especially state, control as Foucault had described it, but rather through individualised procedures of government which are supported but not directly executed by the state. In this perspective, bioethics as a practice can be described as a form of liberalised and individualised biopolitics. Memmi (2003) argues that bioethics is a new form of biopolitics that is particularly marked by the delegation and individualisation of government. She observes a shift in forms of government which she calls "conditional decriminalisation" (Memmi, 2003, p. 645). Especially with regard to the administration of birth and death, Memmi detects the installation of a "government through speech" (Memmi, 2003) that is marked by the replacement of punishment by guidance. German as well as French abortion law can serve as examples. Both mandate that women seeking an abortion present their wish before a doctor or counsellor in a particular manner.[6] They have to offer good reasons for their wish and prove that their decisions are consciously made and are the reasonable result of counselling and rational self-reflection. While constructed as a private matter and personal decision, the wish to have an abortion has to be integrated into the expert-guided framework of counselling discourse. Provided, she adheres to this process, the decision is delegated to the individual woman. Abortion has been subjected under a regime of rational and expert-guided individual agency and decision making at the expense of any other way of dealing with (unwanted) pregnancy. The personal decision has become a demand supported and institutionalised by the state. Thus, Memmi (2005) speaks of "delegated biopolitics" (*la bio-politique déléguée*) when it comes to the control and government of one's own bodily existence. We can add that this delegated biopolitics functions not through punishment or force but through "the regulated choices of individual citizens" (Rose, 1996, p. 41) that depend upon expert-guided self-reflection, speech and decision making. While the decision to have an abortion is up to the woman's personal conscience and self-determination, it is embedded in a request to self-government: Guided by an expert, the woman is asked to reflect her life, balance her options and make a decision that she takes the responsibility for – at the expense of an exclusion of activities (or inactivities) that do not comply with the requirements of rationality, self-reflection or decision making, such as for example, having an abortion without undergoing counselling outside of a decision-making process of balancing pros and cons. Control and government of bodily existence is realised via the stimulation and simultaneous control of speech, or what Weir (1996) has called "guided self-government". The language and method offered for self-government is the language of ethics: It is the language of (individual) conscience, beliefs, values and responsibility. Rather than suggesting or providing a strict ban on biomedical practices, the ethics regime supports a form of regulation that allows and fosters individual decision making surrounded by expert guidance and supervision.

We find a similar tendency to emphasise the autonomy and decision-making competence of concerned individuals who take part in biomedical practices or more generally 'take their lives in their hands' also at the level of recommendations or statements of ethics bodies. Examples would be informed consent to genetic tests after genetic counselling or the writing of a living will. In its statement "The advance directive", the German National Ethics Council, states that

> self-determination presupposes the capacity for volition. The individual is held capable of making-responsible decisions for himself [sic!]. At the same time he bears the onus of decision. (German National Ethics Council, 2005, p. 23)

While the council does not believe that the validity of living wills depends on expert advice taken by its maker, it nonetheless recommends that expert advice is taken before the will is drawn up (German National Ethics Council, 2005, p. 64). A recently published brochure on 'how to write a living will' by the German Ministry of Justice (Bundesministerium der Justiz, 2006, our translation) provides text modules as "rough guiding post and suggestions for the description of one's own situation and personal conception" and suggests to discuss the content of the will with a doctor. The ministry states that everyone, however, should be aware that writing a living will is a

> process of personal consideration of questions related to disease, suffering and death. This examination is necessary in order to raise awareness, that a living will – as an expression of the right to self-determination – embraces also responsibility for the consequences resulting if the will is realized. (ibid., our translation)

Self-determination is inseparably bound to self-reflection, the "capacity of volition" and responsibility. Individuals are asked to 'tell their story', (possibly) seek doctor's advice and think about what they consider to be a good death and decide which dying options they want and which they do not want. The practice of writing a living will is an invitation to reflect one's own life and death, one's beliefs, wishes and needs; to balance different options and to make a responsible decision through which they are granted self-determination and autonomy.

The more general background normative principles of the ethics regime are informed consent, voluntary (moral) action, autonomy, individual choice and responsibility. These are, however, not free of charge but have to be earned in a guided self-reflection process.

PUBLIC EXERCISES IN BIOETHICS

Next to those dimensions of the ethics regime that are directed at guiding self-government regarding individual bodily existence that opens up spaces for individual decision making, there is a second dimension directed at guided participation in bioethical debate. The emphasis on freedom, autonomy and self-determination is accompanied by a tendency to publicise and proliferate ethical debate, to include more and more, especially hitherto non-involved, people and educate them in the ways of how to speak in an 'ethical manner'. Public education in bioethics is a tool to foster guided self-government in the field of biomedicine and bioethics. Although to different degrees, we can observe a tendency towards what we call the *ethicisation* of the public in Germany as well as in France. In the following section, we will discuss different examples of how the ethics regime contacts the public and invites participation in bioethics debate while at the same time providing a frame for the organisation of the debate.

Include the Public

We can observe the tendency to publicise and proliferate ethical debate, not the least in the fact that most ethics commission, including the French *Comité Consultatif National d'Ethique pour les sciences de la vie et de la santé* (CCNE) and the German National Ethics Council (*Nationaler Ethikrat*, NER), are formally charged with making public their statements, recommendations or discussion as well as stimulating and organising public debate and raising awareness of 'ethical aspects of the life sciences'. "As part of its mission", the French CCNE "organises annually a public conference on ethical issues in the field of health and life sciences" and publishes its *Avis*, opinions, and sometimes recommendations (CCNE, 2006). At the annual public meetings, the so-called *Journées annuelles d'éthique,* opinions already published, as well as 'open' topics, are presented to the audience (Interview F II, CCNE, 2005; Interview F IV, CCNE, 2005). In this way a debate between members and participants is to be stimulated (Interview F IV, CCNE, 2005). The publication of the positions reached by the CCNE, along with the expansion of "biological and medical information" (Interview F IX, CCNE, 2006, our translation), should also encourage debate. The effects of such debate include the criticism that the positions provoke from the public (Interview F IV, CCNE, 2005). Didier Sicard, the current president of the CCNE, confirms this assessment in his suggestion that the committee should be called the "national advisory committee for unsettling ethics" (Sicard, 2001, our translation). The French Bioethics Law of 2004[7] provides for, through the CCNE, so-called *espaces éthique*, 'ethical spaces', at the regional and sub-regional levels, which represent a possible expansion of the space for ethical discussions in order to reach a wider public (Interview F IV, CCNE, 2005). The role of the *espaces éthiques* is to assist in the organisation of public debates and to facilitate the informing and advising of citizens in bioethical questions in the area of health (Assistance Publique Hôpitaux de Paris, 2006). The *Agence de la biomédicine*,[8] also constituted through the Bioethics Law of 2004, is charged with the production of a "dialogue between society, the public authorities, and biomedical practitioners and researchers", in order "to facilitate reflection on scientific developments" (Douste-Blazy, 2005, our translation). Whether it is a matter of provoking criticism, unsettling ethical conceptions in the public realm, or setting up of 'ethical spaces', it should serve the initiation and/or the broadening of ethical debates.

The German National Ethics Council, according to the decree on its establishment,

> ... shall organize the social and political debate and ensure that all the relevant groups are involved. It shall provide citizens with information and material for discussion (e.g. exhibitions, publications, internet forums, etc.). Every year the National Ethics Council shall hold at least one public conference on ethical issues. (Draft Decree, 2001, §2(1))

While these public events also serve the information of the boards "on the situation of the social debate" (Draft Decree, 2001, §2(5)), as well as they might inspire "reflection within the ethics board" itself (Interview F II, CCNE, 2005, our translation), a more important function is to induce a reflection process within participants: In the opinion of a former member of the CCNE, the role of the committee ideally lies in making citizens "mature to reflect for themselves" (Interview F IX, CCNE, 2006, our translation). In this respect, the German National Ethics Council wrote,

> *Everyone* must be able to form an impression of the prospects and risks of the new technologies, as a basis for arriving at his or her own judgement on the associated ethical issues. To this end, the Ethics Council will seek to facilitate understanding of the

presuppositions and consequences of current problems. (German National Ethics Council, 2001, p. 7, emphasis added)

Thus, next to the initiation, the *organisation* and *structuring* of public debate is a further function of these events. The former chair of the German NER said that next to discussions within the board itself, "the maybe more relevant function of such a body would be to communicate to the public the problem areas that are at the centre of its work" (Interview G, NER, 2005, our translation).

Integrate Non-Involved People and Guide Rational Reflection

A second aspect in the proliferation of ethical debate is the integration of particularly *non-involved* people. The *Journées annuelles d'éthique* are distinctive in their integration of school pupils into the debate. Students make presentations on bioethical themes and take part in discussions with members of the CCNE and other participants at the meetings. The students are considered by the committee as future citizens, who ought to practice bioethical reflection (Interview F IV, CCNE, 2005). Their reflections are seen as useful by the committee, as *"richesse pour le future"*,[9] because their "naïvety" can provide the inspiration for new questions within the committee, and because they are considered to be 'multipliers', who will convey reflections to their parents and carry them forward in discussions with their families (Interview F IV, CCNE, 2005). The students are given a twofold function: First, they carry the ethical debate into their families, thus reaching a wider circle of people, and secondly, they serve as 'sources of inspiration' for future debates of the CCNE. The German Council also organises *Schülerforen* (school forums) directed at "young people between 16 and 19" which it regards to be an important target group for its work because "they are at a stage where they develop their moral concepts and measures for their further lives, as well as they are open-minded and unbiased towards new issues" (Nationaler Ethikrat, 2006, our translation). At this stage, according to the NER, school plays an important role not only concerning knowledge transfer but also, and more importantly, concerning the 'development of personality' and 'personal morality'. Therefore, the NER had decided to "trigger and guide bioethics-discourse in schools" (ibid.). It is precisely their "naïvety", their open-mindedness and their undeveloped morality that make school children a target for the ethics regime: As participants in bioethical debate they are *supposed to* not be interest driven or biased or not have a certain position towards the respective issues under discussion.

Next to those bioethics exercises initiated by the national ethics boards, since about the mid-1990s, in many European countries so-called citizen's conferences on bioscientific issues have been organised in order to foster the participation of the wider public in ethical debate, many of them being discourse experiments. Germany already had two of these conferences: one on genetic diagnosis (*Streitfall: Gendiagnostik*),[10] more precisely on preimplantation genetic diagnosis (PGD), in 2000 and one on stem cell research in 2004. Both issues had been widely and very controversially debated in the German press and public. However, the participants invited had to be particularly un-involved in the issues and not be members of the many socio-politically interested groups or initiatives that dealt with these issues in Germany. Participants were addressed and were to take part as *individuals* and not as, for example, representative of certain organised interests. The focus of these conferences, thus, was not to debate different existing or controversial views or interests and to find a consensus or compromise among them, but rather to initiate a discussion among uninterested individuals. They were attempts to activate discussion among people who until then had *not* thought about these issues. The goal of the first German citizens conference was to initiate dialogue, to initiate public opinion building processes, to test the method 'consensus conference', to reduce information deficits within the public through new ways of knowledge transfer and to complement expert discussions with a "qualified contribution of citizens" (Zimmer & ISI, 2002, our translation). Similarly, the goal of the stem cell research conference was to invite participants to "broaden their experiences and knowledge" on a "higher level of cognition", as one of the organisers said in his opening speech.[11] Rather than focussing on contents and substantial outcomes, these events centred on the discursive format and the process itself as well as on effects and cognitive results within participants, which were also the main issues in the evaluation report (Zimmer & ISI, 2002).

Since a few years, German policy makers place increasing emphasis on the initiation and organisation of broader public bioethics exercises. In May 2006, the German Federal Ministry of Research published funding guidelines for "discourse projects on ethical, legal and social questions in the modern life sciences" (Bundesministerium für Bildung und Forschung, 2006, our translation). The projects considered for funding should be dealing with issues that directly "derive from research or application in the life sciences" and should address especially "the young generation". The projects should "contribute to objective and unbiased information ... support qualified opinion building of the respective target groups and process it in a publicly visible discourse" (ibid., our translation). The ministry wants to fund discourse projects that "are directed at a qualified development and consolidation of bioethical discourse processes" (ibid., our translation) conducted by experienced discourse specialists, who have to explicitly prove their competences as regards conducting discourse events.

In France there are now ongoing attempts to introduce greater numbers of citizen's conferences (Callon et al., 2005; Île de France, 2006; Lipinski, 2006). The "qualified opinion-formation" is guided not by discourse experiments, as in Germany, but rather through the CCNE. At the *Journées annuelles d'éthique* of the CCNE, the students, who present on topics that are fixed in the programme of the meeting, are given confirmation that they have reflected 'correctly': "You have understood the difficulties and the problematisation" and it is simultaneously asserted that there can be no conclusive solution, because in ethics such conclusiveness "can never be reached".[12] What becomes clear from the quotations is that the CCNE adopts the function of guiding students in the development of the capacity for 'correct' and continual reflection, and the method of argumentation, of the 'future citizens' (Interview F IV, CCNE, 2005), in which finding a conclusive answer is not the goal.

In France, as compared to Germany, processes of guided self-reflection are more directly initiated by the CCNE via its *Journées anuelles d'éthique*, which are 'ritually' held once a year and which additionally also serve the inspiration of the CCNE itself. In Germany we find more divers institutions and processes of bioethical debate, such as consensus conferences conducted by the Hygiene Museum Dresden and discourse projects initiated by the Ministry of Research and Education. The ethics regime in France is rather concentrated on the 20-year-old CCNE, which in public is often called '*comité de sages*' (committee of the wise) that provides 'qualified' reflection and which seems to be more central in the French ethics regime than the NER is in Germany.

Public exercises in (bio)ethics are usually not directed at teaching participants about what is morally right or wrong as regards biotechnological issues. They are also not directed at finding a consensus among participants, a common substantial answer to the question as to how should we deal with these issues. Indeed, a consensus is usually considered impossible or irrelevant.[13] Rather, exercises in bioethics are directed at practicing certain ways of reflection and argumentation, including the exclusion of certain arguments.

For example, one overlooked objection by a student at the *Journées annuelles d'éthique* was that on the grounds of over-production, the issue was not the further technical development of genetically manipulated plants, but rather it was above all a question of distribution. Similarly overlooked was an extremely emotional contribution from a vehement animal rights activist among the members of public, who wanted to speak not about the scientific utility of animal experiments, but rather about the personal relationship between man and animal.[14] That these two contributions were ignored clearly shows that discussions about scientific development itself are not integrated into the ethical debate. At the same time, both contributions failed to show themselves as moderate and reasonable with respect to other arguments, a pre-condition for acceptance within the ethical frame.

Public bioethics exercises are supposed to educate participants in forms of reflection and discussion on the basis of the appropriate information. What do these events teach the participants? First of all they teach participants that they have to deal with, reflect and talk about these issues, on the basis that biotechnological developments will take place (whether we want it or not) and that these are the starting point for discussions. The question as to whether or not biotechnological development *should* take place at all does not appear. Participants learn to accept that even the most gruesome (possible future) developments, such as cloning or hybrid creation, embryo research or embryo selection, are worth to engage with. Secondly, participants learn that each (even the most troublesome) perspective is worth the deliberation, that everyone has to have an opinion on each and every issue, and that each and every opinion is equally valid and has to be taken into account. Thirdly, these events teach participants ways of obtaining the 'appropriate knowledge' provided by experts, besides certainly teaching that it needs expert knowledge in order to be able to evaluate biomedical developments. Last but not least, participants are taught the ways of deliberating in an ethical manner by (discourse) experts. The most important dimensions in this respect are modesty, tolerance, being informed and the ability and willingness to balance diverse viewpoints: the ability "to get along and understand each other" (Interview F IX, CCNE, 2006, our translation) or what the German NER calls a "culture of mutual respect ... in which all arguments are objectively examined" (German National Ethics Council, 2001, p. 11). So-called 'fundamentalist' assertions or arguments that 'lack' the appropriate knowledge base, for example, are easily excluded from the deliberation as 'irrational' or 'undemocratic'. Thus, it gets extremely difficult, if not impossible, to take up a clear-cut position, especially one against new biomedical developments. The acquisition of the appropriate knowledge and of the appropriate ways of deliberation are the only accepted prerequisites for the formation of a personal judgement.

What we are witnessing here is the invitation of everyone to engage in ethical deliberation and start to reflect upon his or her own perceptions of the issues, however, in an organised and rational manner guided by experts. We are witnessing the incitement to test one's beliefs or judgements on the issues within a certain rational pattern of deliberation and, what is more, to *have* an opinion in the first place, which however is always tentative. Within the ethics regime, in principle, each and every one is regarded as requiring scientific as well as *ethical* education based on the assumption of scientific ignorance and a lack of *ethical* competences within the public. 'Ethical' in this sense refers to the mode of thinking and talking about biotechnological issues, or in the terms of governmentality, a *mentality* that guides and organises reflection and discussion.

CONCLUSION

While there are certainly differences in scope, organisation or design of the ethics regimes in Germany and France, we can, however, observe a tendency to foster guided self-government as regards bioethical issues in both countries. Despite differences in centrality and presence of the national ethics bodies themselves within the respective ethics regimes, as regards what we have describes as guided self-government in bioethics policy, we find corresponding developments in both countries, which were the focus of this paper.

From a governmentality perspective we can analyse the activation and proliferation of (bio)ethical discourse as a form of discourse *stimulation*, as a form of integrating subjects into the expert-guided process of rational reflection and self-reflection. For Foucault, the stimulation of discourse, as opposed to its repression, was one of the most powerful tools to integrate subjects into the nexus of power/knowledge (Foucault, 1981) and it is, as it were, a prerequisite for releasing subjects into the world of liberal self-government – at the level of individual bodily existence as well as at the level of debates on bioethics policy more generally. As has been shown in the second part of this paper, the ethics regime promotes and guides individualised forms of government concerning bodily existence. This comes along with incitements to self-reflection and self-government: Self-determination is the offer that comes at the cost of self-reflection and responsibility.

Within the ethics regime, in both countries more and more people are invited to become knowledgeable and to participate in organised ethical debates, to reflect their own standpoints in an expert-guided discussion so as to come to rational individual decisions or judgements regarding not only their personal lives but also bioscientific development in general. However, excluded from ethical debates are questions regarding techno-scientific development itself; the question discussed is not whether we want techno-scientific development to proceed, but indeed its 'progress' is the starting point for discussion – granting the ongoing of discussions on 'the ethical aspects' of it. The public bioethics exercises discussed above address (possible) participants as hitherto non-involved, 'naïve' or 'open-minded' *individuals* who are/have to be educated in the appropriate forms of reflection and argumentation. This individualisation implies the exclusion of particular speaker positions: such as that of a representative of a certain organised interest or socio-political position as well as of certain arguments, such as those which include a more general interrogation of techno-scientific development itself. The ethics regime implies an incitement to constantly reflect upon one's individual – tentative – beliefs or judgements, within a certain rational pattern on the basis of a particular knowledge which participants are supposed to learn to accept as *the* pattern or mode of thinking and speaking about these issues. In this sense, the ethics regime provides a *mentality* for guided self-government, actively initiating and simultaneously framing a reflection process. The ethics regime provides a frame for the production and organisation of discourse rather than a substantial normative orientation for action.

However, we cannot necessarily assume a one-to-one relationship between the goals of the exercises and the ways individual participants respond to them. There are certainly several ways of responding to the invocations of the ethics regime. Nonetheless, those utterances which are supposed to be heard in public have to comply with the requirements of the regime. In a personal discussion with the authors, a participant of the German–French Summer School on Bioethics (2004, in Berlin) brought the interaction of stimulation and channelling the discourse to the point:

> You have to think all the time, but you can not influence the direction of your thinking anymore.

NOTES

1. We speak of an ethics, rather than a *bio*ethics, regime, as we can observe a proliferation of ethical discourses and institutions in other (policy) fields also such as economics, food issues or issues concerning so-called development aid.

2. In this paper we use the notion of 'government' in a broad sense referring to what Michel Foucault has called "the conduct of conduct".

3. The research project 'Ethical Governance? Knowledge, Values and Political Decision-Making in Germany, France and Great Britain' at the University of Hanover, Germany, is funded by the German Federal Ministry of Research and Education. For further information see: http://www.sciencepolicystudies.de, Retrieved December 9, 2006.

4. We have argued elsewhere (Herrmann, 2006) that 'ethics' discourses have been strategically initiated in the 1980s in Germany with regard to genetic technologies in order to prevent the heavily politicised notion of risk. However, ethics did not necessarily totally replace the concept of risk, which is still an important notion in the negotiation of biotechnology conflicts.

5. In fact, those cases where recommendations were directly implemented into regulation are rather the exception. In order to keep this paper to a decent length, we can unfortunately not go into more detail regarding this point. For further discussions cf. Braun (2006).

6. The German Abortion Act prohibits abortion, however, on a case-by-case basis the act rules that women are not liable to punishment if they underwent counselling.

7. French Bioethics Law 2004: http://www.legifrance.gouv.fr/WAspad/UnTexteDeJorf?numjo=SANX0100053L, Retrieved August 20, 2004.

8. See: http://www.agence-biomedecine.fr/fr/index.asp, Retrieved October 10, 2006.

9. Member of the CCNE on November 16, 2004, at the *Journées annuelles d'éthique* (November 16–17, 2004), Université Paris V René Descartes, Grand Amphithéâtre, Paris. (Sabine Könninger (SK) attended the conference.)

10. Cf. http://www.buergerkonferenz.de/pages/start2.htm, Retrieved September 1, 2006.

11. Svea Luise Herrmann (SLH) attended the conference.

12. A member of the CCNE November 17, 2004, at the *Journées annuelles d'éthique* (November 16–17, 2004), Université Paris V René Descartes, Grand Amphithéâtre, Paris (our translation). (SK attended the conference.)

13. Even *if* the result of the public conference is a (consensual) statement on a particular development or practice, these papers do not have any impact on the decision-making processes. It is usually the discursive process itself that is at the centre.

14. Audience contributions at the *Journées annuelles d'éthique* (November 16–17, 2004), Université Paris V René Descartes, Grand Amphithéâtre, Paris. (SK attended the conference.)

REFERENCES

Assistance Publique Hôpitaux de Paris. (2006). Loi relative à la bioéthique. Retrieved May 10, 2006, from http://www.espace-ethique.org/fr/actualite.php#loi_bioethique

Bacchi, C. L. (1999). *Women, policy and politics: The construction of policy problems*. London/Thousand Oaks/New Delhi: Sage.

Beck, U. (1992). *Risk society: Towards a new modernity*. London: Sage.

Braun, K. (2006, May 25–27). Framing self-government. Liberalism in the bioethics regime in the light of Schmitt and Foucault. Paper presented at the Conference "The politics of ethics and the crisis of government. Contested technologies, the language of ethics and the transformation of governance in Europe and North America," University of Washington, Seattle, WA.

Bundesministerium der Justiz. (2006). Patientenverfügung. Leiden, Krankheit, Sterben. Wie bestimme ich, was medizinisch unternommen werden soll, wenn ich entscheidungsunfähig bin? Retrieved October 12, 2006, from http://www.bmj.de/media/archive/1338.pdf

Bundesministerium für Bildung und Forschung. (2006). Richtlinien zur Förderung von Diskursprojekten zu ethischen, rechtlichen und sozialen Fragen in den Lebenswissenschaften. Retrieved September 4, 2006, from http://www.bmbf.de/foerderungen/6156.php

Callon, M., et al. (2005). Democratie locale et maîtrise sociale des nanotechnologies. Les publics grenoblois peuvent-ils participer aux choix scientifiques et techniques? La Métro. Retrieved October 12, 2006, from http://sciencescitoyennes.org/article.php3?id_article=1387

CCNE. (2006). Founding documents. Paris. Retrieved November 20, 2006, from http://www.ccne-ethique.fr/english/start.htm

Dean, M. (2001). *Governmentality: Power and rule in modern society.* London/Thousand Oaks/New Delhi: Sage.

Douste-Blazy, P. (2005). Discours. Inauguration de l'Agence de la Biomédecine. Saint-Denis. Retrieved October 10, 2006, from http://www.sante.gouv.fr/htm/actu/33_050510pdb.htm

Draft Decree. (2001). Draft decree submitted to Cabinet on 25 April 2001. Establishment of a National Ethics Council. Retrieved February 23, 2006, from http://www.ethikrat.de/_english/about_us/decree.html

Foucault, M. (1981). *The history of sexuality* (Vol. 1). London: Penguin.

Foucault, M. (1991). Governmentality. In: G. Burchell, C. Gordon & P. Miller (Eds), *The Foucault effect: Studies in governmentality* (pp. 87–194). Hemel Hempstead: Harvester Wheatsheaf.

German National Ethics Council. (2001). *The import of human embryonic stem cells: Opinion.* Berlin: Nationaler Ethikrat Deutschland.

German National Ethics Council. (2005). *Patientenverfügung. The advance directive. La testament de vie. La instrucción del paciente.* Berlin: Nationaler Ethikrat Deutschland.

Gordon, C. (1991). Governmental rationality: An introduction. In: G. Burchell, C. Gordon & P. Miller (Eds), *The Foucault effect: Studies in governmentality* (pp. 1–52). Chicago: University of Chicago Press.

Herrmann, S. L. (2006). *Bioethics policies in Germany: From conflict prevention to conflict management.* Paper presented at the Conference "The politics of ethics and the crisis of government. Contested technologies, the language of ethics and the transformation of governance in Europe and North America," May 25–27, University of Washington, Seattle, WA.

Île de France. (2006). La conférence de citoyens sur les nanotechnologies: Explorons les enjeux de l'infiniment petit. Conférence de presse du 10 Octobre. Retrieved November 22, 2006, from http://espaceprojets.iledefrance.fr/jahia/webdav/site/projets/users/JLACHKAR/public/communiqu%C3%A9%20du%2010-10-06.pdf

Interview F II, CCNE. (2005). Interview with a former member of the Comité Consultatif National d'Ethique (1983–2005), November 13, 2005, Paris.

Interview F IV, CCNE. (2005). Interview with the (Deputy-) Secretary General of the Comité Consultatif National d'Ethique (1986–), November 14, 2005, Paris, Comité Consultatif National d'Ethique.

Interview F IX, CCNE. (2006). Interview with a former member of the Comité Consultatif National d'Ethique (1983–2000), January 25, 2006, Paris.

Interview G, NER. (2005). Interview with a member of the German National Ethics Council (2001–), October 27, 2005, Berlin, German National Ethics Council.

Lipinski, M. (2006). Pourquoi une conférence de citoyens régionale sur les nanotechnologies? Retrieved November 21, 2006, from http://espaceprojets.iledefrance.fr/jahia/Jahia/NanoCitoyens

Memmi, D. (2003). Governing through speech: The new state administration of bodies. *Social Research, 70*, 645–658.

Memmi, D. (2005, January 7–8). La Bio-politique déléguée. Paper presented at *Colloque "Le politique vue avec Foucault."* Paris.

Nationaler Ethikrat. (2006, August). Informationen und Nachrichten aus den Nationalen Ethikrat: VZK 64247, No. 11, p. 7. Retrieved September 1, 2006, from http://www.ethikrat.org

Rein, M., & Schön, D. (1993). Reframing policy discourse. In: F. Fischer & J. Forester (Eds), *The argumentative turn in policy analysis and planning* (pp. 145–166). Durham/London: Duke University Press.

Rose, N. (1996). Governing 'advanced' liberal democracies. In: N. Rose, T. Osborne & A. Barry (Eds), *Foucault and political reason: Liberalism, Neo-Liberalism and rationalities of government* (pp. 37–64). London: UCL Press.

Rose, N. (1999). *Powers of freedom: Reframing political thought.* Cambridge: Cambridge University Press.

Rose, N. (2001). The politics of live itself. *Theory, Culture, and Society, 18*, 1–30.

Rose, N. (2005, February 2). Will biomedicine transform society? The political, economic, social and personal impact of medical impact of medical advances in the twenty first century. In: *Clifford Barclay Lecture,* Hong Kong Theatre, London School of Economics.

Sicard, D. (2001). Erfahrungsberichte. Ethikräte in Frankreich und der Europäischen Union. In: *Berliner Dialog zu Biomedizin* (pp. 10–15). Berlin: Friedrich-Ebert-Stiftung.

Weir, L. (1996). Recent developments in the government of pregnancy. *Economy and Society*, 373–392.

Zimmer, R. & Fraunhofer Institut für Systemtechnik und Innovationsforschung (ISI). (2002). Begleitende Evaluation der Bürgerkonferenz "Streitfall Gendiagnostik." Retrieved September 1, 2006, from http://www.isi.fraunhofer.de/t/projekte/buergerkonf.pdf

CUTTING RISK: THE ETHICS OF MALE CIRCUMCISION, HIV PREVENTION, AND WELLNESS

Ananya Mukherjea

In this paper, I critically examine the history of the public health debate surrounding whether male circumcision should be promoted as a preventative measure against HIV transmission and consider the practical ethics of the procedure *as a public health instrument*.[1] Those promoting circumcision to prevent HIV transmission – a move endorsed by former US President Clinton in August 2006 and validated by the joint United Nations/World Health Organization initiative on AIDS (UNAIDS) in March 2007 – mainly advocate its adoption in those parts of the global South that currently have high transmission rates but no established tradition of circumcising boys. The debate of whether this would be sound practice or not, whether it is *the best fix currently available in certain communities or not*, and what the attendant risks and benefits would be has been unfolding since at least 2000, when the director of UNAIDS gave the issue a special, and cautious, mention in that year's epidemic report. In the previous year, 1999, Halperin and Bailey published a paper in *Lancet* suggesting that male circumcision could prevent HIV infection, and that article and its media coverage brought the issue to the attention of many HIV/AIDS researchers, activists, and service providers, including me.

In 2006, three randomized, controlled studies – conducted in South Africa, in Kenya, and in Uganda – found that HIV-negative men who underwent

Bioethical Issues, Sociological Perspectives
Advances in Medical Sociology, Volume 9, 225–243
Copyright © 2008 by Elsevier Ltd.
ISSN: 1057-6290/doi:10.1016/S1057-6290(07)09009-2

circumcision as part of the studies were between 30 and 60% less likely than their uncircumcised counterparts to contract HIV from vaginal sex with a woman. The South African study – which ended and was reported first – found 20 seroconversions among the men in the "intervention" group who received circumcisions at the beginning of the trial, as opposed to 49 seroconversions among the men who did not (Bailey et al., 2007; Gray et al., 2007). This yielded the 60% reduction number, which is the statistic most cited now, in the UNAIDS recommendations of March 28, 2007, and in much of the media coverage of this development. No conclusive studies have been done on how circumcision might impact men who primarily engage in anal sex as the insertive partner, and it does not seem to keep HIV-positive men from transmitting the virus to their receptive sexual partners. These 2006 findings were followed, in early 2007, by a caution that recently circumcised men who are already infected have an increased chance of infecting their sex partners (see *Washington Post*, March 7, 2007). Kahn, Marseille, and Auvert qualified in the Public Library of Science medical journal on April 2, 2007, that compensating for increased risk behavior among HIV-positive men who are circumcised would somewhat lessen the estimated benefits of male circumcision, but that this was offest by other factors. Nevertheless, the results of the South African, Kenyan, and Ugandan studies are noteworthy and were compelling enough to cause their researchers to call off the latter two investigations early in order to give the men in the control group the option to be circumcised immediately rather than later.

The fulcrum of this argument is the still somewhat uncertain science[2] suggesting that circumcised men are significantly less likely to contract HIV, as well as other sexually transmitted infections, than are men with intact foreskins. I contend, however, that the issue is *a heavily racially and culturally inflected one*, which cannot be easily decided through the application of somewhat unclear clinical-scientific rationales and, further, which cannot replace the real need for thorough social and behavioral changes to slow the spread of HIV, in the long-term as well as the immediate future, and to address the existing pandemic. Except in the situation of North America in the twentieth century, boys have been circumcised, almost exclusively, on the basis of religious or cultural traditions – whether practiced by Jews, Muslims, or less populous tribal groups such as the nomadic herders of central Australia. As such, circumcision is a purification ritual; it is a rite onto a path toward a traditionally circumscribed manhood. In this capacity, the rite is accompanied by culturally bounded expectations of male behavior with respect to hygiene and sexuality. *It is a practice conducted within a cultural and moral context, as is the decision not to circumcise boys.* Throughout history, and certainly throughout the twentieth century, circumcision has served not only as a marker of socially bounded manhood within a group but also as a marker of an individual who is decidedly out-of-group.[3]

The question of male circumcision as a public health measure, more generally, is an old one extending back, in the modern United States, to Henry Simes, John Kellogg, Lewis Sayre, and the other health advisors of the turn of the twentieth century who collapsed moral hygiene with bodily hygiene and found that male circumcision served both purposes for the social integrity of the new America (see Glick, 2006 and Gollaher, 2001, for sample accountings of this history). This history has always brought together the trajectories of race, ethnicity, gender, and contested moral precepts, especially as the questions of moral and bodily hygiene have been crucial to discussion of the ritual within Jewish and Muslim communities. The case of the HIV/AIDS pandemic is no different, although it is a defining element of our current age and, as such, highlights other flashpoint ethical questions for a sustainable approach to a contemporary, global pandemic even as it further complicates the varied meanings of circumcision and masculinity.

Particularly in an environment in which many members of socially and economically marginalized communities suspect the motivations of those major nations and transnational institutions that advise them on the management of the disease or the treatment of the ill, it is crucial to carefully consider the ethno-political ramifications of any new proposal. This is particularly true when a key element of male circumcision as HIV prevention that its proponents emphasize – the *cheapness* of the procedure – is one that is touted all too often with reference to the global South and, pointedly, not nearly as frequently with reference to the global North.[4,5] In their book *Global AIDS: Myths and Facts*, Irwin, Millen, and Fallows repeatedly point to the dangers and offenses of raising cost-effectiveness as a primary directive in determining HIV/AIDS policies for southern Africa, south and southeast Asia, and Latin America (see Irwin, Millen, & Fallows, 2003, esp. pp. 59–96 and 115–134). Not only does such an emphasis create unsound and unfair policy, but it also creates resentment among governing and community bodies that need to cooperate to adequately address what has long been a very transnational pandemic.

This is an especially poignant issue, given that the vast majority of AIDS deaths that occur today are due to poverty – perhaps as much a lack of food as of antiretroviral therapy (ART) – and promised money that appears too belatedly. It also seems increasingly unnecessary as foundations such as the Global Fund to Fight AIDS, Tuberculosis, and Malaria; the UNAIDS funds; and the Gates Foundation are bringing in billions of US dollars for treatment, anti-stigma work, and other responses to HIV/AIDS that were previously considered to be unjustifiable money drains. Paul Farmer, in deliberating the ethics of medicine and public health in his book *Pathologies of Power*, writes, "Without a social justice component, medical ethics risks becoming yet another strategy for managing inequality ... a failure to understand social processes leads to analytic failures, with significant implications for policy and practice." (Farmer, 2005, pp. 201–208). The implementation of physical, behavioral, cultural changes must take into account how specific communities will absorb and adjust to those changes. The results of widespread implementation might be quite different from what they are in the test run of a fairly localized surgery.

ETHICS, WELLNESS, AND LIABILITY

The question of ethics has accompanied all discussion of male circumcision and HIV: How can trials be run ethically? How could circumcision be promoted and provided ethically? Is it ethical to provide medical circumcision and payment to under-resourced test subjects? Would it be ethical to not do so? Two comprehensive and widely read papers ("Circumcision and HIV prevention research: An ethical analysis," *Lancet*, 2006, and "The first randomised trial of male circumcision for preventing HIV: What were the ethical issues?," *PLoS Medicine*, 2005) addressed the ethical issues of these investigations from the perspective of scientific liability, and many of the opponents of male circumcision, for this or other reasons, call their viewpoint a human rights matter. In this paper, I draw from social science and from the harm reduction movement to propose an ethic of wellness, built on causing the least harm and contributing to the most knowledge. This approach to the ethical question is linked to, but distinct from and sometimes at odds with, the traditional canon of medical ethics or bioethics.

Barry Hoffmaster writes in the introduction to his edited volume *Bioethics in Social Context*:

> Bioethics has been preoccupied with making judgements about troublesome moral problems and justifying those judgments, with doing what has aptly been called 'quandary ethics ...' [and], in this view, is situated in rationality and generality. It prescinds the messy details and attachments that give our lives meaning and vigor, the nagging contradictions that make us squirm and struggle, and the social, political, and economic arrangements that simultaneously create and constrain us .... [Social scientists] engage in *descriptive ethics* when they investigate and interpret the *actual moral beliefs, codes, or practices of a society* ... [the ultimate goal being] a bioethics that is

more attuned to the particular and more sensitive to the personal – a bioethics that is *more humane and more helpful.* (Hoffmaster, 2001, p. 1–2) (emphasis mine)

This gives us a fuller sense of what the practical uses of bioethics may be, and I am concerned here with practical matters. One reason I choose not to use this paper to ally myself with those critics of circumcision as HIV prevention who oppose the practice altogether is that I find those arguments do not adequately address the urgency of the HIV/AIDS pandemic, with over 39 million people infected globally and a projection of 18 million AIDS orphans by the end of the decade, in sub-Saharan Africa alone (UNAIDS Epidemic Report, 2006; Council of Foreign Relations report, 2006). My concern is that the promotion of male circumcision as prevention will further reduce the availability of condoms, the regular use of condoms, peer education programs, the autonomy of receptive sexual partners to protect themselves from infection, and the ability of individual ethnic groups to determine the intimate practices that they consider hygienic and desirable. I fear, too, that it will overshadow basic, non-radical needs that are at least as important, such as increasing food aid. For male circumcision to be an ethical, practical, and favorable public health tool, the three randomized controlled studies reported in 2006 would be immediately followed by extensive, non-intrusive ethnographic, descriptive research on the real-world health effects of circumcision and knowledge about it.

In December 2006, UNAIDS released a statement on the link between circumcision and HIV risk reduction, repeatedly noting that the effective and safe deployment of this research into public health practice must be accompanied by continuous attention to the ethics and humanity of the practice (UNAIDS, December 13, 2006). I believe such consideration must take place with respect to lived circumstances and social and political realities, not in the logical vacuum of bioethical think tanks or vis à vis the legal liabilities of clinicians. Even in their article on what medical researchers are strictly obliged to do in order to fulfill their basic ethical obligations to trial participants, Lie, Ezekiel, and Grady (2006, p. 2) cite, "the fundamental ethical requirement for any person to do what they can to help others in need." Determining what others need, though, and what one can do to provide it, is more easily said than done.

A last ethical consideration here is that of human rights, considered in terms of individual security and autonomy. Also in *Pathologies of Power*, Paul Farmer writes that it is important to seek a new agenda for health and human rights, one which assumes "that social and economic rights must be central" and which is "inspired by the notion of a preferential treatment of the poor, is coherent and pragmatic, and informed by careful scholarship" (Farmer, 2005, p. 238). He also quotes Jonathan Mann and Daniel Tarantola, noting that AIDS "has helped catalyze the modern health and human rights movement, which leads far beyond AIDS, for it considers that promoting and protecting health and promoting and protecting human rights are inextricably connected" (quoted in Farmer, 2005, p. 234). The current HIV/AIDS pandemic is absolutely a human rights matter, and I wish to underscore the fact that it is the receptive partners in sex who have always been more at risk for HIV infection, who are more stigmatized by HIV-positive status, and who have the least recourse to actively protecting themselves from the virus. Rates of HIV infection are growing more rapidly among heterosexual women than among heterosexual men and in sub-Saharan Africa, 59% of all adults living with HIV are female (UNAIDS Epidemic Report, 2006). In an opinion piece published in *PLoS Medicine* on January 31, 2007, Kalichman, Eaton, and Pinkerton write, "avoiding the sexual dissatisfactions of condom use and the desire to have more sex partners are likely to be significant motivations for men to seek circumcision ... . It is difficult to imagine a convincing public health message that effectively influences men to undergo circumcision and continue to consistently use condoms." Noting that circumcised men in the South African trial had more sexual contacts than uncircumcised men, they observe, "This suggests that, in the short term at least, circumcision would reduce the incidence of HIV among men, but increase the incidence among women, translating to increased prevalence among women, which in turn translates to greater risk to men." (Kalichman et al., January 31, 2007).

Another issue that received attention at the 2006 AIDS Congress – though much less than circumcision did – was that of microbicides. If circumcision might provide an important margin of protection for the insertive partner in sexual intercourse – ideally, in turn, preventing him from later infecting his receptive partners – then the application of microbicides might provide protection for the receptive partner. Microbicides would be available as gels or creams that could be applied vaginally or rectally,[6] without necessitating consultation or cooperation with the penetrative sex partner. They could prevent a range of STDs including HIV infection, and, in some cases, could also prevent pregnancy at the same time that they provide lubrication crucial for protecting against tears, lesions, and pain. Clearly, an uninfected insertive partner cannot infect anyone else, but the risk of contracting HIV through being penetrated has always been the greater one, by far, which is why outspoken critics like Cindy Patton and Paula Treichler have long called for putting protection in the hands of women, sex workers, and men who have sex with men. Yet, with the exception of the relatively unknown, unavailable, and unused "female" condom and the mistaken promotion of Nonoxynol-9, the primary modes of preventing HIV transmission – most prominently, of course, *consistent and correct* condom usage – have lain, for the past 25 years, in the hands of insertive men who may or may not want to, or know how to, comply. How, then, can prevention efforts *best* help these men to protect their partners and, thus, also themselves?

The development of microbicidal gels, foams, and sponges has been a contested issue since the first suspicions in the early 1980s that a virus causes AIDS. Nonoxynol-9, for a long time, has been the only microbicide approved by the US Food and Drug Administration (FDA), and it was promoted as protective against HIV until quite recently. Since 2000, however, claims that some gay and feminist activists had long been making – that Nonoxynol-9 is so harsh and indiscriminate a microbicide that it breaks down epithelial cells, actually making many users more prone to infections – have been verified.[7] Much of the research that led to a critical article in the British medical journal *Lancet* in 2002 was derived from trials on female sex workers in South Africa, Benin, Côte d'Ivoire, and Thailand (*Lancet,* 2002). In 2005, the Microbicide Development Act was introduced in the US House of Representatives. In January 2007, a trial of another microbicide, cellulose sulfate, which was being conducted in Benin, India, South Africa, and Uganda, was halted before completion because a higher number of women in the test group were seroconverting than those in the placebo group (WHO, UNAIDS statement, January 31, 2007). Regardless of these setbacks, microbicidal research, overall, has been slow, dampened by caution by some like the FDA, who argue that their development will make people less likely to use condoms, *which would be unjustifiably risky.*

The questions surrounding the use of circumcision and microbicides are similar. How practically effective can these means be in the real world, in the contexts of established relationships, casual encounters, or commercial sex? If they are incompletely effective, is the risk of people being less willing to use condoms so great that these other methods become public health liabilities? Are prevention planners already so disheartened about the likelihood of promoting condom use under any circumstance that such a risk would be worth taking anyway? This last question gains greater prominence as the number of condoms that the United States makes available domestically and internationally has diminished steadily over the past three years and since the President's Emergency Plan for AIDS Relief (PEPFAR) continues to focus its efforts on faith-based, abstinence-oriented campaigns. Major funders and policy makers who continually encounter failure and inefficacy in the pandemic have long been freighted with pessimism and, thus, short-term and worst-case thinking in the face of its dangers. What stands out to me, then, is that circumcision is repeatedly endorsed in recent years as a cheap, effective solution, while research on microbicides seems to remain more controversial and prospective. Male circumcision is a known quantity for many, but I wonder how it might affect the identities, perceptions, and decisions of those for whom it is neither familiar nor simple. To make some guesses, let me return to how this controversy emerged.

MEDICALIZATION AND EDUCATION

In the United States, which has had the second highest rate of circumcision in the global North since the 1930s (falling just behind Israel, where male circumcision has an explicitly religious rationale, and well ahead of any other nation), the popularization of male circumcision was justified largely on the grounds of moral motivations couched in the language of clinical medicine (Van Howe, 1999). The individual-health implications of the procedure were not firmly grounded and were secondary to the social-health implications, regarding the idealized American family, throughout the several decades following World War I. A primary justification for circumcision, in US medical discourse, was the claim that, in reducing the natural lubrication of the penis' shaft, it would make masturbation more difficult for boys and, in supposedly reducing sensation in the penis, it would lower the male sex drive, thus undermining the urge to have extra-marital or pre-marital, or otherwise deviant, sex. Circumcising boys promised an effective means to controlling their sexual urges and of enforcing dominant sexual mores throughout a nation. Sayre, Simes, and Kellogg urged that circumcision and a reduction in masturbation could ameliorate conditions ranging from imbecility to depression to lameness (again, see Glick, 2005, and Gollaher, 2000, for two accounts of this history).

It was in this context, too, that the circumcision of young boys was biomedicalized, taken out of the hands of ethnic communities and put into the hands of physicians aided by standardizing technology such as the Gomco clamp or Plastibell. This new method of surgery, popular in North America since the 1940s, changed the procedure such that a complete excision of the entire prepuce superceded the earlier, ritualized removal of a part of it. This biomedical removal of the entire prepuce, in infancy, at puberty, or in adulthood, is the operation at issue with respect to HIV, and I argue its history makes this procedure as cultural (in this case, American and modern) a matter as any other cirucmcision. It is medical circumcision practiced by a biomedical expert in biomedically sanitary conditions with a biomedical implement like the Gomco clamp that is proposed in this debate about HIV, but such surgery, for being medical, is not without a profound cultural context.

Of course, whether circumcision does reduce sensation is impossible and, likely, irrelevant to judge in this debate. Rather, popular authors of social standards have had to concede the point and turn away from the drive to control masturbation, and in 1971, the American Academy of Pediatrics stated that there are no medical indications for circumcising boys. According to the American Academy of Pediatrics, in 2005, nearly 70% of American infant boys were circumcised, as compared to just under 25% of all boys worldwide. Some studies have demonstrated that men with foreskins are more likely to contract and transmit human papilloma virus (HPV)[8] and, thus, also more likely to contribute to HPV-related vaginal, cervical, and anal cancers in their sex partners. In a paper published in the *New England Journal of Medicine* in April 2002 (Castellsagué et al., 2002), researchers found, through a control study of 3,790 women and their male sex partners, that there is a "moderate but non-significant" decrease in instances of cervical cancer for women whose sex partners were circumcised. The American Cancer Society, though, has been reluctant to verify this association, stating in 1998 that "circumcision is strongly associated with other socioethnic practices that, in turn, are associated with lessened risk,"(ACS, April 11, 1998) and that the regular use of condoms is much more directly associated with a reduction in HPV-related cancer risk. Overall, though, there is little substantial evidence of variance in cancer rates between populations that do circumcise and those that do not, once high-risk sex has been controlled for.

Further, the promotion of so radical an intervention – one which requires a permanent and surgical alteration to the intimate physical person rather than behavioral or motivational changes – contains within it an underlying despair at the potential efficacy of educational programs. Again, I want to be clear that my argument is not against circumcision per se as an atrocity or necessarily wrong because I remain unconvinced that boys or men, *within their cultural contexts*, sustain measurable harm for being, or not being, circumcised. So many men are circumcised as infants or at adolescence, and so many more never are, yet few members of either group seem to later feel that the presence or lack of a foreskin has been a serious advantage or disadvantage in terms of health or pleasure *precisely because this decision whether to circumcise a boy or not is normalized within communities.*

My emphasis remains on not distancing circumcision from its cultural meanings in our eagerness to hail it as a magic bullet against this disease. There are serious ethical questions surrounding male circumcision, but they concern the repositioning of the surgery in biomedical terms, which can misleadingly seem politically and culturally neutral, rather than in ethnic ones.

Education, arguably the most hopeful and least invasive of HIV-prevention methods, flounders when public health workers conclude that men and women cannot be adequately counseled to make informed decisions regarding their own health. But I think it is true that public health education campaigns – including the extremely well-funded ones like the Kaiser Foundation programs – have demonstrated limited and localized success, which undergirds the argument that focusing too heavily on them comprises a misuse of funds and capability. These limitations can, in part, be explained by the minimal funding, attention, and prioritization given to innovating, developing, and testing HIV prevention work overall, for different groups of people at different phases of the pandemic. They may also be due to the social and economic divide that often exists between health-care workers and those populations most vulnerable to HIV infection.

The few success stories – particularly among gay men in North America in the 1980s and 1990s and among sex workers in India since the mid-1990s – demonstrate what prevention can achieve in these cases where members of communities with deep knowledge of their own needs and circumstantial challenges took on the work of stunting the epidemic among themselves. The success of Thailand's state-sponsored, long-term, and comprehensive prevention and education program demonstrates what vigorous government commitment can achieve. Catherine Campbell, in 'Letting Them Die': Why HIV/AIDS Programmes Fail, writes that education campaigns are crucial but that they must be dynamic and participatory, and must give people practical and flexible options for protecting themselves if they are to work. Catchy slogans are occasionally very effective,[9] but Campbell writes that creating productive community-based prevention plans depends

> ... very heavily on the extent to which local attempts by marginalized groups are supported and enabled by the efforts of more powerful constituencies, at the regional, national, and international levels, and the development of health systems and organizational infrastructure to coordinate joint efforts. (Campbell, 2003, p. 195)

Effective education, then, must be a continuous, intensive, multi-agentic effort, and few prevention efforts have had the funds or stamina to sustain such a structure.

In their article on the ethical obligation of the researchers running the circumcision trials, Lie et al. respond to the frustrations of providing effective education.

> The obligation [to provide counseling to trial participants] seems to derive not from the method's proven effectiveness, but from the principle of informed consent and the disclosure of relevant information as part of this process. Risk reduction counseling is part of the obligation to provide information about risk behavior, rather than an attempt to implement a behavioral intervention with a known or quantifiable reduction in risk of HIV infection. *As with condoms, it is left to the participants to decide whether to act on this information* (from Lie et al., 2006, emphasis mine).

Such formalistic informing is not the sort of coordinated, partnered education of which Campbell writes, but it does stand in for "education" when time and resources are tight. This is not the kind of education that is likely to fully inform a man of all the limitations of circumcision as a health measure. Especially, as circumcision begins to be promoted to prevent HIV, existing education funding, development, and provision must be stepped up, not relaxed, to make it a more beneficial move than a risky one.

CULTURE, MASCULINITY, AND WOMEN

Major HIV/AIDS organizations in the UK, where male circumcision declined after the 1930s while it rose in the United States, such as the Terrence Higgins Trust and the National AIDS Trust have taken a more cautious approach to the 2006 findings, emphasizing that adult circumcision should always be entirely voluntary and accompanied by extensive education about its limitations (see Terrence Higgins Trust *Issue*, July 2006, and National AIDS Trust, February 2007). If it is relevant to consider questions of culture when deciding to circumcise or not in the global North – as the American Association of Pediatrics has shown we do and as shown by the rates of circumcision throughout the European Union, where the HIV epidemic is also extensive – then these questions also pertain to southern and eastern Africa. This is especially true because it is quite easy to argue, as Catherine Campbell and Cindy Patton and many others have done so well, that the worldwide failure to use condoms consistently and correctly is due, in large part, to the issue of masculinity and the negotiation of sexual pleasure as, primarily, a man's terrain.

In particular, it is often an issue of a masculinity colored by economic scarcity and political marginalization, and by exaggerated ethnic identity seen as a balance to these problems. Campbell has written of the reluctance of migrant South African mine workers to use condoms with the prostitutes they patronize because they find the prophylactics demeaning, implying poor hygiene and lower class status as well as impinging on the intimacy *and* domination of the sex act. These are not straightforward navigations of risk analysis, cost-effective protection, and mid-range or long-term thinking. These are immediate and emotional navigations of economically, culturally circumscribed gender relations. A thorough understanding of how male circumcision can be deployed to best effect and least possible harm will take into careful account how the procedure, and the culturally contextualized penis it renders, is an element of these sorts of gender relations, which determine not only infection risks but also what pleasure or security the receptive sex partner feels.

In discussing the well-being of the partners of the men at the center of this debate, I do not mean only the wives and "future mothers" frequently invoked in this discourse but, as well, the invisible girlfriends, sex workers, and male partners who conspicuously have been left out of much of this conversation. In particular, men who have sex with men, unattached but sexually active women, and those men and women who do sex work have always occupied a strange and dangerous territory in public health discourse. Their health, wellness, families, and interests rarely receive adequate attention; but they are often placed in the spotlight when considering "dangers" to more broadly legitimated populations. Women's concerns in the HIV/AIDS epidemic, more generally, have historically received less attention from medical and public health authorities. At the 3rd International Conference on AIDS, in 1987, members of the International Women and AIDS Caucus protested that "... women are largely invisible except in two roles: as vectors for transmission either perinatally or (putatively) through prostitution" (reprinted in Crimp, Ed. 1991, p. 168). These two roles remain the prominent ones for women in AIDS transmission discourse, particularly for women of the global South.

Fixing the "future" of the nation (or the planet or the people) as the main reason for curtailing the spread of disease implies that the daily, immediate suffering of people, today, is less important an issue than the larger-scale consequences for whole societies; and, in terms of ecological and economic disaster, one does see this argument. While some of the earlier works on the connection between male circumcision and HIV risk (Cameron et al., 1989) drew data on men who visited commercial sex workers, the welfare of those sex workers was not highlighted. There is an embedded and implicit hierarchy of which lives are savable – or worth saving – and which are not. The concern, in focussing on the factor of the foreskin, was how to prevent transmission of the virus to men and, thereby, to their *wives* and, thus, to future generations, to children. Now, too, a sticking point in planning the implementation of circumcision promotion is the fact that circumcisions are most safely performed on very young boys but that circumcising babies today will not yield appreciable population-level benefits for 12–20 years.

There is also the question of the day-to-day comforts and needs of commercial sex workers and the implications for them if newly circumcised men, who now lack the crucial lubrication a foreskin provides, feel that condom use is rendered entirely unnecessary. General knowledge about how HIV is transmitted and how it causes AIDS is still sporadic. The *2006 UNAIDS Report on the Global AIDS Epidemic* found that "none of the 18 countries in which young people were surveyed by the Demographic Health Survey/AIDS Indicator Survey between 2001 and 2005 had knowledge levels exceeding 50%" (UNAIDS, 2006, p. 13). No cost-effective surgery can do the work of the large-scale and ongoing education that is needed. In this light, it is particularly important to give receptive sexual partners much more agency. Proponents of the circumcision proposal assert that circumcision could prevent infections that are occurring now, regardless of existing education and condom distribution programs, and I agree that this is an important point. It is not my intent to argue against *any* avenue of prevention that might prove more efficacious than those currently employed. Again, my concern is that the promotion of male circumcision as a barrier to HIV infection will lead to an erosion of other programs, to a greater diminishment of the social sense of urgency around the epidemic, and to a larger number of infections rather than fewer.

THE MEDIA AND REPRESENTATION

Peter Conrad, in a 2001 article on the ethical implications of imprecise or inaccurate reportage of genetic findings, writes that science journalism's focus on covering new and positive findings published in just a few major medical journals "suggests that science reporting presents a very selective slice of biomedical research" (Conrad, 2001, p. 91). Specifically, science journalism for the popular press tends to simplify complicated information, to fail to report negative findings (such as the lack of a correlation), and to seldom follow up and report when a study cannot be replicated or is disproved. Further, science journalism too often focuses on a vague future – "A cure is around the corner!" – granting what seems like a tested foundation to what might be an unfounded hope. Conrad avers that such writing, more than unprofessional, is unethical. In proclaiming premature, partial, or reduced information to be confirmed fact, headlines and soundbites disseminate misinformation and influence public opinion about responsibility and blame with regard to health and sickness.

Conrad examines reportage of the so-called breast cancer gene and finds that, throughout the 1990s, headlines in major newspapers repeatedly heralded the certain finding of "a" gene that "caused" breast cancer and that definitive testing for the gene would be available shortly. He asks, "Why should this apparent journalistic shorthand matter?" and gives us several reasons (Conrad, 2001, p. 103). Among them is that after-the-fact disconfirmation or qualification of invalidated or incomplete studies happen infrequently or quietly so that, in the meantime, the "cultural residue" of the initial idea continues (Conrad, 2001, p. 106). Further, a focus on unifactorial "causes" for disease shifts the responsibility for illness from the society to the individual.

I want to apply Peter Conrad's careful argument to this circumcision–HIV debate. Reportage of positive correlations between circumcision and reduced tranmission rates have been announced strongly and definitively over the past several years: "Circumcision Cuts AIDS Rates;" "Circumcision Associated with Lower HIV Incidence;" and the BBC at least used qualifying quotes, "Circumcision 'Reduces HIV Risk." The association seems a foregone conclusion, and the matters of confounding factors, the need for more evidence outside clinical trials, the limitations of protection, or the earlier inconclusive studies are mentioned briefly and usually toward the ends of such articles. Again, the BBC coverage stood out for consistently highlighting complicating issues.

Further, the cultural barriers to the propagation of circumcision to prevent HIV transmission begin to seem a minor, structural obstacle. Compare this mass media influenced perspective to the multifaceted UNAIDS statement of December 2006, which is positive and hopeful about the correlation between circumcision and HIV risk, but tempered in its analysis, recommending that

[Potential policies must account for] cultural and human rights considerations associated with promoting circumcision; the risk of complications from the procedure performed in various settings; the potential to undermine existing protective behaviours and prevention strategies that reduce the risk of HIV infection; and the observation that the ideal and well-resourced conditions of a randomized trial are often not replicated in other service delivery settings. (WHO, UNAIDS statement, December 13, 2006)

With respect to the shifting of responsibility for illness from the social to the individual, this is particularly problematic for a disease often contracted through stigmatized or taboo behavior and for subjects who might be racially, ethnically, or economically marginalized. I am unconvinced that male circumcision really can be a voluntary surgery if it is made to seem that it is an essential safeguard against HIV and if the subjects are already considered implicitly responsible for tranmission – because of over-active sexual appetites, under-active intellects, or whatever other racist character- istics have historically been attributed to men of color. For example, Susan Pietrzyk cites a 1922 British colonial law, which required Africans in Zimbabwe to submit to a medical exam to qualify for employment, the assumption being that simply being African was associated with disease (Pietrzyk, 2005). If it is true that male circumcision offers a way to significantly reduce rates of HIV infection in the coming decades, that hope would be undermined by the oversimplification of, or miseducation about, the individual limits and community-level consequences of the surgery in this capacity.

The problem of the HIV/AIDS pandemic coincides clearly with severe economic inequity and major lapses in the public health systems of countries, cities, and provinces that do not, in the United States for example, or cannot, in Haiti for another example, effectively promote holistic, whole-society wellness standards. This fact has been thoroughly researched and clearly written in highly accessible form by Paul Farmer (1999), Laurie Garrett (2001), Paula Treichler(1999), Simon Watney (1994), and many others. For safer-sex campaigns in poor nations to have a measurable effect, they require a kind of attention and effort they have not been able to garner. Given this, the promotion of circumcision may well eclipse continuing safer sex work. If the assumption is that poor men or Black men cannot, or will not, use condoms, lowering their risk factors will not further induce them to do so. What happens if the procedure said to lower risk factors actually does not do so? And what might be the negative results of effectively pathologizing uncircumcised men and their penises? Might this not contribute to the further reduction of a public health crisis to problematic individuals?

Indeed, we are left with a series of important questions, which demand attention in the international debate about circumcision and HIV. (1) Which populations do we choose to prioritize as the ones that we can save or should try to save? While microbicides were tested on female sex workers, some of who contracted HIV during the trials, the potential benefits of circumcision to a community have not been thoroughly tested with respect to the sex partners of the men in question. Throughout the history of the pandemic, it has been clear that receptive sex partners are at a greater risk for infection, but there have been few advances made that allow them to actively protect themselves. This is particularly true for all those whose livelihoods might depend on being sexually available to men who have, at least relatively, more power than they have. (2) What are the ethno-political and racial implications/ ramifications of this policy? How will circumcision promotion affect existing gender roles and gender relations within communities? And will it affect how those communities understand and identify themselves vis à vis others? And, relatedly, (3) from a global political economic perspective, is it risky in terms of further alienating groups already very alienated by the national-corporate major AIDS institutions? Another topic of conversation at the 2006 AIDS Congress was South African President Mbeki's unorthodox and dangerous stance on handling the massive HIV/AIDS epidemic in his country and his medical minister's unfounded theories that home remedies can help those with AIDS as much as the more expensive antiretroviral therapies. Mbeki counters domestic and international critics by denouncing them as imperialist, calling the epidemic one of poverty more than of any specific virus. While his stance is extreme and unjustifiable, Mbeki's perspective that the transnational NGOs, public health agencies, and foundations convey cultural and economic imperialism is not an isolated one. Those who plan and implement prevention policies are helpless without the full cooperation of local governing bodies – both at the state and at the community level – and being seen as imposing cultural imperatives does not facilitate cooperation. (4) Will existing prevention methods, such as innovative, evolving education programs and the widespread provision of quality condoms and the knowledge to use them correctly, continue to receive funding and attention and, in fact, be accelerated and promoted alongside circumcision?

A more radical intervention does not automatically promise more radically beneficial effects. Male circumcision, no matter how coldly clinical an issue it may seem, is inextricable from its ancient cultural contexts and from its modern one – that of twentieth century, American medicine. A program to promote circumcision that is produced without much more investigation, reflection, and discussion must be prepared, at least, to be held accountable for its possible human consequences.

NOTES

1. This paper only addresses male circumcision's potential utility as a public health practice to manage the HIV/AIDS pandemic, not the general moral rightness or wrongness of the surgery. My argument is a *sociological* one based in a concern for social welfare and practical ethics.

2. I call the science uncertain because while a correlation seems clear now, the cause for that correlation remains less clear. For example, the concentrated presence of Langerhans cells in the prepuce is given as a key reason for why circumcision reduces the risk for behaviorally heterosexual men to contract HIV from their female sex partners (see Halperin & Bailey, 1999). These cells seem to provide a receptor site that is particularly well suited to HIV, and Langerhans cells are densely concentrated in the vaginal, anal, and preputial linings, making these tissues more vulnerable to HIV infection. More recently, this has been cited as a reason why women are far more likely to contract HIV from male sex partners than those male partners are to contract HIV from them (see Miller & Miller, 2007). However, others argue that it is not the Langerhans cells that make the prepuce more vulnerable but rather, the fact that the space between the foreskin and the rest of the penis holds vaginal secretions in place long enough to make infection more likely to occur and Olivier Schwartz, in March 2007, published a piece in *Nature* arguing that Langerhans cells produce a substance called Langerin that "consumes" HIV, actually preventing infection and accounting for what is a fairly inefficient rate of transmission (the enormous number of HIV infections in the world today may speak more of the frequency of "high-risk" activity in the world than of the efficiency of HIV transmission). Despite the significance of the 60% risk reduction rate that was drawn from the South African Orange Farm study, the number of subjects from that study who seroconverted was small (fewer than 80). Ideally, more research would be done, but this is ethically difficult because such studies would depend on subjects becoming infected with HIV.

3. There are many studies of inter-ethnic violence that demonstrate how the presence or lack of a foreskin has served as a marker of an embraced co-group-member or a reviled enemy. Urvashi Butalia's ethnographic record of inter-religious violence following the partition of India and Pakistan – *The Other Side of Silence* – provides us many such examples (Butalia, 2000). See also, Peter Aggleton's social history of circumcision in the May 2007 issue of Reproductive Health Matters.

4. See, for example, the December 2006 article published by Kahn, Marseille, and Auvert (Auvert was the lead researcher of the South Africa study), called "Cost-Effectiveness of Male Circumcision for HIV Prevention in a South African Setting."

5. To fully consider the relevance of this global North/South divide in policy and practice, it is also worth noting that almost all the male circumcision clinical trials have been conducted in southern Africa and in South Asia, which fits the pattern of the testing of most new and risky medicines and medical procedures.

6. WHO, as of early 2007, only formally acknowledges that microbicides might be helpful for women who engage in vaginal intercourse with men, but the issue earlier came to light in the context of the predominantly gay epidemic of North America 20 years ago.

7. Nonoxynol-9 is, however, still the only microbicide approved by the FDA and is commonly available in the United States.

8. A vaccine to protect girls and women from acquiring HPV is now available, sparking another debate about whether to make that vaccine mandatory or not and what effect distributing the vaccine might have on widely socially accepted sexual standards.

9. South Africa's Treatment Action Campaign's popularization of the "HIV Positive" t-shirts that destigmatize HIV testing are a good example of this as are the seductive advertising campaigns featuring attractive models that are aimed at eroticizing condom use as a lifelong message for adolescent boys and young men.

242 ANANYA MUKHERJEA

ACKNOWLEDGMENTS

I am grateful for the suggestions by the editors of this volume. This paper has also benefited greatly from the comments of the following individuals: Jeffrey Bussolini, Patricia Clough, Melissa Ditmore, Ariel Ducey, Hester Eisenstein, Peter Hoffman, Laura Kaehler, Penny Lewis, Lorna Mason, Gina Neff, Michelle Ronda, Neil Smith, Ida Susser, Craig Willse, Betsy Wissinger, and Salvador Vidal-Ortiz. I had the opportunity to present part of this paper at the American Sociological Association's annual meeting as well. All of the paper's shortcomings, of course, are my sole responsibility.

REFERENCES

Aggleton, P. (2007). "Just a snip"? A social history of male circumcision. *Reproductive Health Matters*, *15*(29), 15–21.
Bailey, R. C., Moses, S., Parker, C. B., Agot, K., Maclean, I., Krieger, J. N., Williams, C. F. M., Campbell, R. T., & Ndinya-Achola, J. O. (2007). Male circumcision for HIV prevention in young men in Kisumu, Kenya: A randomised controlled trial. *Lancet*, *369*, 643–656.
Cameron, D. W., Simonsen, J. N., D'Acosta, L. J., Ronald, A. R., Maitha, G. M., Gakinya, M. N., Cheang, M., Ndinya-Achola, J. O., Piot, P., Brunham, R. C., et al. (1989). Female to male transmission of Human Immunodeficiency Virus type 1: Risk factors for seroconversion in men. *Lancet*, *2*, 403–407.
Campbell, C. (2003). *Letting them die: Why HIV/AIDS prevention programmes fail.* Bloomington: Indian University Press.
Castellsague, X., Bosch, F. X., Munoz, N., Chris, J. L. M. Meijer., Shah, K. V., Silvia de Sanjosé, P. H., Eluf-Neto, J., Ngelangel, C. A., Chichareon, S., Smith, J. S., Herrero, R., Moreno, V., Franceschi, S., et al. (2002). Male circumcision, penile human papillomavirus infection, and cervical cancer in female partners. *New England Journal of Medicine*, *346*(15), 1105–1112.
Cellulose sulfate microbicide trial stopped. (2007, January 31). Statement of the World Health Organization and UNAIDS, http://www.who.int/mediacentre/news/statements/2007/s01/en/index.html
Cleaton-Jones, P. (2005). The first randomised trial of male circumcision for preventing HIV: What were the ethical issues? *PLoS Medicine*, *2*(11).
Crimp, D. (Ed.). (1991). *AIDS: Cultural analysis: Cultural activism.* Cambridge: MIT Press.
Farmer, P. (1999). *Infections and inequalities: The modern plagues.* Berkeley: University of California Press.
Farmer, P. (2005). *Pathologies of power: Health, human rights, and the new war on the poor.* Berkeley: University of California Press.
Garrett, L. (2001). *Betrayal of trust: The collapse of public health.* New York: Hyperion.
Glick, L. B. (2006). *Marked in your flesh: Circumcision from Ancient Judea to Modern America.* New York: Oxford University Press.
Gollaher, D. (2001). *Circumcision: A history of the world's most controversial surgery.* New York: Basic Books.

Gray, R. H., Kigozi, G., Serwadda, D., Makumbi, F., Watya, S., Nalugoda, F., Kiwanuka, N., Moulton, L. H., Chaudhary, M. A., Chen, M. Z., Sewankambo, N. K., Wabwire-Mangen, F., Bacon, M. C., Williams, C. F. M., Opendi, P., Reynolds, S. J., Laeyendecker, O., Quinn, T. C., & Wawer, M. J. (2007). Male circumcision for HIV prevention in men in Rakai, Uganda: A randomised trial. *Lancet, 369,* 657–666.
Halperin, D., & Bailey, R. (1999). Male circumcision and HIV infection: 10 years and counting. *Lancet, 354,* 1813–1815.
Hoffmaster, B. (2001). *Bioethics in Social Context.* Philadelphia: Temple University Press.
Kahn, J. G., Marseille, E., & Auvert, B. (2006). Cost-effectiveness of male circumcision for HIV prevention in a South African setting. *PLoS Medicine, 3*(12), 517.
Kahn, J. G., Marseille, E., & Auvert, B. (2007). Circumcision for HIV prevention: Authors' reply. *PLoS Medicine, 4*(3), 146.
Kalichman, S., Eaton, L., & Pinkerton, S. (2007). Circumcision for HIV prevention: Failure to fully account for behavioral risk compensation. *PLoS Medicine, 4*(3), 138.
Lie, R. K., Ezekiel, E. J., & Grady, C. (2006). Circumcision and HIV prevention research: An ethical analysis. *Lancet, 368,* 522–525.
Pietrzyk, S. (2005). AIDS and feminisms. *JENDA: A Journal of Culture and African Women Studies,* 7.
Treichler, P. (1999). *How to have theory in an epidemic: Cultural chronicles of AIDS.* Durham: Duke University Press.
UNAIDS/06.29E. (2006, December). *AIDS epidemic update.* (English original).
Van Howe, R. S. (1999). Circumcision and HIV infection: Review of the literature and meta-analysis. *International Journal of STD and AIDS, 10,* 8–16.
Watney, S. (1994). *Practices of freedom: Selected writings on HIV/AIDS.* London: Rivers Oram Press.

FURTHER READING

Auvert, B., Taljaard, D., Lagarde, E., Sobngwi-Tambekou, J., Sitta, R., Puren, A., et al. (2007). Randomized, controlled intervention trial of male circumcision for reduction of HIV infection risk: The ANRS 1265 trial. *PLoS Medicine, 2*(11), 298.
Moses, S., Bailey, R. C., & Ronald, A. R. (1998). Male circumcision: Assessment of health benefits and risks. *Sexually Transmitted Infections, 74,* 368–373.
UNAIDS. (2007, February 26). Male circumcision (3-part series). http://www.unaids.org/en/MediaCentre/PressMaterials/FeatureStory/20070226_MC_pt1.asp

GENOMICS, GENDER AND GENETIC CAPITAL: THE NEED FOR AN EMBODIED ETHICS OF REPRODUCTION

Elizabeth Ettorre

In this paper, I explore the social complexities of genetic technologies with special reference to biomedical prenatal practices. I hope to establish gender and the body as key contextual and theoretical sites in what I see as a complex exploration. The aim of my paper is to show how the field of reproductive genetics can benefit from a feminist perspective and how gender, the body and ethics go hand in hand. My paper will not focus on the new reproductive technologies (NRTs) which I term 'pre' prenatal technologies (i.e. in terms of the site for foetal development). NRTs include a variety of techniques such as in vitro fertilisation (IVF) *in conjunction with* superovulation, ultrasound, laparoscopic egg retrieval and embryo transfer as well as gamete intrafallopian transfer (GIFT). For the purpose of this paper, I am most interested in the techniques geneticists and obstetricians employ in determining the fate of 'fertile' pregnant women's foetuses. Geneticists and obstetricians working in the field of prenatal screening and prenatal diagnosis use molecular genetics tests, including blood sample analysis, amniocentesis, chorionic villus sampling as well as diagnostic ultrasound. I define prenatal genetic technologies as those which are used for foetal analysis and can be either non-DNA based (i.e. unrelated to

Bioethical Issues, Sociological Perspectives
Advances in Medical Sociology, Volume 9, 245–261
Copyright © 2008 by Elsevier Ltd.
All rights of reproduction in any form reserved
ISSN: 1057-6290/doi:10.1016/S1057-6290(07)09010-9

genetics – such as ultrasound scanning) or DNA based (i.e. related to genetics, blood or serum collection – such as chorionic villus screening, maternal serum screening or amniocentesis). My primary focus in this paper is on DNA-based prenatal techniques. However, both non-DNA- and DNA-based practices are used in conjunction with each other in the search for foetal abnormalities. Some experts see non-DNA-based procedures as genetic technologies because these tend to be linked procedurally in reproductive medicine. Beyond the procedural level, prenatal technologies are ethically the most difficult applications of genetics (Henn, 2000).

In this context, Ruth Schwartz Cowan commenting on the thalassemia prenatal screening program in Cyprus has said: 'We need to understand the consequences of genetic programs way more clearly than we do. There's too much rhetoric and too little information about what is actually happening, what could be happening and what the consequences of any of the programs are' (quoted in Guterman, 2003, p. A22).

While genetic technology is related to NRTs (i.e. the genetic composition of eggs, sperm and embryos are monitored before implantation), prenatal screening and prenatal diagnosis tend to be focused on fecund, already pregnant women. All of these practices can be seen as assisting the birth of a 'normal', 'non-afflicted' baby/child.

Here, my assumption is that prenatal genetic technologies have unintended consequences which tend to remain invisible in the field of reproductive genetics. That the female reproductive body is the focal point of these powerful and diverse technologies is often a hidden or subverted concern. This process is carried out under the assumed, benevolent gaze of physicians with their own meanings, values and behavioural norms. Set within the context of 'genetic governmentality' (i.e. the development, regulation and application of new genetic technologies) (Kerr & Franklin, 2006, p. 40), reproductive genetic technologies have emerged from within a medical system and thus scientific culture whose members have identified traditionally with social progress and humane goals (Foucault, 1973; Turner, 1987). Very often, unintended consequences, as we shall see, subvert 'social progress' and make these goals unachievable.

While there are disparate discourses concerning the desirability of prenatal genetic technologies amongst feminists and pregnant women themselves (Lupton, 1994), these technologies have been found to have less than calming effects upon pregnant women (Green, 1990). Indeed, their effects are often invidious (Rothman, 1994; Dragonas, 2001). To understand the importance of developing a feminist perspective is to recognise the powerful interplay between genomics, modern reproductive medicine, foetal diagnosis, gendering processes and women's bodies. My paper is divided into three inter-related discussions. First, to set the scene for an understanding of the social complexities of genetic technologies, I examine the complex workings of prenatal politics. Second, I demonstrate how the mix of prenatal politics, genetics and gender creates threats to female embodiment. Third, I outline what embodied ethics in this field means and why this type of feminist ethics is needed. I conclude with the contention that given that prenatal genetic technologies are gender biased, they need re-visioning (See Clarke & Olsen, 1999). Those of us working in the field need to construct new perceptions about their use and how women's embodied experiences are shaped by these practices.

PRENATAL POLITICS, GENETIC CAPITAL AND COMMODIFICATION

Prenatal comes from the Latin words 'prae' and 'natalis' meaning 'before' and 'to be born', respectively (Concise Oxford Dictionary, 1995). This word is semiotically loaded because 'prenatal' connotes the time before being born. The word itself signifies the foetus (who is 'before being born') not the pregnant body within whom the foetus grows. If medical experts working within the discipline of reproductive medicine concentrate more on the foetus and its health than the pregnant woman, they take this meaning to heart. Experts argue that 'a multidisciplinary approach to the foetus is essential part of antenatal screening' (Malone, 1996, p. 157), a view suggesting that the foetus, more than a pregnant woman, is the physician's main focus during the prenatal period.

The workings of reproductive genetics expose the long-standing feminist unease that the medicalisation of reproduction, pregnancy and childbirth has, more often than not, been against the interests of pregnant women, making them objects of medical care rather than subjects with agency and rational decision-making powers. Indeed, women's reproductive power has consistently been grounded in the ambiguity of their wombs (Duden, 1991, p. 8). Bordo (1993, p. 88) contends that the ideology of the woman-as-foetal-incubator pervades women's experience of pregnancy. Pregnant women are neither subjects nor treated as such, while their foetuses become 'super subjects'. This representation of women as objects of mechanical surveillance rather than active recipients of prenatal care is an obvious message of the photograph displaying the first ultrasound device used in

Glasgow, Scotland, in 1957 (see Oakley, 1984, p. 159). This photograph shows a woman lying on her back on a gurney with a 2 ft^2 ultrasound box supported above her, touching her pregnant stomach. Oakley's (1984, p. 159) 'apropos' caption is 'diagnosing the tumor of pregnancy'. Accordingly, many prenatal technologies objectify women and uphold this ideology of woman-as-foetal-incubator.

While prenatal politics are more foetus-directed than pregnant-women-directed, women bear the brunt of damaging beliefs and painful procedures. Pregnant women are more done to than the doers, as the well-being of their foetuses are appraised over time through various technical procedures. Prenatal politics operate in the discursive spaces of knowledge and practices generated by the universalising system of reproductive genetics. DNA, reproductive material, foetuses, gendered bodies and reproductive functions are surveyed and managed in a multiplicity of ways with the effect that pregnant women are required to take 'security measures' (Hubbard, 1986) necessary for 'successful' reproduction. When pregnant women choose what is generally seen by physicians as the 'correct' prenatal behaviour, their choices are constructed more by the power conferred on physicians when using these technologies than by women's own embodied experiences (Doyal, 1995, p. 141).

Intersecting with genomic governmentality and the subsequent ways that expert knowledge and scientific discourse are drawn upon in the construction of identity (Bunton & Petersen, 2005, p. 2), prenatal politics set reproductive limits upon both the internal and the external problems of the body in our modern consumerist culture with the result that women's, more than men's, bodies are restrained. For example, the science of genetics becomes an ideal way of bringing together what Turner (1992, pp. 58–59) has referred to as the external bodily problems of representation (i.e. commodification) and regulation and the interior ones of restraint (i.e. control of desire, passion and need) and reproduction. Through reproductive genetics, pregnant bodies experience self-imposed restraint through a type of *reproductive asceticism.* This refers to pregnant women's self-regulation or self-discipline which directs them towards the use of reproductive technologies in order to ensure normal babies. As these technologies become routinised, pregnant women begin to accept prenatal screening under the rubric of older non-controversial medical practices and routine prenatal care (Press & Browner, 1997).

When pregnant bodies undergo these invasive tests, this austere self-disciplining of reproductive asceticism can be viewed and experienced as necessary for the overall, external regulation of 'fit' populations in consumer culture. In this type of disciplinary regime, the female body emerges as a reproductive resource or provider of 'good babies'. We now in the social sciences speak of the body as a comprehensive form of physical capital, a possessor of power, status and distinctive symbolic forms – integral to the accumulation of resources (Shilling, 1993, p. 127). The pregnant body in reproductive genetics can be seen as women's physical capital. In turn, women's physical capital becomes inexorably linked with their genetic capital (i.e. genes or genetic makeup), as they encounter the regulatory practices of reproductive genetics. In this feminised regimen, women enact a morality of the body which upholds the external population's standard – the desire for conventional (i.e. non-diseased, genetically normal) offspring and the need for citizens who are fit to be born. Genetic capital not only determines whether or not a particular woman's body should be viewed as a reproductive resource but also is central to constructing a genetic moral order. Thus, when physicians speak of affected offspring, risk pregnancies and genetic disorders, and utilise technologies to rid wombs of 'non-viable foetuses', they are actively supporting the population's desire and society's supposed need for fit bodies as well as firmly establishing the link between physical and genetic capital. In this context, 'viable foetuses' become problematic and indeed expensive if they are born prematurely, disabled or with genetic disorders. Here, the effects of linking physical capital with genetic capital become clear. Through prenatal politics, biomedical discourses transform women's wombs into highly managed social spaces – sites of discourses about 'good' genes, women-as-foetal-incubators, 'good enough' foetal bodies and disability.

As a consequence of prenatal politics, pregnant women can be seen to practice reproductive asceticism. They consume reproductive genetics for the foetus, the reproductive product, and attempt to gain knowledge of its quality. In effect, the medical workforce facilitates the commodification of reproduction through the use of prenatal technologies that impart knowledge about the status of foetuses. On the one hand, the concepts such as high risk/low risk, afflicted/non-afflicted and carrier/non-carrier are traditional diagnostic categories, underpinning women's reproductive behaviour and choices. On the other hand, through the commodification of reproduction, these same concepts are constructed as descriptions of 'embodied foetuses' with economic labels. Simply, given that impairment excludes any 'future' child from taking part in normal society (Davis & Watson, 2002, p. 159), this has economic implications as this 'child' will also be stigmatised as non-productive. These 'embodied' descriptions conjure up various types of foetal body images in the minds of pregnant women, their significant others (i.e. partners, families, etc.), medical experts and society. Low-risk, non-afflicted and 'non-genetic disease carrier' foetal bodies are viewed as more valuable both economically and physically in terms of what these potential social bodies can produce and how they are able to contribute to society.

Economic relationships are introduced into human reproduction (Overall, 1987, p. 49) because defective foetuses are viewed as prospective, burdensome human beings with a price tag on their heads as well as defective products. Normal foetuses are represented as potential human beings – productive products with a future full of prolific energy. Generally, reproductive technologies evidence a capital-intensive approach to medicine, or 'cost benefit analysis approach' (Rothman quoted in Guterman, 2003), treating reproductive care as well as reproduction as commodities. Thus, in a context where gender inequality is already present, the negative effects of these technologies upon women, especially the less privileged, should not be surprising (Gimenez, 1991, pp. 335–336).

Given that the 'products' of women's reproductive activities (i.e. conception, pregnancy and birth) can be ranked according to this system of child quality control, women themselves are ranked as 'good' or 'bad' reproducers. Undeniably, we have experienced a reproductive revolution – this technological upheaval in which a diverse series of medical advances have been allowed to insinuate and spread biomedical values (about 'good' genes, disability, women-as-foetal-incubators and 'high quality' bodies, etc.) more indirectly (Lee & Morgan, 1989, p. 3). While biomedicine has a tendency to 'fracture social experience' particularly those of pregnant women (Annandale & Clark, 1996), reproductive genetics, emerging from this self-same biomedicine, may also rupture pregnant women's experiences in a far-reaching way. Prenatal technologies have clear social dimensions and values, upholding a reproductive morality. For pregnant women, this usually means that they are drawn into a moral discourse about good foetuses and bad foetuses as well as their good or bad reproducing bodies.

While the technologies of reproductive genetics may have the potential for great benefits, and may create possibilities for medical advances and opportunities to make choices about the health of future generations, these technologies are value laden and experts make moral verdicts about foetuses. Nicholas (2001, p. 46) contends that all genetic technologies are constructing a new moral landscape and culture, disrupting long-established social understandings of how the world 'is', the meaning of the family, the place of humans in the biosphere and the role and responsibilities of the authorised knowledge makers of Western culture. Indeed, through the lens of these technologies, much of the social world is collapsed into an ultra-Darwinian model in which biological imperatives predominate (Shakespeare & Erikson, 2000).

TECHNOLOGY, GENDER AND 'BROKEN BODIES'

Over the past 300 years, biomedical scientists have owned, developed and managed the study of the body. They have been the main proselytisers on how this 'machine' works. Indeed, the biomedical discourses on the body have become entrenched in contemporary cultures as our bodies have been, time and again, shaped by notions embedded in Cartesian dualism. Living bodies have been treated as no different from a piece of equipment, while this powerful and far-reaching discourse has consistently obscured considerations of sentient bodies. Since the late 1980s, sociologists (Turner, 1996, 1992; Frank, 1995; Williams & Bendelow, 1998; Nettleton & Watson, 1998) have begun to position bodies centrally to studies in sociology, specifically the sociology of health and illness. At the same time, specialists in biomedicine continue to invent ways to make bodies more accessible for their perusal, while altering the boundaries of these bodies through various procedures such as organ transplants and limb and skin grafts and through exploring more possibilities of xenotransplantation.

Turner (1992, pp. 165–166) contends that the uncertain status of the body in human cultures, the contradictory relationship between nature, society and the body, and the social role of illness in human cultures, all act as a symbolic map of the political and social structure, and are the province of medical sociology. Indeed, bodies are growing to be more compliant and more disciplined as they progress from being healthier or sicker.

While the concepts of health and illness are culturally and socially defined, all cultures have known concepts of these terms. These terms differ from culture to culture in relation to how ailing and well bodies become visible as well as the intensity of the 'scopic drive'. The scopic drive is the biomedical quest to make the unseen visible in the biotechnological world (Braidotti, 1994). Whether sick or healthy, bodies are viewed as empirical objects to be quantified, classified, visualised and disciplined through biomedicine. Thus, through this biomedical gaze, bodies are treated as 'things' to be studied and not as embodied, living and moving subjects with agency.

Alongside this scopic drive produced by biomedicine, an authoritative need arises among experts to categorise 'abnormal', 'irregular', 'odd' or 'deviant' bodies, situate them in biology and patrol these bodies in public spaces. Urla and Terry (1995, p. 1) argue that since the nineteenth century, the somatic territorialising of deviance has been an important component of a larger effort of the State including scientists, lawmakers and the police to organise social relations according to categories denoting health versus pathology, normality versus abnormality and national security versus social danger. As a result of these multifarious practices, bodies have been marked as deviant and normal bodies, and social relations have been organised according to these bodies. Nevertheless, before cultural conceptions of normal and abnormal, conformity and non-conformity or health and pathology can be constructed, an assemblage of bodies upon which these conceptions can be inscribed needs to exist. Specifically, qualified biomedical experts using their convincing discourses and scientific practices perform the distinctive process of inscribing bodies as healthy or diseased. This process of inscription includes the pressing of technology into the service of medicine.

Modern biotechnology has been described as an ambiguous mix of knowledge and engineering, science and technology, nature and culture, possibilities and risks, and hopes and fears (Nielsen, 1997, p. 102). Technological medicine produces simultaneously great expectations as well as more arenas for uncertainty (Freund & McGuire, 1999, p. 222), and the union between the medical profession and biotechnology has empowered the profession as well as helped to create lucrative returns on many biotechnological investments, especially in the global genomics industry (Rabinow, 1999). As the concept of biotechnology developed, it was seen to integrate the contemporary idea of manufacturing with visions of humanity (Bud, 1993, p. 52). The stuff of biology became the raw material for medical exploration and, in some instances, exploitation and death (Jones, 2000). Biotechnology has had a major impact on present-day notions of reproduction. Wajcman (1991) argues that in no other area of social life is the relationship between gender and technology more forcefully disputed than in the sphere of human biological reproduction. Indeed, 'technological fixes' have been increasingly applied to pregnant, female bodies.

In this context, I use the metaphor of 'broken bodies' to suggest that women's bodies have become psychologically, emotionally and morally damaged as their bodies confront these technological fixes. The implication is that bodies are real material objects (Urla & Terry, 1995) whose disposition is of great concern to society as a whole. Bodies figure in moral considerations as both generators of ethical issues as well as sites for embodied ethics (Russell, 2000, p. 102). Specifically, pregnant bodies have become the province of experts (Lee & Jackson, 2002, p. 115) who subject these bodies to minute scrutiny of the medical gaze as well as technologies which visualise, assess and record their intimate workings. Longhurst (2001, p. 84) argues that within popular culture, pregnant women occupy a borderline state as they disturb identity, system and order by not respecting borders, positions and rules. Their subjection to medical expertise and subsequent technologies is consistent with Western ways of thinking about the body. Viewed as social and moral actors, Western subjects must be separated from their bodies. We have become disembodied, and because morality is highly mediated by gender, morality has been based on the exclusion of female bodies from full moral agency. Through moral agency, one experiences oneself as a contributor in the process of evolution towards greater autonomy and connectedness (Tomm, 1992, p. 108). Clearly, women, especially pregnant women, have lost out. Any person whose unique experiences have been largely omitted from the dominant culture (e.g. women, the poor, Black and ethnic minority women, lesbians and gay men, the disabled, etc.) will sense this loss. It is a distortion to think that generic persons exist in moral situations or that gender is irrelevant to moral deliberations (Warren, 1992). Making morals is an embodied experience as well as a deeply gendered process.

Thus, women experience a fragmented morality of the body. In moral terms, their bodies are not whole but they have become fragmented or broken. Sharpe (2000) argues that the application of reproductive technologies and other biotechnologies mark a paradigmatic shift in our understanding of the body. Bodies become commodified and fragmented. Furthermore, as we saw earlier, a hidden morality surrounds pregnant bodies. On the one hand, pregnant bodies are appropriated into a series of gendered narratives – mythological, biblical, classical humanist, anthropological and teleological. On the other hand, these gendered narratives help to discipline the cultural threat posed by reproductive bodies (Newman, 1996) and are hostile to female subjectivity (Klassen, 2001). We need to challenge this type of hidden morality and ensure that pregnant bodies remain whole, sentient bodies. These bodies can remain whole only if, as Ahmed (2004) contends, embodied emotions work to ally individuals (e.g. pregnant women) with collectives (e.g. other pregnant women) and help them in dealing with the intensity of their attachments.

Recognising the fragmentation of women's bodies psychologically, emotionally and morally and bringing in whole bodies back to our work, sociological or otherwise, has been made possible by the efforts of women bringing in themselves back. The traditional neglect of the body reflected a masculinist stance that naturalised bodies and legitimated control of male over female bodies. Feminist scholars have documented the types of regulation, restraint, provocation and resistance experienced by gendered bodies. Witz (2000, p. 2) contends that our disembodied sociological heritage includes a history of 'her excluded body' (i.e. in patriarchy, women's bodies are excluded from full social agency) and 'his abject body' (i.e. in patriarchy, men are the 'horrible' bodies who victimise women). She cautions that the recuperated body in sociology is in danger of being the abject male body – a warning that we must heed.

While recognising the need to recover the lived experiences of both the excluded and the abject body, I am aware that all sorts of activities in which we are involved as social beings are embodied activities. With Frank (1995), I suggest that social scientists become aware that what bodies experience, suffer, bear, desire and consume should be the foundation stones for our work. Here, I contend that these embodied experiences should also enlighten our understanding of reproductive genetics.

The Need for Embodied Ethics

We must ensure that the stories we, as sensitive and gender aware sociologists, tell reflect the lives of the people we study. This type of professional behaviour is ethical work. Frank (1991, 1995) has argued that there is a need for an ethics of the body, shaping the sociology of the body. He equates ethics with a social science that empathises with people's suffering. For him, only an empathic social science that witnesses suffering is worthy of our attention. He wants sociologists to give careful consideration to bodies in order to bear witness to what people suffer. So for me as a feminist sociologist interested in reproductive genetics, ethics means offering true reflections that are empathetic as well as attentive to reproductive bodies. Ethics means that I do not consider these issues in a gender, race and class neutral manner. Rather, I argue that considerations of these differences and others (i.e. sexuality, ability, age, etc.) in reproductive genetics are crucial to maintain an ethics of the body as well as to uphold care and justice (Mahowald, 1994, p. 67) in society. Furthermore, feminist ethics needs to love and embrace otherness as well as value becoming, flux and instability (Ahmed, 2002, p. 559). How will we develop an ethics of the body that is attentive to our diverse, embodied realities?

On another level, ethics is defined as 'rules of conduct'. But ethics can also be defined as 'the science of morals' (Concise Oxford Dictionary, 1995). From a feminist viewpoint, care must be taken when we speak of ethics in the context of women's embodied moral lives, given that contemporary social practices encourage discrimination against us and the suppression of our moral views (Browning-Cole & Coultrap-McQuin, 1992). I argue that all advancements within reproductive genetics should be framed by feminist perspectives on bioethics (see Holmes & Purdy, 1992).

Viewed as ethical, beneficent medical practices, regulatory techniques are played out on pregnant bodies through the science of reproductive medicine. Within biomedical knowledge, benevolence is the virtue of being disposed to act for the benefit of others, while beneficence is the moral obligation to do so. Both terms can be linked to paternalism (Beauchamp & Childress, 1994). When the pregnant body enters into this moral equation and becomes a material site of medicine's paternalistic moralising and technological explorations, problems emerge. For example, physicians may override pregnant women's autonomy vis a vis prenatal genetic technologies and may justify their actions. They do this when they advocate the use of these technologies to avoid harm. In their eyes, avoiding harm means avoiding the birth of a disabled baby. On another level, reproduction increasingly comes to be constructed as a matter of consumption and the foetus a commodity (Taylor, 2000). When this happens, pregnant women are judged by how well they reproduce, and giving birth to a 'perfect baby' becomes the goal of reproduction.

Here, I argue that medicine needs healing. The feminist project of healing medicine utilises 'epistemic empathy', offering oppressed groups help and insights based on gender-sensitive theories and practices (Holmes, 1992, p. 3). Certainly, the practice of mixing prenatal techniques with the judgements of individuals, including both physicians and their female patients, demands a rigorous, moral formula upon which future research and service development must be based (SGOMSEC, 1996).

Is it fair that some women condemn themselves to shame because they do not measure up to society's image of what it means to be a good reproducing mother? Is it just that they experience their bodies as psychologically, emotionally or morally damaged? The obvious answer is no. That these questions need to be asked demonstrates that reproductive genetics has profound ethical implications. If women's reproductive processes continue to be ranked according to genetic information or 'reproductive success', the field of genetics needs to become more gender sensitive than it is at present and we need to see that gender, bodies and ethics go hand in hand.

Spallone et al. (2000) argue that the use of prenatal genetic techniques demands a socially informed ethics which provides a way of allowing a sense of social responsibility, rooted in an understanding of the effects of new technologies, to replace the one-dimensional requirement for quality control and technical expertise. Given the above, an ethics of the body and feminist ethics are inter-related. In earlier work (Ettorre, 2002), I have shown how experts in reproductive genetics while they articulate, construct and reproduce their positions of authority, also fulfil important social and scientific roles as interpreters of genetic knowledge. Experts represent specialists: reproductive invigilators, fulfilling the cultural need in the population for genetic supervision and 'know how'. In this invigilation process, they embody educators, surveillors and storytellers whose role it is to reinforce and legitimate a genetic moral order. Experts' ethics are disembodied ethics, and in fulfilling a need for embodied ethics, we should recentre women's experiences within reproductive genetics.

Embodied ethics are responsible ethics framed by and through embodied relationships. When medical experts deal with pregnant bodies, these experts should be aware that these pregnant bodies are not only gendered but also can become morally judged as good or bad reproducers. Embodied ethics takes as its starting point the corporeal experiences of moral, gendered individuals. With regard to reproductive genetics, this starting point is crucial if women's bodies are to become whole, not damaged. Embodied ethics has been absent from this field. Indeed, consistency (Kuhse & Singer, 1999) and factual accuracy, not embodiment and emotion, have been the traditional requirements of defensible bioethical positions. In the field of reproductive ethics, moral analysis and rational argument are used to bring about moral agreement (Bayles, 1984, p. 3). Emotions have not been part of the equipment to discern moral answers (Little, 1996).

A feminist approach to ethics and specifically bioethics challenges this overly rationalised view of morality. A feminist approach to bioethics evaluates medical practices in terms of the impact of such practices on women (Lebacqz, 1991) and their bodies, and helps experts to recognise that gender matters. This approach insists that women's varied experiences should be taken into account (Rothenberg, 1996) – experiences, I would add, that are corporeal. Embodiment must be a key issue in feminist approaches to bioethics. Similar to Witz (2000) we should be more concerned with how women's bodies (in this case, pregnant bodies) are controlled and broken through patriarchal practices rather than problema-tising embodiment per se. Thus, I would contend that embodied ethics with special reference to reproductive genetics makes moral appraisals of the impact of a variety of medical practices and technologies on pregnant bodies. Simply, women's bodies and their corporeal experiences should be the starting point for any ethical evaluations; these gendered bodies and experiences should not be taken for granted.

In conclusion, when pregnant women encounter reproductive genetics, their experiences are shaped by all the social inequalities that embed them in society such as class, race, ethnicity, sexuality, etc. To be truly sensitive to these bodies, those of us working within reproductive genetics should develop a focused gender dimension in our work. All technologies affect our conceptions of femininity and masculinity (Wajcman, 1991; Stabile, 1994); technologies are feminised and masculinised as they take shape, and technologies are shaped by gender (Rudinow Saetnan, 1996). The sorts of technologies used in reproduction are designed for women's bodies and have profound consequences for gender relations during pregnancy and beyond (Faulkner, 2001). The promise and allure of these technologies for the future of science and medicine tend to overshadow experts' need to reinforce dualistic thinking, especially with regard sex and gender (Ettorre, Rothman, & Steinberg, 2006).

The injection of biology into social relationships through genetics allows more attention than ever before to the workings of the 'female' human body in reproduction (Franklin, 1993) as well as this gendered body, situated in other areas of social relationships (Martin, 1992). I have viewed these developing discourses on the interplay between nature and human biology as raising important issues around the discourse on the body. At the intersection of surveillance medicine and reproductive genetics is a focus on the female body – interacting within the community, the site of genetic capital and a material entity where scientists are able to 'see' the structure of the material of genes(DNA) – as well as the growth of the foetus. But, this physical body, the original site for foetal (Newman, 1996) and/or genetic investigations, is shaped by gender. It is a pregnant body – a gendered, female body. Through the medical gaze, this body becomes less than body, as it is 'relegated to foetal environment' (Degener, 1990, p. 90).

That a pregnant woman's genetic capital may be ranked in this gender-biased context suggests that female more than male bodies are subject to a reproductive morality. The imposition of a genetic moral order during reproduction separates pregnant bodies into good and bad reproducers. Some pregnant bodies experience their reproductive potential as shameful in comparison to other pregnant women. A body reproducing badly becomes a new form of embodied transgression for women. Bad reproducers are viewed morally as those with 'bad genes' and who dare to allow 'bad genes' or 'gene mistakes' come into this world.

I have shown in this paper the need to re-vision women's experience of reproductive genetics. Re-visioning means letting go of how we have seen in order to construct new perceptions (Clarke & Olsen, 1999). Thus, we need to let go of our damaging images and ideas about gendered bodies as bad reproducers in order to construct new perceptions about them and their embodied experiences within reproductive genetics. I have attempted to inject new ideas on gender and the body into an analysis of reproductive genetics. I have argued that our Western ethics have excluded female bodies from full moral agency during pregnancy and, this exclusion has resulted in a fragmented morality of the female body. As more prenatal technologies are being deployed, critical scholars need to place themselves at their 'foetal work stations' (Haraway, 1997, p. 35), make visible the multiple sites of contestation in the new genetics and expose some of the repressive dynamics of reproductive genetics. We need to actively expose not only how these repressive dynamics work but also the affective, embodied dimensions of these dynamics. More importantly, we need to remember that pregnant women's reproductive rights are a matter not only of helpful interventions and technologies but also of social justice and human rights (Merali, 2000).

REFERENCES

Ahmed, S. (2002). This other and other others. *Economy and Society, 31*(4), 558–572.
Ahmed, S. (2004). Collective feelings or the impression left by others. *Theory, Culture and Society, 21*(2), 25–42.
Annandale, E., & Clark, J. (1996). What is gender? Feminist theory and the sociology of human reproduction. *Sociology of Health and Illness, 18*(1), 17–44.
Bayles, M. D. (1984). *Reproductive ethics.* Englewood Cliffs, NJ: Prentice-Hall, Inc.
Beauchamp, T. L., & Childress, J. F. (1994). *Principles of biomedical ethics.* New York and Oxford: Oxford University Press.
Bordo, S. (1993). *Unbearable weight: Feminism, Western culture and the body.* Berkeley: The University of California Press.
Braidotti, R. (1994). *Nomadic subjects: Embodiment and sexual difference in contemporary feminist theory.* New York: Columbia University Press.
Browning-Cole, E., & Coultrap-McQuin, S. (Eds). (1992). *Explorations in feminist ethics: Theory and practice.* Bloomington: Indiana University Press.
Bud, R. (1993). *The uses of life: A history of biotechnology.* Cambridge: Cambridge University Press.
Bunton, R., & Petersen, A. (2005). Genetics and governance: An introduction. In: R. Bunton & A. Petersen (Eds), *Genetic governance: Health, risk and ethics in a biotech era* (pp. 1–27). London: Routledge.

Clarke, A. E., & Olsen, V. L. (1999). Revising, diffracting, acting. In: A. E. Clarke & V. L. Olesen (Eds), *Revisioning women, health and healing: Feminist, cultural and technoscience perspectives*. New York: Routledge.

Concise oxford dictionary (9th edn.). (1995). Oxford: Clarendon Press.

Davis, J., & Watson, N. (2002). Countering stereotypes of disability: Disabled children and resistance. In: M. Corker & T. Shakespeare (Eds), *Disability/postmodernity: Embodying disability theory* (pp. 159–174). London: Continuum.

Degener, T. (1990). Female self-determination between feminist claims and 'voluntary' eugenics, between 'rights' and ethics. *Issues in Reproductive and Genetic Engineering*, *3*(2), 87–99.

Doyal, L. (1995). *What makes women sick: Gender and the political economy of health*. Houndsmill: Macmillan.

Dragonas, T. (2001). Whose fault is it? Shame and guilt for the genetic defect. In: E. Ettorre (Ed.), *Before birth*. Ashgate.

Duden, B. (1991). *The woman beneath the skin: A doctor's patients in eighteenth century Germany*. London: Harvard University Press.

Ettorre, E. (2002). *Reproductive genetics, gender and the body*. London: Routledge.

Ettorre, E., Rothman, B. K., & Steinberg, D. (2006). Feminism confronts the genome: Introduction. *New Genetics and Society (Special Issue, Feminism confronts the genome)*, *25*(2), 133–141.

Faulkner, W. (2001). The technology question in feminism. *Women's Studies International Forum*, *24*(1), 79–95.

Foucault, M. (1973). *The birth of the clinic*. London: Tavistock Publications.

Frank, A. (1991). For a sociology of the body: An analytical review. In: M. Featherstone, M. Hepworth & B. Turner (Eds), *The body: Social and cultural theory*. London: Sage.

Franklin, S. (1993). Postmodern procreation: Representing reproductive practice. *Science as Culture*, *3*(17), 522–561.

Frank, A. (1995). *The wounded storyteller: Body, illness and ethics*. Chicago: University of Chicago Press.

Freund, P. E. S., & McGuire, M. B. (1999). *Health, illness and the social body: A critical sociology* (3rd edn.). Upper Saddle River, NJ: Prentice-Hall.

Gimenez, M. (1991). The mode of reproduction in transition: A Marxist-feminist analysis of the effects of reproductive technologies. *Gender and Society*, *5*(3), 334–350.

Green, J. M. (1990). *Calming or harming? A review of psychological effects of fetal diagnosis on pregnant women*. London: The Galton Institute.

Guterman, L. (2003). Choosing eugenics: How far will nations go to eliminate a genetic disease? *The Chronicle of Higher Education*, May 2, A22–A26.

Haraway, D. (1997). The virtual speculum in the new world order. *Feminist Review*, *55*, 22–72.

Henn, W. (2000). Consumerism in prenatal diagnosis: A challenge for ethical guidelines. *Journal of Medical Ethics*, *26*, 444–446.

Holmes, H. B. (1992). A call to heal medicine. In: H. B. Holmes & L. Purdy (Eds), *Feminist perspectives in medical ethics*. Bloomington: Indiana University Press.

Holmes, H. B., & Purdy, L. (Eds). (1992). *Feminist perspectives in medical ethics*. Bloomington: Indiana University Press.

Hubbard, R. (1986). Eugenics and prenatal testing. *International Journal of Health Services*, *16*(2), 227–242.

Jones, J. (2000). The tuskegee syphilis experiment. In: P. Brown (Ed.), *Perspectives in medical sociology* (3rd edn.). Prospect Heights, IL: Waveland Press Inc.

Kerr, A., & Franklin, S. (2006). Genetic ambivalence: Expertise, uncertainty and communication in the context of new genetic technologies. In: A. Webster (Ed.), *New technologies in health care: Challenge, change and innovation* (pp. 40–56). Houndsmill, Basingstoke: Palgrave Macmillan.

Klassen, P. E. (2001). Sacred maternities and postmedical bodies: Religion and nature in contemporary home birth. *Signs: Journal of Women in Culture and Society, 26*(3), 775–810.

Kuhse, H., & Singer, P. (1999). Introduction. In: H. Kuhse & P. Singer (Eds), *Bioethics: An anthology*. Oxford: Blackwell Publishers.

Lebacqz, K. (1991). Feminism and bioethics: An overview. *Second Opinion, 17*, 11–25.

Lee, E., & Jackson, E. (2002). The pregnant body. In: M. Evand & E. Lee (Eds), *Real bodies: A sociological introduction* (pp. 115–132). Houndsmills, Basingstoke: Palgrave.

Lee, R., & Morgan, D. (1989). A lesser sacrifice? Sterilization and mentally handicapped. In: R. Lee & D. Morgan (Eds), *Birthrights, law and ethics at the beginnings of life*. New York and London: Routledge.

Little, M. O. (1996). Why a feminist approach to bioethics? *Kennedy Institute of Ethics Journal, 6*(1), 1–18.

Longhurst, R. (2001). Breaking corporeal boundaries: Pregnant bodies in public places. In: R. Holliday & J. Hassard (Eds), *Contested bodies* (pp. 81–94). London: Routledge.

Lupton, D. (1994). *Medicine as culture: Illness, disease and the body in Western societies*. London: Sage.

Mahowald, M. B. (1994). Reproductive genetics and gender justice. In: K. Rothenberg & E. J. Thomson (Eds), *Women and prenatal testing: Facing the challenges of genetic testing*. Columbus, OH: Ohio State University Press.

Malone, P. S. J. (1996). Antenatal diagnosis of renal tract anomalies: Has it increased the sum of human happiness? *Journal of the Royal Society of Medicine, 89*(3), 155–158.

Martin, E. (1992). *The woman in the body: A cultural analysis of reproduction*. Boston: Beacon Press.

Merali, I. (2000). Advancing women's reproductive and sexual health rights: Using the international human rights system. *Development in Practice, 10*(5), 609–624.

Nettleton, S., & Watson, J. (Eds). (1998). *The body in everyday life*. London: Routledge.

Newman, K. (1996). *Fetal positions: Individualism, science and visuality*. Stanford, CA: Stanford University Press.

Nicholas, B. (2001). Exploring a moral landscape: Genetic science and ethics. *Hypatia, 16*(1), 45–63.

Nielsen, T. H. (1997). Modern biotechnology – sustainability and integrity. In: S. Lundin & M. Ideland (Eds), *Gene technology and the public: An interdisciplinary perspective*. Lund, Sweden: Nordic Academic Press.

Oakley, A. (1984). *The captured womb: A history of the medical care of pregnant woman*. Oxford: Basil Blackwell.

Overall, C. (1987). *Ethics and human reproduction*. Boston: Allen and Unwin.

Press, N., & Browner, C. H. (1997). Why women say yes to prenatal diagnosis. *Social Science and Medicine, 45*(7), 979–989.

Rabinow, P. (1999). *French DNA: Trouble in purgatory*. Chicago: University of Chicago Press.

Rothman, B. K. (1994). *The tentative pregnancy: Amniocentesis and the sexual politics of motherhood*. London: Pandora.

Rothenberg, K. (1996). Feminism, law and ethics. *Kennedy Institute of Ethics Journal*, 6(1), 69–84.

Rudinow Saetnan, A. (1996). Contested meanings of gender and technology in the Norwegian ultrasound screening debate. *The European Journal of Women's Studies*, 3(1), 55–75.

Russell, R. (2000). Ethical bodies. In: P. Hancock, B. Hughes, E. Jagger, K. Paterson, R. Russell, E. Tulle-Winton & M. Tyler (Eds), *The body, culture and society: An introduction* (pp. 101–116). Buckingham, UK and Philadelphia, USA: Open University Press.

SGOMSEC (Scientific Group on Methodologies for the Safety Evaluation of Chemicals). (1996). *Proceedings of the 12th SGOMSEC workshop*, Rutgers: New Jersey.

Sharpe, L. A. (2000). The commodification of the body and its part. *Annual Review of Anthropology*, 29, 287–328.

Shakespeare, T., & Erikson, M. (2000). Different strokes: Beyond biological determinism and social constructionism. In: H. Rose & S. Rose (Eds), *Alas, poor Darwin* (pp. 229–248). New York: Harmony Book.

Shilling, C. (1993). *The body and social theory*. London: Sage Publications.

Spallone, P., Wilkie, T., Ettorre, E., Haimes, E., Shakespeare, T., & Stacey, M. (2000). Putting sociology on the bioethics map. In: J. Eldridge, J. MacInnes, S. Scott, C. Warhurst & A. Witz (Eds), *For sociology*. Durham: Sociology Press/British Sociological Association.

Stabile, C. A. (1994). *Feminism and the technological fix*. Manchester: Manchester University Press.

Taylor, J. S. (2000). Of sonograms and baby prams: Prenatal diagnosis, pregnancy and consumption. *Feminist Studies*, 26(2), 391–418.

Tomm, W. (1992). Ethics and self-knowing: The satisfaction of desire. In: E. Browning-Cole & S. Coultrap-McQuinn (Eds), *Explorations in feminist ethics: Theory and practice*. Bloomington: Indiana University Press.

Turner, B. (1987). *Medical power and social knowledge*. London: Sage Publications.

Turner, B. (1992). *Regulating bodies: Essays in medical sociology*. London and New York: Routledge.

Turner, B. (1996). *The body and society* (2nd edn.). London: Sage.

Urla, J., & Terry, J. (1995). Introduction: Mapping embodied deviance. In: J. Terry & J. Urla (Eds), *Deviant bodies: Critical perspectives on difference in science and popular cultures*. Bloomington, IN: Indiana University Press.

Wajcman, J. (1991). *Feminism confronts technology*. University Park: Pennsylvania State University Press.

Warren, V. L. (1992). Feminist directions in medical ethics. In: H. B. Holmes & L. Purdy (Eds), *Feminist perspectives in medical ethics*. Bloomington: Indiana University Press.

Williams, S., & Bendelow, G. (1998). *The lived body: Sociological themes, embodied issues*. London: Routledge.

Witz, A. (2000). Whose body matters? Feminist sociology and the corporeal turn in sociology and feminism. *Body and Society*, 6(2), 1–24.

PART IV: RE-IMAGINING BIOETHICS: EXPANDING THE BORDERS OF BIOETHICAL INQUIRY AND ACTION

Why does bioethics need to be re-imagined? And what would a re-imagined bioethics look like and do? These questions are at the heart of this section. The bioethics enterprise in the United States has taken a very particular form, as many sociological commentators have pointed out. At the center of bioethics is autonomy as the dominant feature of the bioethics landscape. This emphasis on autonomy has its roots in American individualism, as well as the congruent history of bioethics and the civil rights movement in the United States. With autonomy at the center of the frame, many other features of the landscape loom large: attention to the individual as the epicenter of the bioethical dilemma, a concordant emphasis on rights, an enduring inattention to the social relationships in which individuals are embedded, the institutions that constrain individual action, and the social structures that channel individual lives, and, finally, the heavy weight accorded to the provision of information to enable patient-directed decision making as the ultimate ethical duty of the clinician. Relegated to the background – indeed more often than not barely visible on the far horizon – are welfare, care, justice, kin, culture, and society itself. While the sociological critique of bioethics for this peculiarly narrow and microscopic view is not new, the three chapters in this section prove that it remains as relevant as ever. More importantly, they demonstrate how expanding the borders of bioethics to encompass the social context actually affords us a stronger vantage point to assess the moral significance of our actions.

A second sociological critique of bioethics targets the assumption that the four principles are universal and applicable in any situation, anywhere. According to the dominant view, the principles in effect constitute the map by which any bioethical terrain may be traversed. Yet as the still-flourishing controversy over research ethics in developing countries demonstrates, the map that contemporary American bioethics provides can, at best, sometimes lead us far astray of our own ethical goals; at worst, it may take us down a path that veers dangerously close to the worst historical abuses of research subjects. These three essays remind us that only by attending to the local topography can we avoid missteps and dead ends. Tausig, Subedi and Subedi in particular suggest that bioethics, like politics, is local, that is to say, patterned by prevailing social conditions.

Moreover, all three chapters concern one of the most favored topics of contemporary American bioethics: the human genome. Chaufan deconstructs the debate over a diabetes gene. Tausig, Subedi and Subedi report on a research project to uncover a genetic susceptibility to helminthic infection. Shostak and Rehel likewise describe efforts to decontextualize human subjects by emphasizing the role of genetics in determining risk status. Genetics has a checkered history when it comes to the gap between the ideal and the actual, the promised and the real. But genetics – or genomics as it is now known – has been a central preoccupation of bioethics more or less from the field's inception. The prime status of genetics within bioethics is a reflection of the fact that the two more or less co-evolved (Jonsen dates "the birth of bioethics" from the promulgation of the Nuremberg code in 1947, while Watson and Crick discovered the structure of DNA in 1953). But there are many other parallels between genetics and bioethics: the focus on the individual (what could be more individualized than a person's genome?), the romance with technological possibilities, and a preoccupation with the liberating value of more and more information. These three papers, in particular Chaufan's and Shostak and Rehel's, point out the blindspots in bioethics' fascination with the genome. Not surprisingly, this critique is related to the first: an undue focus on the individual (the genome), to the exclusion of the social (the environment).

What *would* a re-imagined bioethics look like? The three chapters in this section offer us a view into that landscape. First, they insist that we widen our angle of vision to include the past as well as the future. Bioethics typically operates as a forward-looking enterprise, one that emphasizes novelty (for instance, how to cope with emerging technologies) while often overlooking the perennial dilemmas that bedevil medicine. Yet these authors demonstrate that context matters, in multiple ways. Not only do we need to understand the current social situation, we also need to trace the trail by which we arrived at this particular ethical juncture: How have historical and cultural forces landed us where we are? Each paper is centrally concerned with not only "what to do" in a given situation, but also how we got there in the first place. What features of the social system led us to this particular configuration? For most bioethicists, the social landscape remains virtually uncharted, because it is simply out of the frame, irrelevant. These three papers insist that we understand that social landscape before we even begin to contemplate the ethics of the situation. They argue that we cannot "do ethics" without first comprehending something of the social forces that shaped whatever terrain we find ourselves in, however familiar, however alien. C. Wright Mills' sociological imagination, with its insistence on seeing the connections between personal troubles and public issues – is apparent in this reframing.

In order to accomplish this reframing, these authors shift our focus away from the personal and towards the public. Significantly, these three papers all owe an intellectual debt to Link and Phelan's foundational paper on "social conditions as fundamental causes of disease." The distribution of health and illness in any society is inextricably related to the distribution of resources and opportunities in that society. Since medicine – whether in the form of clinical care or biomedical research – is centrally concerned with changing that distribution of health and illness (even if it does so only at the margins), so must bioethics be concerned with the social distribution of resources and harms. Politics is not just medicine writ large, as Virchow famously argued. Politics is also bioethics writ large. Here these authors encourage us to grapple with the political economy that shapes each of these instances of "bioethics," whether the impact of social stratification in Chaufan's chapter, the "90–10 gap" in Tausig, Subedi and Subedi, or environmental racism in Shostak and Rehel.

Finally, precisely because they take matters of political economy to be fundamentally ethical concerns, these authors insist that we engage seriously with the most neglected of the four principles, justice. That justice receives short shrift in much of bioethics is commonly acknowledged. What these chapters do is to begin to show us both why this happens and why it matters so much. The authors show us in Tausig, Subedi and Subedi's words "subjects embedded in pathogenic social and economic environments" and make the case that charting those pathogenic environments ought to be part and parcel of the bioethics endeavor. Justice involves distributional issues – that is, who gets what – but not just who gets the rare heart transplant, but also who gets to live where, next to the toxic dump or on the other side of town. These issues are typically seen as outside the purview of bioethics.

How do these papers achieve this re-imagining of bioethics? Each shows us a different feature of this new bioethical terrain. Chaufan forcefully challenges bioethics to take seriously not only the manifestation of disease at the individual level, but also the distribution of disease in society. Thus, she not only foregrounds justice, but she also socializes it. It is not enough, she argues, for bioethicists to consider what is just in any given clinical scenario. Rather, justice centrally concerns the distribution of disease – who gets sick in the first place, not just what to do after that person is sick and in need of care. Bioethics has traditionally been preoccupied with questions of *who lives* and *who dies* – that is to say, with our coming in and our going out. Chaufan reminds us that what happens to us in between the two landmark events of our lifespan matters too; *who gets sick* (and from what causes) ought to be a matter of bioethics as well. She asks, "Should bioethics concern itself with how the distribution of social power, rights and burdens shapes patterns of health and disease in human populations?" Using the rising incidence of type 2 (non-insulin-dependent, or so-called adult-onset) diabetes among children, she charts the ways in which both the biomedical and the public discourse about this disease not only blame the victim, but also distort our sense of solutions to this epidemic, "contributing to the problem of diabetes by misrepresenting it." Chaufan focuses on debates about the genetics of type 2 diabetes, arguing that to posit diabetes as a genetic disease is to mistake biology for genes, social circumstance for physiological fate. She argues that "disparities are not mere differences, but differences that are avoidable, unnecessary and unjust." Her chapter exhorts us to remember that disease disparities are rooted not in genetic differences among population groups, but in social injustice.

In their investigation of a biomedical research project situated in rural Nepal, Tausig, Subedi and Subedi also confront the ways in which social context determines illness. Like Chaufan, they contend that reliance on the individual biomedical model constrains the ability of bioethics to make a difference in resource-poor settings, like that of the Nepalese village they report on. They tackle head-on the vexed matter of research ethics in settings marked by inadequate health care and extreme poverty. They categorize current positions within bioethics around this much-debated issue as, on the one hand, universalistic, and on the other, relativistic. According to the first, exemplified by the Helsinki Declaration, there is but one model of bioethics governing research regardless of locale. A human subject in Helsinki is no different from a human subject in Katmandu. In contrast, the relativist position, as captured in the CIOMS accord, argues that ethics is local and culturally specific. As Tausig, Subedi and Subedi show, each of these arguments is a way of *thinking* about the ethics of engaging human research subjects, but neither provides much of a template for *doing* research involving human subjects. In their view, that is because both "formulate research ethics in individualistic, patient-centric terms rather than in aggregate population and structural terms." They use the Jiri Helminth Project to illustrate how biomedical researchers might ethically engage human subjects in locales that are almost unimaginably deprived by Western standards. Most significantly (and perhaps paradoxically), this approach treats individuals *as communities*. The researchers involved in the Jiri Helminth Project find that the ethical way to treat their Jirel subjects is not to single them out for special treatment, but rather to raise the level of care offered to the entire Jirel village, regardless of formal participation in the research trial. Like Chaufan, this paper explicitly links bioethics not only to social justice, but also to public health. Moreover, Tausig, Subedi and Subedi suggest expanding the meaning of beneficence, from the provision of good at the individual, clinical level, to the provision of good to the group *qua* group.

Like the two papers that come before, the chapter by Shostak and Rehel critiques the prevailing bioethical model of individualism, noting a troubling synergy between ways of conceptualizing the individual in bioethics and nascent ways of conceptualizing the individual in environmental science. They are particularly interested in "what constitutes human subjects." In bioethics, as in science, the human subject "exists largely independent of social context ... inhabiting an imagined social world in which autonomy, equality, and agency are more or less equally available to all." Shostak and Rehel point out that "dimensions of human subjectivity remain under theorized in bioethics" – and in particular that bioethical notions of the human subject tend to obscure the social factors that shape human vulnerability. Likewise, they delineate the ways that contemporary environmental health scientists work to "bring the human in," arguing that, paradoxically, molecularization in environmental health science actually brings the human subject into sharper focus. In shifting away from their reliance on animal models, environmental health scientists open "the black box of the human body." Yet another consequence of this molecularization is the shift from regulating toxic chemicals in the environment to regulating the behavior of genetically susceptible individuals. Shostak and Rehel problematize this shift by reminding us that toxic waste does not just happen; it is locally – and inequitably – situated, and it is minority populations who are most likely to bear "the burden of environmental exposures." In shifting their focus towards "the black box of the human body," environmental health scientists run the risk of neglecting to map where exposures occur, what social agglomerations are disadvantaged, and the "intersecting forms of inequality" that accrete in some bodies, leaving others unscathed.

Shostak and Rehel mount perhaps the most radical challenge to bioethics in this section. They suggest that at precisely the moment of a major paradigm shift in environmental health science when bioethics might be most relevant, it also threatens to lead environmental health scientists farthest astray. As in Chaufan's analysis, Shostak and Rehel show us how leaving context out leaves us pointing the finger at the victim, in this case the genetically at-risk individual who failed to manage his exposure to a toxic environment.

So, what then, in these authors' eyes, is a re-imagined bioethics good for? Chaufan argues that a re-imagined bioethics reveals a path towards social change and social justice. "Reframing would be the beginning of social change," in her words. Tausig, Subedi and Subedi provide a map out of the ethical quagmire that has dogged biomedical research in less-developed countries. Shostak and Rehel take us inside the social structure of ethical implications, arguing that what is a "challenge" for bioethics is in fact "an opportunity for sociology." Each of the chapters in this section argues for expanding the borders of bioethics by engaging the sociological imagination. These authors demonstrate how sociologists can serve as the advance scouts in what has heretofore been terra incognita for bioethicists. The lens shifts from the microscopic to the panoramic, taking in the configuration of the situation in toto, rather than in disconnected pieces. These three chapters suggest that we need to ask different questions both in and of bioethics. In bioethics we must ask, how does the social world in which individuals are embedded shape our understanding of what counts as ethical dilemmas? And of bioethics, we must ask, how can this way of thinking about the world become an instrument for the achievement of social justice?

Elizabeth Mitchell Armstrong
Editor

WHAT DOES JUSTICE HAVE TO DO WITH IT? A BIOETHICAL AND SOCIOLOGICAL PERSPECTIVE ON THE DIABETES EPIDEMIC

Claudia Chaufan

ABSTRACT

Since World War II, rates of type 2 diabetes (henceforth diabetes) have skyrocketed, leading to talk of an "epidemic," believed to result from formerly "adaptive" genotypes colliding with "affluent" postindustrial societies – largely their food excesses and physically undemanding jobs. Hence, experts describe diabetes as a struggle between biology and behaviors – "genes-as-destiny" and "lifestyles-as-choice" – said to have spared no social group. However, racial and ethnic minorities and the poor are affected disproportionately.

In this paper I challenge the "genes–lifestyle" framework and argue that the epidemic, particularly its distribution, is produced not by affluence but by poverty. The cumulative effect of malnutrition or hyperglycemia during pregnancy, of stunting in young children, of structural constraints over healthy lifestyles, and of the lack of a right to adequate medical care, which are all the results of poverty, leads to diabetes and its complications, and to disparities in their distribution among social groups. Hence, diabetes disparities are not mere differences

Bioethical Issues, Sociological Perspectives
Advances in Medical Sociology, Volume 9, 269–300
ISSN: 1057-6290/doi:10.1016/S1057-6290(07)09011-0

but differences that are avoidable, unnecessary, and unjust. I also highlight selected conceptual problems of the genes–lifestyle framework that mislead about the potential contributions of genetics to human health.

I conclude that because the roots of the diabetes epidemic lie in inequities in social power, the solutions required are not medical but political, and ought to concern a sociologically informed bioethics. I also conclude that insofar as dominant accounts of the diabetes epidemic ignore or downplay these roots, they will legitimize research and policies that reproduce or even increase diabetes disparities. The paper is part of a larger project on the political ecology of diabetes.

SHOULD WE CARE?

Only recently has the discipline of bioethics come to be recognized as an independent field of inquiry, with an agreed-upon subject matter, body of literature, methods of analysis, and so forth. The word "bioethics" itself as an endeavor different from, and broader in scope than, its more narrowly focused intellectual relative, medical ethics, was coined in the 1970s by the oncologist Van Rensselaer Porter, and in 1978, the *Encyclopedia of Bioethics* defined it as a discipline engaged with "the systematic study of the moral dimensions – including moral vision, decisions, conduct, and policies – of the life sciences and health care, employing a variety of ethical methodologies in an interdisciplinary setting" (Reich, 1995, p. xxi), not only providing a working definition of the field, but also building toward its current social and intellectual status. But bioethics as a *social practice*, i.e., as ethical thinking around issues of life, death, health, and disease, for the purpose of guiding human action, is a much older endeavor. It was after all in Ancient Greece that Hippocrates is credited with having commanded those with the capacity to heal that they would "use (their) power to help the sick to the best of (their) ability and judgment (and) abstain from harming or wronging any man by it" (Lloyd, 1983, p. 67).

What about when this power to heal or harm is exercised by a society as a whole, more specifically, by a set of social, economic, and institutional arrangements that determine to a great extent the distribution of social goods and burdens, and in so doing, enhance or undermine people's capacity to remain healthy or recover from disease? To sociologists interested in the ethical dimension of health and disease, it makes sense to ask, should bioethics concern itself with how the distribution of social power, rights, and burdens shapes patterns of health and disease in human population? Put otherwise, should bioethics use the "sociological imagination," defined by Wright Mills (1959) as the ability to relate history and biography, to understand how the history of a structure of privileges and disadvantages affects the distribution of health and disease, and in so doing, the biography of individuals whose lives are marked by disease? If we take John Rawls' concept of justice – and justice undeniably is, or at least should be, of interest to those concerned with ethics – any concern with justice should include an examination of the principles that organize the distribution of rights and burdens in society, and of their effects on human welfare (Rawls, 1958). This is no easy feat. Aristotle defined justice as giving to each one his or her due – a just person, he said, "does not award too much of what is choiceworthy to himself and too little to his neighbor ... but awards what is proportionately equal; and he does the same in distributing between others" (Aristotle, 1995, p. 397). The problem is that Aristotle left it to us to decide who owes what to whom in complex societies, or which principles we should follow to distribute social wealth equitably, i.e., in accordance with justice.

Whatever the case, sociologists know well the importance of social goods – of power, rights, and burdens – in the production of disease: They have known this for at least 200 years, ever since the work of social reformers like Friedrich Engels showed that it was the appalling conditions of the industrial towns that caused the precarious health of English workers, and not, as was largely believed at the time, their weak morality (Engels, 1968). And yet, from a cursory examination of the table of contents of textbooks in bioethics, it is apparent that the distribution of social goods and its impact on human health is hardly a topic of interest to contemporary bioethics, filled as these tables are with a range of important, yet very limited in scope, topics – the right to live (Is abortion murder? Should we save the life of a gravely impaired newborn?); the right to die (Should physicians help terminally ill patients end their lives?); patient autonomy (How much medical information should be disclosed to patients?); or how to deal with sophisticated medical technologies (Is stem cell research "playing God"? What are the limits of assisted reproduction?). If distributive justice issues figure at all, they address the realm of the unusual (What moral principles should regulate the distribution of organs for transplants?), or, in the United States, the debate, resolved by all other industrialized nations, of whether medical care ought to be treated as a social right or as a commodity whose purchase is left to the discretion and economic capacity of "consumers." And even then, these issues figure only as an afterthought, typically in the last chapters.

In this essay, I do not attempt to explain the conspicuous absence, in the field of bioethics, of a concern with the distributive justice of basic social goods and with the implications of this distribution for human health. Rather, I make the case that the distribution of social goods deserves the attention of bioethicists at least as much as questions of autonomy or of sophisticated medical technologies do. Why? Because this distribution literally produces patterns of health and disease, obviously acting through and upon physical bodies, and can do so since the moment of conception – type 2 diabetes, which I use as a case study to develop my thesis, is a case in point.[1] If this distribution is unjust, and there are good reasons to believe it is, then the unequal distribution of disease that ensues is unjust as well – indeed a measure of social injustice – and should figure therefore not merely in the table of content of textbooks in bioethics but also in public debates about how, as a society, we, as Hippocrates commanded, "use (our social) power to help the sick to the best of (our) ability and judgment (and) abstain from harming or wronging any man by it."

In order to build my case, I review the evidence for the role of poverty and social exclusion in the production of a biological predisposition to type 2 diabetes (henceforth diabetes), drawing from diabetes-relevant medical and policy literature and from my own analysis of public discourses on the diabetes epidemic (Chaufan, 2006). My goal is twofold: first, to show that the "sociological devil" lies in the biological details of diabetes, by which I mean that in the production of a biological, albeit not genetic, predisposition to insulin resistance, the key cellular malfunction underlying diabetes (Reaven, 1988), the structure of opportunities and disadvantages plays a key role, especially crucial during the fetal stage and the first years of life, such that it is virtually impossible to "attack" the current epidemic without attending to its structural roots; second, to draw attention to expert accounts of the problem of diabetes, which overwhelmingly attribute it to an evolved "genetic susceptibility" colliding with "affluent" lifestyles (Bernstein, 2000) and to show that these accounts are plagued with conceptual confusions that muddle the diabetes waters, leaving out much of what is relevant to the disease, and intentionally or not, blaming its very victims.

If my thesis is correct, and dominant accounts of the epidemic are contributing to perpetuating the problem of diabetes by misrepresenting it, then these accounts should be challenged, and the problem reframed, for the sake of human health and of social justice. And if "frames are mental structures that shape the way we see the world ... the goals we seek ... and the institutions we form to carry our policies" (Lakoff, 2004, p. xv), then changing our frames should lead to changing disease-producing institutions and policies. Reframing would be indeed the beginning of social change.

THE MAKING OF A MODERN EPIDEMIC

A few years ago, my interest in the relationship between health and social justice, and my research into racial and ethnic disparities in a "new" clinical form of diabetes, of early onset, led me to Riel, a Canadian boy of mixed German and Native heritage. Riel, who was back then 10 years old, was considered at "high risk" for diabetes at least on three counts: his heredity, his weight, and his sedentary lifestyle. This boy challenged the conventional medical wisdom that I had been schooled in: In Argentina, in 1990, as a diabetes specialist-in-training, I had learned that diabetes affected the young only exceptionally, and only those from very specific racial and ethnic backgrounds, assumed to bear a rare "genetic susceptibility" to the disease. Pima Indians in Arizona were one such case. During our first encounter, Riel's mother, Debra, told me about her struggles with her own diabetes, about a husband lost to heart disease, and about her usually failed attempts to make ends meet. I also learned that she worried because when she was pregnant with Riel, the doctor had warned her that her high blood sugar levels, which she had been unable to control, would affect the baby, although how exactly it was unclear to her. Debra was also concerned about Riel's "spare tire and lack of physical activity." When sharing her concerns with her mother-in-law, an old-age pensioner with limited financial resources, the woman had said: "Let's be honest, Debra, we just don't have the money for any of the food and activities other people can afford to keep their children healthy."

What would have been a medical oddity a mere 20 or 30 years earlier was anything but about the time I encountered Riel, when the words "diabetes" and "epidemic" first "met" each other in a headline of the *New York Times*, heading the news that at a rate of 6% of Americans affected by diabetes, there was "evidence of an unfolding epidemic" (Associated Press, 2001, p. A8). Today, diabetes in the young is no longer rare – quite the contrary, hand in hand with its "twin sister," childhood obesity, it is affecting an increasing number of children and youth who by their 30s or even 20s will already be victims of diabetes complications, such as kidney failure, foot amputations, blindness, and heart disease (Rosenbloom et al., 1999), and already accounts for up to half of the new cases of diabetes among children (Fagot-Campagna, 2001). The cost of diabetes in the United States alone has been estimated to be over 130 billion dollars (1 out of 10 health-care dollars), and counting (American Diabetes Association, 2003). While these costs do not discriminate among different types of diabetes, type 2 diabetes, the true protagonist of the epidemic, accounts for at least 90% of all cases.

"Everybody," it has been suggested, may be affected by diabetes – all races and ethnic groups, all ages, and "the rich and the poor" (Diabetes Research Working Group, 1999, p. 13). It has also been suggested that certain racial and ethnic groups, typically non-white, are particularly "susceptible" to diabetes by virtue of their genetic makeup (Smith, 1992). Indeed, the consensus that while nurture "pulls the trigger" it is nature that "loads the gun" is virtually unanimous; hence, the dominant account, produced by experts (Bernstein, 2000) and reproduced by the media (Maugh, 2000a), states that diabetes strikes only when formerly "adaptive" genotypes collide with the "excesses" of Westernized lifestyles – after all, not all lifestyle-related excesses result in diabetes. In the case of children, lifestyle-related excesses include "junk" food beating less-attractive counter-parts (like broccoli), and video games and television beating outdoor games, play, or sports. Television in turn entices children to consume "junk" through advertising, thus closing the vicious circle of obesity and diabetes (Hansen, Fulop, & Hunter, 2000). If only parents were more "aware" and paid more attention to their children's eating and playing habits! If only schools did their job of educating children in healthy lifestyles! If only children could be encouraged to cut down on fries, befriend broccoli, and stay away from video games!

Yet these facts about diabetes are not the whole story behind the new epidemic: While it is true that rates of obesity and diabetes are increasing among children worldwide, neither condition is affecting all of them equally. Children from racial or ethnic minorities are disproportionately affected (Fagot-Campagna et al., 1999), as are, and have been for over half a century, their adult counterparts, whose rates of diabetes and diabetes complications are two to six times greater than those of whites (American Diabetes Association, 2001). On the other hand, starved or chronically undernourished children, still very common in many parts of the world, seem to have been spared from this "new" childhood epidemic. So much then for diabetes and equality. As to "a disease of affluence," as diabetes is often referred to because of its alleged relationship with the "affluence" of the modern world (Fall, 2001), it is hard to think about the type 2 variety as a disease of the "affluent" if one is to make any sense of stories such as that of Riel and Debra, or of the estimates of the future of the disease: Toward the year 2025 there will be an increase in the prevalence of diabetes of 42% in industrialized nations, *yet of 170% in developing nations*, and within the wealthier nations, it is the lower classes, not the better off, who will be disproportionately affected (King, Aubert, & Herman, 1998). Thus, children and adults at "high risk" are not merely racial or ethnic minorities but also poor, with substantially fewer resources to remain free from diabetes.

(THRIFTY) GENES, LIFESTYLES, AND "PLUMP" POVERTY

To the occasional witness of the public debate on the problem of diabetes, the disease appears as a "mix" of "bad" genes and poor "lifestyle choices" – too much food, and too little exercise (Uusitupa, 2002). In turn, poor lifestyle choices appear to result from idiosyncratic cultures (Martorell, 2005; Hunt, Valenzuela, & Pugh, 1998; Poss & Jezewski, 2002; Tessaro, Smith, & Rye, 2005), psychological vulnerabilities (Heiby, Gafarian, & McCann, 1989), or plain and simple weakness of the will (Bernstein, 2000). This "genes–lifestyle debate" frames the problem of diabetes such that it allows no questions that cannot be answered in terms of either side, which appear different enough to allow for a "debate," yet resemble each other in subtle, albeit fundamental, ways: First, debaters take "biological" to entail "genetic"; second, they assume that "lifestyles" is what *really* matters about "environments" (Filozof & Gonzales, 2000); third, they grant that nature and nurture work *together* to produce diabetes and believe that the weight of their relative causal roles can be adjudicated a meaningful number; and fourth, they never question the existence of "diabetes genes" and suggest that while scientists struggle to find them, the best strategy is to "encourage" individuals to take charge of their health destinies, especially those who have the diabetes genes – which they *must* have, otherwise they would not have developed diabetes. In the case of children, it is families and care-takers that debaters call upon to "take charge" (Cummings, 2005). In the struggle for relative weights – how much corresponds to genes? How much to lifestyles? – much of what is relevant to diabetes gets lost in a sea of conceptual confusions and empirical inaccuracies about genetics, human behavior, and human health.

Let me begin with the "lifestyles" side. This side of the debate claims, with good reason, that lifestyles, basically what people eat and how much they move, have the power to cause or prevent diabetes (Imperatore,

Benjamin, & Engelgau, 2002). And indeed, research has compellingly shown that lifestyles so defined and diabetes go hand in hand, that risk for diabetes can be dramatically reduced with lifestyle modifications, and that genes have little to do with the results, which have been established in studies among Chinese, Finns, and Americans of varied ethnic backgrounds. Back in 1986, in the city of Da Qing, China, 577 individuals with pre-diabetes were randomly assigned to either a control group or one of three treatment groups: diet only, exercise only, or diet and exercise. The reductions in the risk of developing diabetes were of 31, 46, and 42%, respectively (Pan et al., 1997). In Finland, 522 middle-aged overweight subjects with pre-diabetes were randomly assigned to either an intense lifestyle modification program of weight reduction and physical activity or to a control group that did nothing. Those in the intervention group reduced their risk of diabetes by 58% (Tuomilehto, Lindstrom, & Eriksson, 2001).

Finally in the United States, 3,234 persons with pre-diabetes were randomly assigned to a control group, an intervention group with pharmacological treatment, and an intervention group with intensive lifestyle modification support. Compared with the control group, in the group subject to pharmacological intervention alone, risk of diabetes was reduced by 31%, while lifestyle group participants cut down their risk of diabetes by 58%. In all cases, results were achieved through a drastic reduction in insulin resistance, the basic metabolic defect underlying type 2 diabetes. Similarly, major clinical studies showed a dramatic reduction in diabetes complications – of up to 70% – when patients with either type 1 or type 2 diabetes were randomized to groups that followed either "conventional" or "intensive" treatments – the latter including very close medical supervision and diabetes education to support lifestyle changes and self-management of blood glucose (American Diabetes Association, 2002a, b). To note, in all cases, ethnicity, often (and wrongly) used as a proxy for medically meaningful genetic makeup, was irrelevant to the results.

Clearly, the effects of lifestyles on diabetes are beyond dispute. Yet social or economic circumstances may impose insurmountable constraints over healthy lifestyles. And they do indeed. Studies showing that under intensive lifestyle modification programs, medically relevant weight reduction was possible, also showed that in a mere five years those favorable results were no longer present (Swinburn, Metcalf, & Ley, 2001; Wing, Venditti, & Jakicic, 1998). More generally, major efforts to reduce morbidity rates through behavioral changes alone, while leaving the economic and social environments intact, such as the Multiple Risk Factor Intervention Trial, have proved disappointing in the long run (Multiple

Risk Factor Intervention Trial Research Group, 1982, cited in Syme, 1994). A group of primary-care physicians, after three years of dutifully making health promotion of 2,000 patients the center of their practice, became aware that the moment patients were left on their own (without the continuous input of exercise physiologists, dietitians, weekly support groups, and so forth), they returned to their usual state, and that the lower their income and the less privileged their social conditions, the faster their return to "normality" was (Guthrie, 2001). This awareness led the physicians to conclude that "it is not patients who don't understand, but we doctors who don't" and that unless the social and economic pressures faced by "high risk groups" were addressed with the right social policies, "health promotion (will help) no one" (ibid. p. 997).

On the "genes" side, several well-established observations are said to support the existence of genes that influence diabetes: the observations that the disease clusters in racial and ethnic groups; that it "runs in families" (Gloyn, 2003); that the concordance rate among identical twins is greater than among fraternal twins (Gloyn, 2003; Elbein, 2002); that significant correlations have been found between gene variants and diabetic states (Horikawa et al., 2000); and finally, that major single-gene "defects," spontaneously or artificially produced in the laboratory, are associated with elevated blood glucose (Shih & Stoffel, 2002). Evolutionary theories of diabetes have further endorsed the belief that diabetes is a "genetic disease": there exists a "thrifty genotype," goes a popular theory, which gave our Paleolithic ancestors a Darwinian edge when access to food was sporadic, by preventing the loss of valuable glucose through the kidney and increasing the body's efficiency to store calories (Neel, 1999). Those who had this genotype were more likely to survive and reproduce – they were "selected" by the evolutionary pressures of the "feast or famine" conditions of our Paleolithic past – hence, were more "successful" in the "struggle for existence" than less "adaptive" genotypes. Today, surrounded by environments where food is plentiful and the need for exercise minimal, the genotype is no longer advantageous, but "maladaptive." Populations at high risk for diabetes (e.g., Pima Indians, Native Polynesians) are presumed to be direct descendants of bearers of thrifty genes (Neel, 1999; Zimmet, 1979).

A number of caveats plague these explanations and, albeit largely ignored by studies in the genetics of diabetes, these caveats have been exhaustively addressed elsewhere (Lewontin, 1974, 2005; Sober, 2000; Joseph, 2004, 2006; Chaufan, 2007). Hence, I will only review one of them – familial aggregation – and only briefly, mainly to use it as a springboard to address more fundamental conceptual issues in genetics, whose misunderstanding can greatly mislead about the power of genetic knowledge to contribute to human health.

Does the fact that a trait – for instance, a disease – "runs in families" indicate that genes are involved? The short answer is no. A "trait" may run in families, i.e., may be "familial," yet have nothing to do with genes. *Familial* and *genetic* have different meanings – familiality is an *observation* that may or may not be *explained* by the action of genes. Many "traits" run in families for purely social or cultural reasons: language, religion, and social status. Children of English-speaking parents tend to speak English, to hold religious beliefs similar to their parents' (at least when they are young), and, if the parents are well off, to be well off themselves. How do we know that these attributes are not "in our genes"? Because we know the full social history of language, religion, and inherited privilege, and the mechanisms of social and cultural transmission. The problem with familiality, at least for those who wish to attribute it to genes, is that families share *both* genes and environments; hence, familial aggregation by itself, as basic genetic textbooks point out, is genetically uninterpretable – it indicates nothing about the cause or source of the observations (Griffiths et al., 1999). Hence, the claim that a positive family history of diabetes "indicates" that both genes and environments play a role (Gloyn, 2003; Freeman & Cox, 2006) is at best trivially true, and at worst misleading if used to suggest something – typically "disease genes" – that there is simply no evidence for.

A compelling instance of ideology getting in the way of sound science is illustrated by the social history of pellagra. At the turn of the twentieth century, experts believed in a "genetic predisposition" to pellagra, *because* the disease "ran in families" (Kevles, 1995) – Southern families who clearly shared not just their genes but the same impoverished nutrition. The failure of experts to make a connection between poverty, poor nutrition, and disease prevented them for many years to understand the true nature of pellagra, now well recognized as a vitamin deficiency (Rajakumar, 2000). At any rate, as it has been noted, even if such thing as a "genetic predisposition" to pellagra *had* been discovered, it would have been rendered irrelevant by the federally-mandated Word War II program requiring that flour and corn meal, the basic staples of poor families, be enriched with vitamins, and in so doing wiping out the disease in the United States (Joseph, 2000). Yet in our day, the familial aggregation of diabetes is hailed in and of itself, time and again, as providing "evidence" that the disease is "genetic" and as providing good reason to believe that "dissecting the genetics of this complex disorder ... will help to halt the rise in morbidity and mortality associated with [it]" (Gloyn, 2003, p. 122).

The question of labeling a disease "genetic" brings us to probably what is most important about human genetics, and about genetics more generally: A claim that a disease, or any "trait" for that matter, is "genetic" needs to make reference to environmental variables contributing to the said trait – otherwise the claim is biologically empty. Organisms are the product of *both* genes and environments. And although virtually everybody agrees on this truism, its implications for diabetes genetic research are rarely acknowledged in searches of "diabetes genes." Let us explore these implications briefly: A basic distinction in genetics is that between *genotype* and *phenotype*. By *genotype* geneticists refer to the DNA of an organism, i.e., the hereditary material; *genotype* contrasts with *phenotype*, i.e. any structural, functional, or behavioral trait of an organism. Organisms and their phenotypical variations are the non-additive product of their genotype, the sequence of environments they encounter as they develop and grow, and developmental random noise (random molecular motions) (Lewontin, 2000). The "norm of reaction," a property of the genotype that has been known in experimental genetics for close to a century, represents this triadic relationship between genotypes, phenotypes, and environments (Lewontin, 2000; Schmalhausen, 1949).

When, in elaborating the norm of reaction for a given genotype, the variable "environment" is plotted in the x-axis against the variable "phenotype" in the y-axis, it becomes apparent that under different environments the phenotypes for any given genotype vary. It also becomes apparent that, with the rare exception of mutants, the relationship between genotypes and their corresponding phenotypes is not consistent as environments change. Put otherwise, a plant with genotype A may be taller than one with genotype B at sea level but shorter than plant B at 3,000 m of altitude and identical in height to B at 1,400 m. This relationship is illustrated by an experiment where seven specimens from a California herb of the genus *Achillea* were collected from the wild, and three cuttings were obtained from each. Cuttings obtained from a single plant were obviously genetically identical to one another yet different from those obtained from other plants (Lewontin, 2000). Each cutting from the same plant was planted at three different altitudes. The genotype that grew the tallest at sea level was not the tallest at 1,400 or at 3,050 m. Similarly, the one that grew the tallest at 3,050 m was not the tallest at the other levels. In fact, not a single one of the seven genotypes was consistently taller or shorter than all others over the range of environments, and for some genotypes, some environments made no difference to their height (Fig. 1).

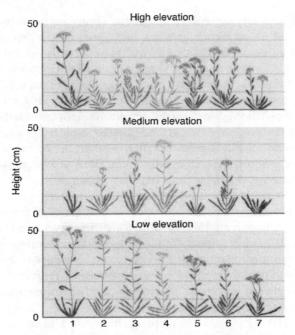

Fig. 1. Parental Plant (Source of Cuttings).

This experiment, illustrating the norm of reaction for height of different genotypes of a simple herb, shows that expressions of the sort "genes for trait X," "genes influencing condition X," or "such and so organism has a genetic tendency to X" are biologically empty until all relevant environments are specified and included in the claim. "Tendencies" do not occur in a vacuum, and a "gene for tallness" at sea level may become a "gene for shortness" at 3,050 m of altitude. It also follows that there is no way to compare two genotypes along any trait, be it length or insulin resistance, unless all environments relevant to the trait are included, and specified. Moreover, finding the relationship between two genotypes under one environment gives no clue as to what the relationship will be under another environment – whether "greater than," "lesser than," or "equal" (Fig. 2).

Norms of reaction have been fairly well studied in experimental plants and animals where genetic and environmental variables are comparatively easy to manipulate – at least in the case of traits that are easy to define and measure, such as height. Yet, elaborating norms of reaction for

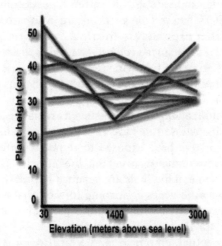

Fig. 2. The Norms of Reaction for Cuttings From Seven Different *Achillea* Plants Grown at Three Altitudes.

complex human traits presents at least three challenges for medical genetic research: first, defining what will count as a "trait"; second, identifying all environments relevant to the development of the trait in question; and third, controlling these environments (empirically, not statistically) to study how they interact with relevant human genes – genes that ought to be identifiable from non-relevant genes; otherwise the whole enterprise would collapse – to produce health or disease.

But of course in human populations, both securing genetically identical "specimens" to "grow" under different environments *and* manipulating these environments throughout the time of the development of the traits of interest is empirically very difficult and ethically out of the question. For this reason we simply do not know the norm of reaction of virtually any interesting and complex human trait (Lewontin, 2000). And for the same reason we cannot know which gene variants influencing such traits are "good" or "bad," assuming that we could agree upon a non-arbitrary definition of "ideal" environment, which, as follows from the *Achillea* example, is a tricky business – what is "ideal" for one genotype may not be so for another one.

Now, if we take these biological facts seriously, the implications for human health and for diseases like diabetes are huge: It is clearly incorrect to claim that some individuals are more "genetically predisposed to diabetes" than others unless *both of them* are compared along a scale of insulin resistance after exposure to *exactly the same range of environments relevant to insulin resistance in the course of its development* – as I have shown so far, and expand on in the following section, in the case of diabetes, these environments are multiple and exposure to them begins very early in life. And if one thing is certain, it is that populations with radically different rates of diabetes and its complications, such as racial and ethnic minorities in the United States, whose rates are two to six times higher than that of whites, are likely to have been exposed to radically different sequences of diabetes-relevant environments over the life course. Of course what is usually *meant* by "some individuals are genetically predisposed to diabetes" is that their idiosyncratic genes contribute to their diabetes *all other things being equal.* But this ceteris paribus clause is precisely the problem that has yet to be resolved, for the reasons stated above.

While these conceptual, empirical, and ethical reasons preclude us from making claims about "diabetes genes," they do not preclude us from making claims about diabetes-protecting environments, and from using our knowledge of them for practical purposes. By this I mean that we do know, and with a substantial amount of detail, which are the human environments where "desirable" (non-diabetic) or "undesirable" (diabetic) phenotypes are likely to appear. For instance, we know that poverty (an environment) and diabetes (an undesirable phenotype) go hand in hand, a knowledge that is confirmed every time somebody cares to measure it (Nicolucci, Carinci, & Ciampi, 1998; Morikawa et al., 1997; Forssas et al., 2003; Bachman et al., 2003; Green et al., 2003; Chaturvedi et al., 1998; Evans et al., 2000) and that is unlikely to be disconfirmed any time soon. As I noted above, we also know that when so-called high-risk individuals are given excellent support to make lifestyle changes, their risk of diabetes drops by more than half, and that excellent medical care dramatically reduces diabetes complications in both the major types of diabetes. Moreover, we have reason to believe that genotypes make no difference to these substantial gains.

Hence, if our goal is to minimize the number of individuals with "diabetic" or "diabetic complications" phenotypes, we seem to know well which environments we should secure. To be sure, doing so might require a redistribution of social resources more radical than anybody is prepared to tolerate, because, for better or worse, there is no single or simple intervention that can secure diabetes-protecting environments over the life course and wipe out the disease, as was the case with pellagra. At any rate, my point is to show that it follows from a well-known and studied concept in genetics, i.e., norm of reaction, that if we wish to eliminate or substantially reduce diabetes and diabetes disparities, it is not knowledge of how to do it that is lacking, even if, as genetic researchers point out time and gain, "the genetic etiology of diabetes remains elusive" (Elbein, 2002, p. 2012).

And yet, a review of over 50 studies on the "genetics of type 2 diabetes" found not a single one that even addressed the question of norm of reaction for insulin resistance (Chaufan, 2006). And expert claims about "diabetes genes" in certain groups, but not in others, proceed unfazed (Thompson Beckley, 2006) and are reproduced uncritically by the media (Maugh, 2000a, 2000b). For example, a recent investigation of the diabetes epidemic by the *New York Times* noted that while diabetes was rampant in East Harlem, it was almost non-existent in the Upper Westside (Santora, 2006). And yet, the report dutifully reproduced expert views that the epidemic in East Harlem was the result of "social factors and genetics" (ibid., A1). Now, it may or may not be true that the genetic makeup of Latinos and African Americans in East Harlem is different enough from the genetic makeup of residents in the Upper Westside in ways that are relevant to the differences between their rates of diabetes. Yet there is no doubt that their respective diabetes-relevant environments are different enough to invalidate any claim, implying that these high rates are caused, in whole or in part, by anybody's special genes – given the conditions of the observation, nothing can be inferred about such genes. The "experiment" that could test a genetic hypothesis would at the very least equalize social environments in both neighborhoods over several generations – at a minimum, it would secure good nutrition and quality medical care of pregnant women and young children, and would provide reasonable access to all residents to healthy lifestyles – and it is yet to be conducted.

This is not to say that genes do not influence diabetes in *some* way. There is no aspect of the human condition that is not influenced by our human genome in some trivially true way: It is *partly* due to my genes that I am able to write an essay that somebody else will publish (also *partly* due to *their* genes) and hopefully others will read and enjoy (also partly due to *their* genes). Chimps cannot write, publish, or read, *partly* because of their genes. But it does not follow from these obvious facts that we can identify specific genes influencing these "capacities" and "target" them independently from relevant environmental components (e.g., years of education).

Likewise, however true it may be that genes contribute to diabetes – a contribution that, as noted above, appears to make no difference to how

successfully individuals respond to quality preventive or treatment interventions – it does not follow that the causal contribution of the alleged genes
can be identified and "targeted" independently from diabetes-producing
environments. Moreover, as diabetes genes are "identified" in North
American Natives (Hegele & Hanley, 1999), Mexican Americans (Horikawa
et al., 2000), or African Americans (Acton et al., 1994), to mention but a
few, it becomes less clear how exactly the information could be applied to
address the impending public health catastrophe of increasing racial and
social disparities in the disease, or how this information would make a
difference to interventions that it would have been wise to have in place
anyway.

THE DIABETES EPIDEMIC AND THE BIOLOGY
OF POVERTY

Given this state of affairs, it would seem reasonable to conclude that the
best hope for defeating diabetes, including its new variety, type 2 diabetes of
early onset, is to focus on raising awareness of the dangers of the disease
through massive health promotion campaigns spreading the healthy lifestyle
gospel and targeted very specially to individuals and families "at risk," while
betting on the abilities of "high risk" children to overcome the social and
financial constraints that defeated their parents. At least this appears to be
the primary public health strategy in the United States these days, as follows
from the frequent press releases of the US Department of Health and
Human Services "encouraging" all Americans to make a personal commitment to eat healthfully and increase their levels of physical activity
(US Department of Health and Human Services, 2002; US Department of
Health and Human Services and USDA, 2005; US Department of Health
and Human Services and National Institutes of Health, 2005; USDA and
USDHHS, 2005), or from well-meaning calls to parents in "high-risk"
communities to educate their children about the benefits of vegetables
(Cummings, 2005). So, is this not the obvious, or even the only, way to go?
    Well, not quite. As compelling medical research has shown, high-risk
status for diabetes may develop way before individuals begin to make
choices, or to "lead" lifestyles, healthy or unhealthy, in any meaningful
sense of the term – that is, in the womb. What is known as the "Barker
hypothesis," "thrifty phenotype hypothesis" (Hales & Barker, 1992),
or "biological Freudianism" (Dubos, Savage, & Shaedler, 2005), i.e., that

abnormal "uterine environments" affect fetal development in ways that predispose to diseases, including diabetes, later in life, has been experimentally demonstrated in animals (McCance & Widdowson, 1953; Benyshek, Johnston, & Martin, 2004) and observed in humans in longitudinal epidemiological studies (Barker, 2003; Ravelli et al., 1998). Malnutrition in pregnant women induces in the fetus the insulin-resistant state that lies at the heart of type 2 diabetes, as indicated by a seminal study conducted among individuals born during the Dutch famine in World War II, which showed that participants with low birth weight born to mothers who had experienced hunger during mid and late gestation, when the pancreas of the baby develops, were more insulin resistant, hence biologically predisposed to diabetes, than the participants with normal birth weight (Ravelli et al., 1998). Another study showed that as birth weight decreased, glucose intolerance, an indicator of insulin resistance, increased, and that individuals with the lowest weight at one year of age had three times the death rates from heart disease as adults than those with normal weight (Hales & Barker, 1992). These outcomes have been interpreted as indicating the effect of interferences with early growth and development, or "fetal programming," programming meaning "a permanent or long-term change in the structure or function of an organism resulting from a stimulus or insult acting at a critical period of early life" (ibid., p. 596).

The programming of insulin resistance resulting from nutritional deprivation during the fetal stage has been replicated experimentally in rats (Benyshek et al., 2004), and is rarely a matter of dispute. And it is also well accepted that its effects do not stop at birth, but continue into the very first years of life. Insulin resistance is also induced by stunting, the failure to thrive due to lack of basic nutrients in early childhood, which currently impairs the adequate metabolic development of at least 200 million children under the age of five throughout the world, and predisposes them to heart disease, obesity, and diabetes (Branca & Ferrari, 2002), independently of ethnic background, as indicated by a study that included children from Russia, Brazil, South Africa, and China, and showed a strong association between stunting and overweight status (an insulin-resistant state) later in life (Popkin, Richards, & Montiero, 1996).

Similarly, high levels of blood glucose when the pregnant woman is diabetic and poorly controlled induce in the fetus vulnerability to diabetes and to other conditions later in life (Freinkel, 1964, 1980; Jovanovic & Pettitt, 2001). The mechanism appears to be the burden placed on the developing pancreas by a uterine environment rich in glucose, as indicated by a study showing that fetuses of diabetic mothers responded to their mothers' elevated blood glucose levels by increasing their own secretion of insulin, hence overworking their fetal pancreases and developing insulin resistance. Later in life, 33% of these children were pre-diabetic, compared to only 3.7% of those whose insulin secretion during their uterine life had been normal. Yet another study of siblings born either before or after their mothers were diagnosed with diabetes showed that the risk of developing the disease increased significantly if the sibling was born *after* the mother had been diagnosed with the disease rather than *before* (Dabelea et al., 2000). These mechanisms, impairment of fetal pancreatic development and early insulin resistance due to malnutrition or poorly controlled diabetes in the mother, or poor nutrition in small children, can combine over generations to produce increasingly high rates of diabetes, such as those observed among so-called high-risk populations, typically, albeit not exclusively, ethnic and racial minorities.

The hypothesis of an intergenerational, non-genetic reproduction of diabetes through a sequence of nutritional mishaps is substantiated by a study examining the nutritional history of a native North American tribe, the Havasupai, in the context of the tribe's political history. In this study, Benyshek, Martin, and Johnston (2001) showed that forced relocations and reservation life in the late nineteenth century and the first half of the twentieth century had affected the nutrition of generations of women who had experienced hunger during their pregnancies, which in turn had affected the glucose tolerance of their offspring. Post–World War I, this tribe was faced with high-calorie diets and little physical activity in the reserves, which compounded the glucose intolerance "wired" in utero and led to very high rates of diabetes, especially among women bearing multiple pregnancies, signaling the beginning of the diabetes epidemic among the Havasupai, and conceivably among many Natives worldwide who experienced similar nutritional and political histories. Currently, argue the researchers, the biological predisposition to diabetes is being reproduced by generations born to poorly monitored diabetic mothers and exposed to the unhealthy lifestyles of the reserves at earlier and earlier ages. More recently, Benyshek et al. (2004) and Benyshek (2006) have tested this intergenerational, non-genetic hypothesis in rats, showing that when compared to a control group (from the same breeding colony, hence with minimal genetic variability) pups born to malnourished dams were low birth weight and glucose intolerant as young adults, and developed diabetes when they became pregnant, delivering a third generation that was insulin resistant and very sensitive to high-calorie diets, and whose insulin resistance was extremely refractory to dietary manipulation. And yet, over

90% of the articles on the etiology of diabetes among Pima Indians in a search in the database of the National Library of Medicine simply ignored these facts and set out to hunt for "diabetes genes" (Chaufan, 2006).

The bottom line is, these mechanisms cause irreversible damage in the development of organs and key metabolic pathways and lead to insulin resistance or pre-diabetes. And all of them are influenced by a structure of opportunities and disadvantages that fosters, or gets in the way of, healthy pregnancies and childhoods. And when these "biologically-wired-for-diabetes" children become the cheap labor of the global economy, their early-developed "susceptibility," that is clearly biological, yet has nothing to do with their genes, makes them all the more vulnerable to the calorie-dense, sedentary environments affordable by the only low-paying jobs available to them, if they are lucky enough to be employed. In fact, this is the case of developing countries, where nutritional deficiencies early in life often combine with calorie "excesses" later in life to produce a host of chronic diseases, including skyrocketing rates of diabetes (Prentice & Moore, 2005). This historical sequence of mechanisms is consistent with the prediction that it is the poor, especially in rural and urbanizing communities in China and India, not the "affluent," who will bear the brunt of the diabetes epidemic in the twenty-first century (Amos, McCarty, & Zimmet, 1997). And their high risk will be produced by early-life mechanisms that cannot be meaningfully construed as the "lifestyles" of small children, let alone of developing fetuses.

Moreover, far from being a "problem" of poor nations alone, it also bedevils the wealthiest nation in the world, the United States, where at least 13 million children live in poverty, four times the child poverty rate of Western European nations (Koch, 2000a). Among them, at least 12 million suffer from, or are at risk of, hunger (Koch, 2000b). The combination of poor fetal conditions, undernutrition at an early age, and constraints on healthy lifestyles, including on a healthy nutrition, at a later stage, is likely to thrust them into the ranks of those affected by the "new childhood epidemic." Vis-à-vis these biological and social facts about diabetes, one wonders why the Congressionally-appointed Diabetes Research Working Group, in its report *Conquering Diabetes: A Strategic Plan for the 21st century*, would have concluded that "the *only* way to reduce the tremendous burden of [diabetes] is through intensified biomedical research" (Diabetes Research Working Group, 1999, p. 1, emphasis added).

Clearly, what might be called "plump poverty," a kind of contemporary poverty characterized by social deprivation in an environment of relative nutritional abundance rarely figures among risk factors for diabetes. Whenever it is referred to in the expert literature, it is rarely recommended as the site for "aggressive" interventions. Rather, mentions to developmental mechanisms of disease production with plausible and well established links with poverty are usually made to "fit" gene–lifestyle type of explanations. For instance, experts may insist that whatever the health status of the mother, fetuses with "bad" genes are more likely to become diabetic (McCance et al., 1994). Or they may grant that a poorly controlled diabetes in the mother may pose risk on the health of the baby, and insist that pregnant women be warned (or, more benevolently, "educated") about such risks, as Debra was, as if warning were what poor pregnant women needed to handle the demands of diabetes, pregnancy, and poverty. Or they may acknowledge that poverty may actually *cause* diabetes, yet reframe this acknowledgment to make fit the explanations that take the status quo, i.e., the existence of poverty, as an unchangeable "given" (Chaufan & Weitz, 2007). For example, an article in a leading diabetes journal that concluded that "(low) socioeconomic status ... can determine a risk [of diabetic complications] not dissimilar from *hard* clinical variables" (Nicolucci et al., 1998, p. 1439) did not call for an "attack" on poverty to resolve the problem, but for "specific *educational* interventions, *targeted* to the socially disadvantaged strata of the population" (ibid.).

While I do not dispute that being educated is important and may even matter to one's health, as it has been pointed out, if the poor of the world were suddenly educated and able to read Kant's *Critique of Pure Reason*, the rank of the unemployed would not ipso facto disappear – although they would be more literate (Lewontin, Rose, & Kamin, 1984). Similarly, it seems unreasonable to expect that education alone will improve the health of the poor when it is poverty itself that led to its deterioration – in fact, it is quite conceivable that both poor health and lack of education indicate poverty status. Yet the assumption that the fundamental problems of the poor lie not in their lack of money but of something else – awareness, motivation, or education – is common in the medical literature, and often leads to the odd belief, exemplified by the quote above, that if the poor have poor health *because* they are poor (and for this reason lack reasonable access to healthy lifestyles, medical care, and so forth), their health can be improved and health disparities eliminated by doing anything and everything *except* eliminating, or at least relieving, poverty (Chaufan & Weitz, 2007).

In sum, the reduced life chances of Riel and his mother are usually, and remarkably, invisible in studies pointing to the developmental origins of adult disease. I am setting aside other notable silences in the expert literature on diabetes – the disease-producing effects of racial discrimination (Williams & Collins, 1995), of the feminization of poverty (Doyal, 1995), and of the many aggregate-level variables (concentration of fast food stores, sidewalks, parks, neighborhood safety) that have been shown to account for a variety of diseases – diabetes among many others – and that cluster disproportionately in poor communities (Berkman & Macintyre, 1997).

INEQUALITIES OR INEQUITIES?

In sum, if one is to gauge the relative importance of genes to the diabetes complex in order to make decisions about the best use of public moneys, it appears that claims about them stretch far beyond what the evidence from the very life sciences warrants, and that they do not deserve the disproportionate amount of diabetes research dollars they currently receive (Chaufan, 2006). As to lifestyles, I am not suggesting that deprived social environments *rather than* "unhealthy" health behaviors explain high-risk status for diabetes. Both are logically and empirically compatible and play a role in the causal chain leading to diabetes and to disease more generally, a feature of human health that has been exhaustively examined and tirelessly theorized in the tradition of social medicine and social epidemiology for at least 200 years (McKeown, 1979; Black, 1996). What appears to be the difference between this tradition and modern epidemiological practice is that the latter conceives of a "web" of causes of disease where the "spider" is invisible (Krieger, 1994). Put otherwise, while it is obvious that multiple factors contribute to disease states and can be construed as "causes," "modern" epidemiologists, in contrast to social or "traditional" ones, believe that the order of factors, which involves a sequence and a history, is unimportant – mere "statistical noise" that can be conveniently parceled out so that each specialist can move on with his or her business.

Yet the sociological approach, that social epidemiology is an instance of, tells us that it is precisely the history and order of disease-producing factors that matter, and shows that putting social and economic equity first will resolve many of the "puzzles" in health disparities, including the current explosion of "adult diabetes" among children. In switching from *equality* to *equity* I assume, as I noted at the beginning, that the social inequalities leading to the current diabetes inequalities are not mere differences but differences that are avoidable, unnecessary, and unjust, and hence rightfully fall under the jurisdiction of bioethics (Daniels, Kennedy, & Kawachi, 1999).

I will not argue for a particular conception of justice, but rather follow Daniels et al. (1999), who apply John Rawls' theory of justice to the analysis of social inequalities in health. Building on their work, I will argue that in addition to the well-established lifestyles leading to diabetes, where people might disagree on the degree of responsibility attributable to those leading those lifestyles, there are two moments in the life course, fetal stage and early childhood, where the mechanisms leading to a biological vulnerability to diabetes depend directly on access to social resources that are beyond the power of the sufferers – fetuses or young children – to do anything about. Because these resources are distributed not merely unequally but inequitably, one result of these differences, i.e., the unequal distribution of diabetes, is a marker of social injustice.

As Daniels, Kennedy, and Kawachi point out, Rawls did not mention health as one of the primary goods that, according to his theory, ought to be equitably distributed.[2] Yet the authors make the case that health is implied by Rawls' conception of justice. Briefly, Rawls argued that for a society to be just, it ought to be organized according to principles of social cooperation that free and equal citizens would agree to. The principles are those of *equal liberty*, *equal opportunity*, and what Rawls called the "*difference principle*," one that would guarantee that inequalities are permissible (i.e., just) only to the extent that they are to the greatest advantage of the worst off. Rawls put further constraints on the citizens engaged in the task of determining the principles of social cooperation that will organize their society, stating that they were to do so under a "veil of ignorance" that would prevent them from knowing, at the moment of choosing, what their lot in life, or even their preferences or dislikes, would be. These principles would then be applied to the distribution of primary goods and to the regulation of political, economic and social institutions.

Social justice, said Rawls, is constitutive of the basic structure of society. By basic structure he meant those social institutions, the effects of whose actions are crucial because they "are so profound and present from the start (of the life of an individual)" (Rawls, 1971, p. 7). According to Rawls, the social positions that people are born into result in inequalities in the distribution of social resources that affect life chances in profound ways and that cannot be attributed to merit. Hence, a politically and socially just system should distribute primary goods in ways that make these initial unjust circumstances more just – in other words, to right what Rawls thought of as the results of the "natural lottery."[3]

How are these matters relevant to health? Daniels, Kennedy, and Kawachi argue that given that Rawls presupposed fully functional, healthy individuals participating in this social contract, that one of the principles of social organization calls for equality of opportunities, and that one of the proposed primary goods that ought to be distributed equitably (i.e., only constrained by liberty and the difference principle) is opportunities, health needs to be factored into the justice equation. Without health, there can be no equality of opportunities. Without health, at least one of the primary goods (opportunities) is undermined. If social arrangements are somehow leading to an inequitable distribution of health burdens – and as I have argued this is the case of diabetes – then inequalities in the current epidemic can be interpreted as indicating social injustice.

Now I can anticipate objections to the view that inequalities in social resources and power cause diabetes. After all, it sounds like those umbrella explanations that embrace too much and explain too little, pushing causes of disease to an infinite regress and failing to provide practical solutions to social problems. To the first objection, let me reply that numerous hypotheses have been developed and successfully tested under one such "umbrella explanation," the "fundamental cause explanation" for health and disease developed by Link and Phelan, showing that it is more than merely plausible that inequalities in social resources and power cause diabetes.

Link and Phelan (1995) have argued that knowledge, power, prestige, and beneficial social connections allow individuals to preserve or restore their health and that of their loved ones whatever the identified risk factors are at any given moment. Because a fundamental assumption of the theory is that knowledge, power, and beneficial social connections enhance individuals' ability to utilize whatever resources are *available* to protect themselves from particular conditions, the theory also predicts that social disparities should decrease or even disappear when such resources do not exist – when a condition is not preventable, not curable, or inevitable – and that patterns of distribution will be reversed over time as new knowledge or medical technologies become available and are applied successfully (Phelan & Link, 2005).

Indeed, when the researchers examined the distribution of highly preventable causes of disease and death, such as ischemic heart disease, chronic obstructive pulmonary disease or pneumonia, and compared it to the distribution of less preventable ones, such as pancreatic or prostate cancer, they found that socioeconomic status made a significant difference to the former and only a minor one to the latter. Moreover, they found that at ages 80 or later, the mortality advantage of high socioeconomic status disappeared (ibid.). As to the prediction that patterns of distribution will be reversed over time once new knowledge or medical technologies become available, this is exactly what happened with diabetes, which today affects the lower classes disproportionately, yet in the past preferred the better off, leading a doctor to claim, as late as 1928, that his patients were all from "prosperous circles" and that diabetes was "a disease of the rich" (von Engelhard, 1995, p. 7). This makes sociological and biological sense, because for most of human history, the poor rarely had the luxury of any kind of "abundance," including the abundance of calories that, combined with other factors, may lead to diabetes. Moreover, the connection between excess calories and diabetes was unknown at a time when elevated body weight was still a sign of prosperity; hence, not even the "prosperous" could benefit from the knowledge we now have.

Clearly, each time the capacity to control disease and death increases, whether with new knowledge or with new medical technologies, so increases the capacity of those with money, power, prestige, and beneficial social connections to use it. Close to 200 years ago, social reformers and social medicine practitioners knew this fundamental fact about human health all too well, which is what led Rudolf Virchow, a physician better remembered for his work on cellular pathology than for his reformist politics, to advocate reform in the workplace, not medical treatment, as a strategy to "conquer" the epidemic of typhus among workers in Upper Silesia (Waitzkin, 2000). In sum, to reconstruct the causal chain leading to diabetes, one does not need to go all the way back to the Big Bang to realize that meaningful claims about diabetes-producing lifestyles need to consider the constraints imposed by structures of privilege and disadvantage on those lifestyles.

As to the second (potential) objection, that this approach I am suggesting may not lead to "practical" solutions, it seems much less practical, even pointless, to call upon individuals to adopt diabetes-free lifestyles as a major public health strategy, as is often the case (National Diabetes Education Program, 2005) if by and large these lifestyles are beyond their reach. Moreover, emphasizing lifestyles leaves out much of what is biologically relevant to the production of diabetes, the very early stages of life. And it is certainly impractical to keep wondering about the emperor's new clothes – those elusive diabetes genes – if, as there is good reason to believe, his clothes are irrelevant to the problem, or worse still, he is naked. At any rate, gene hunts and "change-your-lifestyle" campaigns are not cheap. If money goes where the heart is, then the implications of all of the above for public health policies are huge, because they will translate into priorities that in turn guide social investments.

TREATING THE SYMPTOMS AND MISSING THE DISEASE: THE POLITICAL ECOLOGY OF DIABETES

My encounter with Debra, Riel, and her people have led me to some tentative conclusions about the epidemic of diabetes sweeping the globe and worrying experts and laypeople alike, and about racial and ethnic disparities in the distribution of disease more generally: There may not be that much difference after all among racial and ethnic minorities, or among these and the invisible white poor, vis-à-vis what *really* puts them at risk. For instance, the social and financial constraints against diabetes-free lifestyles that I observed among Mexican Americans in Northern California (Chaufan, 2000) pointed to a more fundamental commonality between them and Debra's people vis-à-vis diabetes than any particular fact about their heredity, behaviors, psyche, or culture. This commonality appears to be shared by low-income Appalachian whites, who are currently joining the ranks of "at-high-risk-for-diabetes" populations, and, to offset this risk, are being "encouraged" to adopt healthier lifestyles (Bailey et al., 2003), even as experts remain oddly silent about idiosyncratic genes (Chaufan, 2006), maybe because "poor whites" is no medical category to look for such genes.

In concluding, I offer the following observations: Today, the biology of diabetes is a "biology of poverty", *produced* by the inequitable distribution of social goods and power whose cumulative effects begin as early as conception: Fetal malnutrition, poorly controlled diabetes during pregnancy, and stunting in small children, all of them products of social exclusion, compound the diabetes-producing effects of a structure of disadvantage and reduced opportunities for health-promoting lifestyles and for access to quality medical care, and explain why diabetes today is not – and cannot be– an "equal opportunity disease," nor one of "affluence." Indeed, to continue to associate diabetes with affluence merely because it requires relative high intake of calories is an anachronism – in our day, excessive calorie consumption is perfectly compatible with poverty – and what is worse, leads to misguided attempts to replace much needed social change with mere band-aids – massive calls for lifestyle changes or elusive promises of genetic miracles – and has serious consequences for human health and for social justice.

The social production of the current epidemic and its unequal distribution among social groups warrants framing diabetes as a "political disease" (Benyshek et al., 2001), and calls for a political ecology framework, i.e., one that is concerned with the social, economic, and political institutions of the human environments where diabetes is emerging, as well as with how these institutions "distribute fundamental rights and duties and determine the division of advantages from social cooperation" (Rawls, 1971, p. 7), a question of social justice that should concern bioethicists. As to sociologists committed to social justice, we are ideally positioned to assume a leading role in this and similar inquiries. Our discipline was born from the union of two concerns: to understand how society works, and to use this understanding for the purpose of producing a better, more just, world. Over the years, we have developed powerful tools of measurement and analysis, and sharpened out theoretical eye, such that we are well equipped to advocate for positive social change.

In diabetes, this change requires at a minimum (1) that maternal and child welfare and health care become top policy priorities (Benyshek, 2005); (2) that medical care be treated as a social right; (3) that prescriptions for "lifestyle changes" only be discussed in the context of "life chances" – those structures of opportunities that have been theorized ad nauseam and whose effects on human health resurface every time somebody cares to measure them (Banks et al., 2006); (4) that the structural causes leading to diabetes be explicitly incorporated and prioritized in public debates about the epidemic; and last, (5) that the implications of these structural causes for social justice be acknowledged. Because diabetes is a paradigmatic "lifestyle-related" disease, this approach can be fruitfully applied to understanding similar conditions, whose roots are embedded in myriad aspects of daily life, hence defy "quick fixes" – a vaccine, one behavioral modification (e.g., quitting smoking), one nutritional supplement (e.g., the case of pellagra), or genetic engineering. All of this can help "conquer" diabetes and many other disease conditions, and decrease health disparities more generally, rather than merely treat the symptoms.

NOTES

1. The focus of this essay is type 2 diabetes, and unless I otherwise specify, all references to diabetes imply this type. The reason is both biological and sociological: Type 1 diabetes, the other major, albeit much less common, type, is biologically different from type 2 in ways that are relevant to a sociological analysis. The fundamental, and initial, metabolic impairment of type 2 diabetes, insulin resistance, is, I argue, sensitive to structural factors in ways that fundamental metabolic impairments of type 1 diabetes are not, at least as far as we currently know. Moreover, it is apparent that type 2 diabetes follows clear socioeconomic lines, which is not the case in type 1 diabetes, and this fact alone deserves a sociological analysis. Now once the diseases are present, complications from poorly treated or untreated

diabetes of *any* type do follow clear socioeconomic lines, and complications disproportionately affect the poor, while the better off are, literally, much better off.

2. Primary goods are those that any member of society, whatever the particularities of that society, would want more rather than less of. Rawls thinks of rights and liberties, powers and opportunities, and income and wealth as *chief* primary goods, and of health, vigor, intelligence, and imagination as *natural* goods, and contends that while the latter are influenced by the basic structure of society, "they are not so directly under its control" as the chief primary goods are (Rawls, 1971, p. 62). But he qualifies his contention saying that this categorization ought to be assumed "for simplicity." Given my belief that there exists a tight, causal connection between Rawls' chief primary goods and natural goods, I am not convinced that the division is correct or even useful for the sake of simplicity. In fact, I suspect that it may obscure precisely what matters about the relationship between these two types of goods for the purpose of social justice.

3. I beg to differ with Rawls about the "naturalness" of this lottery. In fact, I suspect that had Rawls known what we know today about the developmental origins of disease he would have also granted that when it comes to the causes of differences in rates of disease, very little is truly "natural".

REFERENCES

Acton, R., et al. (1994). Genes within the major histocompatibility complex predict NIDDM in African American women in Alabama. *Diabetes Care, 17*(12), 1491–1494.

American Diabetes Association. (2001). *Diabetes 2001 vital statistics*. Alexandria: American Diabetes Association.

American Diabetes Association. (2002a). Implications of the diabetes control and complications trial. *Diabetes Care, 23*, S24–S26.

American Diabetes Association. (2002b). Implications of the United Kingdom prospective diabetes study. *Diabetes Care, 23*, S27–S31.

American Diabetes Association. (2003). Economic costs of diabetes in the US in 2002. *Diabetes Care, 26*(3), 917–932.

Amos, A. F., McCarty, D. J., & Zimmet, P. (1997). The rising global burden of diabetes and its complications: Estimates and projections to the year 2010. *Diabetes Medicine, 14*, S7–S85.

Aristotle (1995). *Aristotle: Selections*. Indianapolis: Hackett Publishing.

Associated Press. (2001). Diabetes as looming epidemic. *New York Times*, New York, p. A8.

Bachman, M. O., et al. (2003). Socio-economic inequalities in diabetes complications, control, attitudes and health service use: A cross-sectional study. *Diabetic Medicine, 20*, 921–926.

Bailey, J., et al. (2003). QSource quality initiative. Reversing the diabetes epidemic in Tennessee. *Tennessee Medicine, 96*(12), 559–563.

Banks, J., et al. (2006). Disease and disadvantage in the United States and in England. *Journal of the American Medical Association, 295*(17), 2037–2045.

Barker, D. J. P. (2003). The developmental origins of adult disease. *European Journal of Epidemiology, 18*, 736–788.

Benyshek, D. C. (2005). Type 2 diabetes and fetal origins: The promise of prevention programs focusing on prenatal health in high prevalence Native American communities. *Human Organization, 64*(2), 192–200.

Benyshek, D. C. (2006). Glucose metabolism is altered in the adequately-nourished grand-offspring (F3 generation) of rats malnourished during gestation and perinatal life. *Diabetologia, 49,* 1117–1119.

Benyshek, D. C., Johnston, C. S., & Martin, J. F. (2004). Post-natal diet determines insulin resistance in fetally malnourished, low birthweight rats (F1) but diet does not modify the insulin resistance of their offsprings (F2). *Life Sciences, 74,* 3033–3041.

Benyshek, D. C., Martin, J. F., & Johnston, C. S. (2001). A reconsideration of the origins of the type 2 diabetes epidemic among Native Americans and the implications for intervention policy. *Medical Anthropology, 20,* 25–64.

Berkman, L. F., & Macintyre, S. (1997). The measurement of social class in health studies: Old measures and new formulations. In: M. Kogevinas, et al. (Eds), *Social inequalities and cancer - UARC Scientific Publications No. 138.* Lyon: International Agency for Research in Cancer.

Bernstein, G. (2000). 1999 presidential address: The fault, dear brutus. *Diabetes Care, 23*(4), 719.

Black, D. (1996). Deprivation and health: Chadwick lecture 1996. *Journal of the Royal College of Physicians of London, 30*(5), 466–471.

Branca, F., & Ferrari, M. (2002). Impact of micronutrient deficiencies on growth: The stunting syndrome. *Annals of Nutrition and Metabolism, 46*(Suppl. 1), 8–17.

Chaturvedi, N., et al. (1998). Socioeconomic gradient in morbidity and mortality in people with diabetes: Cohort study findings from the Whitehall study and the WHO multinational study of vascular disease in diabetes. *British Medical Journal, 316*(7125), 100–105.

Chaufan, C. (2000). To comply or not to comply: In search of the real question. *Clinical Diabetes, 18*(1), 46–47.

Chaufan, C. (2006). *Sugar blues: Issues and controversies concerning the type 2 diabetes epidemic.* Unpublished dissertation. In Sociology (p. 368). Santa Cruz: University of California.

Chaufan, C. (2007). How much can a large population study on gene-environment interactions and common diseases contribute to the health of the American people? *Social Science and Medicine, 65,* 1730–1741.

Chaufan, C., & Weitz, R. (2007). *The elephant in the room: The invisibility of poverty in research on type 2 diabetes.* Under revision in Sociology of Health and Illness.

Cummings, S. B. (2005). At home with diabetes. *Diabetes Forecast (Spanish Edition)* (Fall), 21–25.

Dabelea, D., et al. (2000). Intrauterine exposure to diabetes conveys risks for type 2 diabetes and obesity: A study of discordant sibships. *Diabetes, 49*(12), 2208–2211.

Daniels, N., Kennedy, B. P., & Kawachi, I. (1999). Why justice is good for our health: The social determinants of health inequalities. *Daedalus, 128*(4), 215–251.

Diabetes Research Working Group. (1999). *Conquering diabetes: A strategic plan for the 21st century.* Bethesda: NIH.

Doyal, L. (1995). *What makes women sick: Gender and the political economy of health.* New Jersey: Rutgers University Press.

Dubos, R., Savage, D., & Shaedler, R. (2005). Biological Freudianism: Lasting effects of early environmental influences. 1966. *International Journal of Epidemiology, 34*(1), 5–12.

Elbein, S. C. (2002). Perspective: The search for genes for type 2 diabetes in the post-genome era. *Endocrinology, 143*(6), 2012–2018.

Engels, F. (1968). *The condition of the English working class. 1845.* Stanford: Stanford University Press.

Evans, J. M. M., et al. (2000). Socio-economic status, obesity and prevalence of type 1 and type 2 diabetes mellitus. *Diabetes Medicine, 17*(11), 478–480.

Fagot-Campagna, A. (2001). Type 2 diabetes in children. *British Medical Journal, 322*(17 February), 377–378.

Fagot-Campagna, A., et al. (1999). Type 2 diabetes among North American children and adolescents: An epidemiologic review and a public health perspective. *The Journal of Pediatrics, 136*(5), 664–672.

Fall, C. H. D. (2001). Non-industrialized countries and affluence. *British Medical Bulletin, 60*, 33–50.

Filozof, C., & Gonzales, C. (2000). Predictors of weight gain: The biological-behavioral debate. *Obesity Reviews, 1*, 21–26.

Forssas, E., et al. (2003). Widening socioeconomic mortality disparity among diabetic people in Finland. *European Journal of Public Health, 13*(1), 38–43.

Freeman, H., & Cox, R. D. (2006). Type-2 diabetes: A cocktail of genetic discovery. *Human Molecular Genetics, 15*(2), R202–R209.

Freinkel, N. (1964). The effect of pregnancy on insulin homeostasis. *Diabetes, 13*(3), 260–267.

Freinkel, N. (1980). Of pregnancy and progeny. *Diabetes, 29*(December), 1023–1035.

Gloyn, A. L. (2003). The search for type 2 diabetes genes. *Aging Research Reviews, 2*, 111–127.

Green, C., et al. (2003). Geographic analysis of diabetes prevalence in an urban area. *Social Science and Medicine, 57*, 551–560.

Griffiths, A. J. F., et al. (1999). *Modern genetic analysis*. New York: W.H. Freeman and Company.

Guthrie, C. (2001). Health promotion helps no one. *British Medical Journal, 323*(October 27), 997.

Hales, C. N., & Barker, D. J. P. (1992). Type 2 (non-insulin-dependent) diabetes mellitus: The thrifty phenotype hypothesis. *Diabetologia, 35*, 595–601.

Hansen, J. R., Fulop, M. J., & Hunter, M. K. (2000). Type 2 diabetes mellitus in youth: A growing challenge. *Clinical Diabetes, 182*(2), 52–60.

Hegele, R., & Hanley, A. (1999). Youth-onset type 2 diabetes (Y2DM) associated with HNF1A S319 in aboriginal Canadians. *Diabetes Care, 22*(12), 2095.

Heiby, E., Gafarian, C., & McCann, S. (1989). Situational and behavioral correlates of compliance to a diabetic regimen. *The Journal of Compliance in Health Care, 4*(2), 101–116.

Horikawa, Y., et al. (2000). Genetic variation in the gene encoding calpain-10 is associated with type 2 diabetes mellitus. *Nature Genetics, 26*(2), 163–175.

Hunt, L., Valenzuela, M., & Pugh, J. (1998). Porque me toco a mi? Mexican American diabetes patients' causal stories and their relationship to treatment behaviors. *Social Science and Medicine, 46*(8), 959–969.

Imperatore, G., Benjamin, S. M., & Engelgau, M. (2002). Targeting people with pre-diabetes. *British Medical Journal, 325*(24), 403–404.

Joseph, J. (2000). Potential confounds in psychiatric genetic research: The case of pellagra. *New Ideas in Psychology, 18*(1), 83–91.

Joseph, J. (2004). *The gene illusion: Genetic research in psychiatry and psychology under the microscope*. New York: Algora Publishing.

Joseph, J. (2006). *The missing gene: Psychiatry, heredity, and the fruitless search for genes*. New York: Algora Publishing.

Jovanovic, L., & Pettitt, D. J. (2001). Gestational diabetes mellitus. *Journal of the American Medical Association, 286*(20), 2516–2518.
Kevles, D. (1995). *In the name of eugenics: Genetics and the use of human heredity.* Cambridge and London: Harvard University Press.
King, H., Aubert, R., & Herman, W. H. (1998). Global burden of diabetes, 1995–2025: Prevalence, numerical estimates, and projections. *Diabetes Care, 21*(9), 1414–1431.
Koch, K. (2000a). Child poverty. *CQ Researcher, 10*(13).
Koch, K. (2000b). Hunger in America. *CQ Researcher, 10*(44).
Krieger, N. (1994). Epidemiology and the web of causation: Has anyone seen the spider? *Social Science and Medicine, 39*(7), 887–903.
Lakoff, G. (2004). *Don't think of an elephant: Know your values and frame the debate.* White River Junction: Chelsea Green Publishing.
Lewontin, R. C. (1974). Annotation: The analysis of variance and the analysis of causes. *American Journal of Human Genetics, 26*, 400–411.
Lewontin, R. C. (2000). *Human diversity.* New York: W.H. Freeman and Company.
Lewontin, R. C. (2005). The fallacy of racial medicine: Confusions about human races. *GeneWatch,* 18(4), 5–7, 17.
Lewontin, R. C., Rose, S., & Kamin, L. K. (1984). *Not in our genes: Biology, ideology and human nature.* New York: Pantheon Books.
Link, B., & Phelan, J. (1995). Social conditions as fundamental causes of disease. *Journal of Health and Social Behavior, 35*, 80–94.
Lloyd, G. E. R. (1983). *Hippocratic writings.* London: Penguin Classics.
Martorell, R. (2005). Diabetes and Mexicans: Why the two are linked. *Preventing Chronic Disease (serial online),* Accessed on Jan 2005, Available from URL: http://www.cdc.gov/pcd/issues/2005/jan/04_0100.htm
Maugh, T. H. (2000a). Mutated gene tied to diabetes in some groups. *LA Times,* Los Angeles, p. A-1.
Maugh, T. H. (2000b). Gene discovery gives clue to diabetes' ethnic disparity. *San Francisco Chronicle,* San Francisco, p. A5.
McCance, D. R., et al. (1994). Birth weight and non-insulin dependent diabetes: Thrifty genotype, thrifty phenotype, or surviving small baby genotype? *British Medical Journal, 308*(9), 942–945.
McCance, R. A., & Widdowson, E. M. (1953). The effect of undernutrition upon the composition of the body and its tissues. *Acta Medica Scandinavica, 146*(1), 45–46.
McKeown, T. (1979). *The role of medicine: Dream, mirage or nemesis?* New Jersey: Princeton University Press.
Morikawa, Y., et al. (1997). Ten-year follow-up study on the relation between the development of non-insulin-dependent diabetes mellitus and occupation. *American Journal of Industrial Medicine, 31*(1), 80–84.
Multiple Risk Factor Intervention Trial Research Group. (1982). The multiple risk factor intervention trial-risk factor changes and mortality results. *Journal of the American Medical Association, 248*, 1465–1476.
National Diabetes Education Program, National Institutes of Health, and US Department of Health and Human Services. (2005). *National Diabetes Education Program Updates Campaign Empowering Older Adults to Manage Their Diabetes.*
Neel, J. (1999). When some fine old genes meet a "new" environment. In: A. Simopoulos (Ed.), *Evolutionary aspects of nutrition and health.* New York: Karger.

Nicolucci, A., Carinci, F., & Ciampi, A. (1998). Stratifying patients at risk of diabetic complications: An integrated look at clinical, socioeconomic and care-related factors. *Diabetes Care, 21*(9), 1439–1444.

Pan, X.-R., et al. (1997). Effects of diet and exercise in preventing NIDDM in people with impaired glucose tolerance. *Diabetes Care, 20*(4), 537–544.

Phelan, J., & Link, B. (2005). Controlling disease and creating disparities: A fundamental cause perspective. *Journal of Gerontology, 60B*(Special Issue II), 27–33.

Popkin, B., Richards, M., & Montiero, C. (1996). Stunting is associated with overweight in children of four nations that are undergoing the nutrition transition. *The Journal of Nutrition, 126*(12), 3009–3016.

Poss, J., & Jezewski, M. A. (2002). The role and meaning of susto in Mexican Americans' explanatory model of type 2 diabetes. *Medical Anthropology Quarterly, 16*(3), 360–376.

Prentice, A. M., & Moore, S. E. (2005). Early programming of adult diseases in resource poor countries. *Archives of Disease in Childhood, 90*, 429–432.

Rajakumar, J. (2000). Pellagra in the United States: A historical perspective. *Southern Medical Journal, 93*(3), 272–277.

Ravelli, A. C. J., et al. (1998). Glucose tolerance in adults after prenatal exposure to famine. *The Lancet, 351*(January 17), 173–177.

Rawls, J. (1958). Justice as Fairness. *The philosophical review, 67*(2), 164–194.

Rawls, J. (1971). *A theory of justice.* Cambridge: The Belknap Press of Harvard University Press.

Reaven, G. M. (1988). Banting lecture: Role of insulin resistance in human disease. *Diabetes, 37*(December), 1595–1607.

Reich, W. T. (1995). Introduction. In: W. T. Reich (Ed.), *Encyclopedia of bioethics.* New York: Simon and Shuster MacMillan.

Rosenbloom, A. L., et al. (1999). Emerging epidemic of type 2 diabetes in youth. *Diabetes Care, 22*(2), 345–354.

Santora, M. (2006). In diabetes fight, raising cash and keeping trust. *New York Times,* New York, p. A1.

Schmalhausen, I. I. (1949). *Factors of evolution.* Chicago: University of Chicago Press.

Shih, D. Q., & Stoffel, M. (2002). Molecular etiologies of MODY and other early-onset forms of diabetes. *Current Diabetes Reports, 2*(2), 125–134.

Smith, U. (1992). Life style and genes–the key factors for diabetes and the metabolic syndrome. *Journal of Internal Medicine, 232*, 99–101.

Sober, E. (2000). *Philosophy of biology. Dimensions of Philosophy Series.* Boulder: Westview Press.

Swinburn, B. A., Metcalf, P. A., & Ley, S. J. (2001). Long-term (5-year) effects of a reduced-fat diet intervention in individuals with glucose intolerance. *Diabetes Care, 24*(4), 619–624.

Syme, S. L. (1994). The social environment and health (Health and Wealth). *Daedalus, 123*(4), 79–86.

Tessaro, I., Smith, S., & Rye, S. (2005). Knowledge and perceptions of diabetes in an Appalachian population. *Preventing Chronic Disease, 2*(2), 1–9.

Thompson Beckley, E. (2006). Gene gives new insight into diabetes. *DOC News, 3*(June), 1–11.

Tuomilehto, J., Lindstrom, J., & Eriksson, J. (2001). Prevention of type 2 diabetes mellitus by changes in lifestyle among subjects with impaired glucose tolerance. *The New England Journal of Medicine, 344*(18), 1343–1350.

US Department of Health and Human Services. (2002). *HHS launches first national diabetes prevention campaign. "Small Steps, Big Rewards" aims at stemming rapid rise in diabetes across US.* Washington D.C.: US Department of Health and Human Services.

US Department of Health and Human Services and National Institutes of Health. (2005). *NIH News: The national diabetes education program supports take a loved one for a checkup day.* Bethesda: NIH News.

US Department of Health and Human Services and USDA. (2005). *New dietary guidelines will help Americans make better food choices, live healthier lives.* Washington D.C.: US Department of Health and Human Services.

USDA and USDHHS. (2005). *Finding your way to a healthier you: Based on the dietary guidelines for healthier Americans.* Washington D.C.: United States Department of Health and Human Services.

Uusitupa, M. (2002). Lifestyles matter in the prevention of type 2 diabetes. *Diabetes Care, 25*(9), 1650–1651.

von Engelhard, D. (Ed.) (1995). *Diabetes: Its medical and cultural history.* Berlin: Springer-Verlag.

Waitzkin, H. (2000). *The second sickness: The contradictions of health care in capitalist systems.* Lanham, Boulder, New York and Oxford: Rowman & Littlefield Publishers, Inc.

Williams, D. R., & Collins, C. (1999). US socioeconomic and racial differences in health: Patterns and explanations. *Annual Review of Sociology, 21*(1), 349–386. doi:10.1146/annurev.so.21.080195.002025.

Wing, R. R., Venditti, E., & Jakicic, J. M. (1998). Lifestyle intervention in overweight individuals with a family history of diabetes. *Diabetes Care, 21*(3), 350–359.

Wright Mills, C. (1959). *The sociological imagination.* London and Oxford: Oxford University Press.

Zimmet, P. (1979). Epidemiology of diabetes and its macrovascular manifestations in pacific populations: The medical effects of social progress. *Diabetes Care, 2*(2), 144–153.

SOCIOLOGICAL CONTRIBUTIONS TO DEVELOPING ETHICAL STANDARDS FOR MEDICAL RESEARCH IN VERY POOR COUNTRIES: THE EXAMPLE OF NEPAL

Mark Tausig, Janardan Subedi and Sree Subedi

ABSTRACT

This chapter discusses guidelines that specify the ethical standards for medical research in very poor countries in order to show how a sociological explanation of illness causation and health care access can offer some additional insight into the refinement of those guidelines. There has been considerable discussion on the proper ethical standards to apply given the context of extreme poverty and inadequate health care infrastructure that characterizes poor countries. Our analysis is intended to suggest that a sociological explanation for illness causation provides a clear justification for including the social context when specifying ethical guidelines and also clarifies the issues that must be addressed. This perspective is particularly sensitive to inequalities in health and access to health resources among

Bioethical Issues, Sociological Perspectives
Advances in Medical Sociology, Volume 9, 301–322
Copyright © 2008 by Elsevier Ltd.
All rights of reproduction in any form reserved
ISSN: 1057-6290/doi:10.1016/S1057-6290(07)09012-2

medical research subjects, and therefore addresses core issues of justice and beneficence.

Recent discussion and concern related to the ethical standards that circumscribe medical research in poor countries has focused attention on the limits of existing standards that are applied to such research (Macklin, 2004). In particular, the issues of beneficence and justice (standards of care) are difficult to specify within a social context of extreme poverty, social inequality, and poor institutional infrastructure. Also, issues of informed consent and the use of control groups that provide no intervention or sub-standard care have provoked considerable discussion. On the one hand, the social, economic, and political contexts are clearly related to the potential for research subjects to benefit from the research, their ability to provide informed consent and the definition of control conditions, while on the other hand, it is hard to hold researchers accountable for this context when designing research protocols and outcome assessments. The potential problems raised by such issues have been addressed largely by extending ethical protections that apply to medical research in developed countries. For example, the *Declaration of Helsinki* (WMA, 2000) has been amended to include residents of very poor countries as special populations who are entitled to increased protection and security. Similarly, *The International Ethical Guidelines for Biomedical Research Involving Human Subjects* (CIOMS, 2002), and the positions taken by the National Bioethics Advisory Commission and the Nuffield Council on Bioethics define such populations as economically disadvantaged and, hence, also entitled to special protection.

We suggest that this approach is limited because it implicitly makes assumptions about causes of illness (individualistic) and the locus of treatment that discourage a full appreciation of relevant ethical issues. Underlying the evolution of current ethical guidelines has been a belief that health/medical issues should be kept separate from the social context (Fox, 1989). The biomedical explanation for illness regards illness as having individual biological origins and physical consequences. This makes it difficult to understand the role that social context plays in causing illness and how medical institutional structures affect the course of illness. In developing countries the material and social contexts affect health in more obvious ways than in developed countries. We suggest that among other factors which influence the construction of ethical standards for research in poorer countries is the uncritical assumption of a biomedical model that makes it easier to formulate research ethics in individualistic, patient-centric terms rather than in aggregate population and structural terms. This assumption is also consistent with notions of personal autonomy and individualism that are hallmarks of western liberal capitalism and ethical standards for medical research in developed countries. The difficulty is that such an individualistic approach makes incorporating social contextual factors into a health research model difficult. As long as health/medical issues are delimited to exclude the social context, the importance of social factors for developing ethical research standards will continue to be problematic.

The sociological account of illness emphasizes the centrality of social structure as it affects exposure to health-related stressors (in the broadest sense) and access to health-related resources. In this view, health is not simply a function of individual exposure to health-compromising conditions or genetics. Rather, the material and social context are directly related to illness and must, therefore, be incorporated into explanations of illness causation. The model provides an opening toward the resolution of the health–society relationship as it affects ethical guidelines and may be useful to researchers, ethicists, and public health advocates alike.

That guidelines and declarations of principles have been developed for international medical research is an acknowledgement that there are differences in economic, commercial, political, social, and cultural interests and conditions that affect what is judged to be ethical conduct in medical research. Sometimes the differences are recognized only when controversy arises such as happened with the use of a placebo group in maternal-to-child HIV transmission studies conducted in Africa (Lurie & Wolfe, 1997; Varmuss & Satcher, 1997; Angell, 1997). More generally, guidelines have been developed because it is recognized that much medical research performed to benefit citizens and economic interests in the "developed" world uses research subjects living in the "undeveloped/developing world." This has raised significant questions related to justice, benefit, and respect – the three orienting principles for the ethical treatment of research subjects that have guided development of all protection of human subjects research standards.

To provide a perspective on just how different the economic and health conditions can be between developed and poor countries, we briefly compare the United States with Nepal. Nepal is a small, extremely poor country with a population of 23 million. Ninety percent of the population live in rural areas and engage in farming and animal husbandry. Only urban and few rural areas have access to electricity and clean running water. The magnitude of the difference in the wealth of these two countries is enormous. The per capita gross domestic product (GDP) in 2000 for Nepal was $1,224, while in the United States it was $34,677.

In comparison to the United States the health of Nepalese is very poor. Life expectancy in Nepal is 58 years compared to 77 in the United States. Nepal is one of few countries in the world where males outlive females, mainly due to high rates of mortality in childbirth. Infant mortality in Nepal ranges from 100–115 per thousand births compared to 7–9 in the United States. Despite these statistics, the annual population growth rate in Nepal is 2.4% compared to 1.1% in the United States, and the fertility rate in Nepal is 4.6 compared to 2.0 in the US (WHO, 2001).

The health problems in Nepal also differ from those in developed countries. Vitamin deficiencies and micronutrient-related disorders are widespread in Nepal (Gorstein, Shreshtra, Pandey, Adhikari, & Pradhan, 2003; Baral, Lamsal, Koner, & Koirala, 2002; Murdoch, Harding, & Dunn, 1999). Groundwater and well water contamination are significant problems (Shrestha et al., 2003; Khatlwada, Takizawa, Tran, & Inoue, 2002; Rai, Hirai, Ohno, & Matsumura, 1997). In a typical analysis of the health in a Nepali village, Rai et al. (1997) reported that only 32% of households had access to piped water, but even those with this water were not less likely to report gastrointestinal illness. Food-borne illness is also a substantial source of illness in Nepal. Meat, in particular, is a prime source of food poisoning and acquisition of parasites. An Animal Slaughtering and Meat Inspection Act has not yet been implemented in Nepal (Joshi, Maharjan, Johansen, Willingham, & Sharma, 2003).

Finally, socioeconomic status and gender also affect illness rates. Rous and Hotchkiss (2003) reported that income has a direct effect on the likelihood of becoming ill in Nepal. Low social class is also associated with early marriage, complications in childbirth, and maternal mortality (Shrestha, 2002). Women in general, are at substantial risk of birth complications because 90% of births are unattended by skilled personnel (Osrin, Tumbahangphe, & Shrestha, 2002).

The government has also been deficient in extending modern medical services to villages where the vast majority of the Nepali population reside (Subedi et al., 2000). Health posts lack trained personnel, medicines and supplies, and equipment. It often takes villagers days of travel on foot to even reach these health outposts.

This difference in wealth between these two countries translates into differences in health expenditures as well. The per capita expenditure on health in Nepal in 2000 was $12 compared to $4,499 in the United States, and per capita government expenditure on health was $4 and $1,992, respectively. Nepal derives 27.5% of its public health financing from external sources compared to 0% in the United States. The Nepali people pay 64% of health care costs out-of-pocket compared to 15.3% in the United States (all comparisons are from WHO, 2001).

By itself, this description would suggest that medical research conducted in Nepal should be focused on illness and treatment of health issues endemic to Nepal, and with the purpose of improving the health of Nepalese. Indeed, the *Declaration of Helsinki* requires that medical research conducted in a developing country must be related to significant local health problems.

The sociological perspective also strongly suggests that what constitutes ethical behavior in research in Nepal requires understanding that research subjects are embedded in a pathogenic social and economic environment. To sociologists social and economic conditions are "fundamental causes" of illness and must, therefore, be part of the development of ethical standards for health research.

CURRENT GUIDELINES AND THEIR LIMITS

Although there are various starting points for describing the history of the development of ethical guidelines for medical research in poor countries, we will focus on the recent (2000) revision of the *Declaration of Helsinki* and the 2002 version of *The International Ethical Guidelines for Biomedical Research Involving Human Subjects* (CIOMS, 2002). More specifically, we will discuss the critiques and controversies generated by these guidelines as they illustrate the limits of current guidelines. We will suggest that those limits largely reflect disagreements about whether and how to incorporate social and economic contexts into ethical guidelines. Much of the ambiguity and contention in the meaning and operationalization of the guidelines might be better understood from a sociological perspective. This perspective would not necessarily resolve the conflicts, but it would clarify the issues and provide a basis for dialogue.

In 1997, a series of articles raised concerns about the adequacy of existing ethical guidelines for medical research in developing or poor countries (Lurie & Wolfe, 1997; Varmuss & Satcher, 1997; Angell, 1997). The specific issue raised in these articles was with the research design for several studies of maternal-to-child transmission of the HIV virus. Studies had already been conducted in developed countries that demonstrated the efficacy of intravenous administration of AZT for reducing maternal-to-child HIV transmission. In the African studies, the control group was composed of subjects who received no treatment (placebo), while the experimental group received a short course of AZT. The placebo control group design raised issues of ethical standards of care. As well, the fact that the most effective delivery method determined in prior studies could not be reproduced in the African research sites because of expense and health infrastructure, suggested that the research would have little or no benefit within the countries supplying the experimental subjects.

Another issue that has been raised concerns the question of who benefits from the research. It has been suggested that much of the research in poor countries has little local public benefit. Medical research subjects are simply being exploited by Western economic interests. For example, the Pharmaceutical Research and Manufacturers Association argues that, "...the primary purpose of clinical trials is to advance the knowledge of *researchers* and *regulators* so that new treatments and cures can be developed" (PHRMA, 2002). The statement does not mention the research subjects or the general population. The public benefit of pharmaceutical research is often only indirectly available to research participants as the eventual development of new treatments and cures. This is clearly an issue for poor countries when drug trials demonstrate the efficacy of drugs that cannot be afforded by the country hosting the trials (Andrews, 2005).

Medical research projects conducted in poor countries have recently increased in number because it is cheaper to conduct research in poor countries, and because the regulatory climate is less demanding and vigilant (Brennan, 1999; Hofman, 1999). Shah (2002) notes that the number of foreign investigators seeking FDA approvals for drug testing increased 16 times between 1990 and 1999.

Existing guidelines do not address these issues adequately. Indeed, several authors raised the question of whether there was ever an ethical justification for conducting research in poor countries or if ethical standards that prevail in developed countries should be modified to fit conditions in poor countries (Del Rio, 1998; Shapiro & Meslin, 2001). As a result, bodies such as the World Medical Association (publishers of the *Declaration of Helsinki*) and the Council for International Organizations of Medical Sciences (CIOMS, an international, non-governmental organization established by the World Health Organization and UNESCO and publisher of the *International Ethical Guidelines for Biomedical Research Involving Human Subjects*), began a series of discussions intended to update their existing guidelines. As we will see, however, these revisions do not resolve the issues precisely because neither actually incorporates the relevant differences between developed and developing countries into the ethical debate.

The *Declaration of Helsinki* was revised in 2000 and the CIOMS guidelines were revised in 2002 in part to deal with controversies that arose from the revision of the *Declaration*. The differing positions taken by these two sets of guidelines both underscore the continuing points of controversy and suggest why a sociological approach may helpfully contribute to the discussion. The *Declaration* takes what could be called a "universalistic" approach to the problem, while the CIOMS has taken a "relativistic" approach (Tangwa, 2004). Our analysis will suggest that this is a false dichotomy that arises because of an unacknowledged attempt to keep the social context out of the ethical debate. The irony, of course, is that the discussion arises precisely because of the differences in the social, economic, and institutional contexts between developed and developing countries.

The issues of concern that the maternal-to-child HIV research (as well as other research) brought to the fore has to do with two matters. First, what level of care are research subjects entitled to receive? Second, to what extent are researchers obligated to continue to provide access to care after the research is concluded? As our description of the situation in Nepal illustrates, these are difficult matters to specify. In developed countries with well-established health care infrastructures it is much easier for researchers to circumscribe their study in terms of standards of care and access to care. This is so because research subjects often have independent access to health care outside of the research context. Access to the best available care and its continuation can be arranged by tapping into the health care system. But the situation is entirely different in poor countries where the best levels of care may not be available at all or may be prohibitively expensive. In this situation researchers might enter a host country, conduct their research and leave without materially affecting the health either of research subjects or the society in general. Indeed, many clinical drug trials that are now conducted in poor countries evaluate drugs that are not intended for use in the test countries and would be unaffordable, if available (Shah, 2002). In Nepal, a recent drug trial using Nepal army soldiers (including a placebo group) to test a Hepatitis E vaccine was conducted (also raising concerns about informed consent and coercion). The successful trials resulted in approval of the drug for use by the US army and as a "tourist" drug but the vaccine costs $60 and is not affordable by Nepali citizens (Andrews, 2005).

The revised *Declaration* contains two paragraphs that embody the approach we label as universalistic. Paragraph 29 specifies that the effectiveness of new methods should be tested against the *best* current methods. "Best," in this instance, means the best in the world, i.e., what is available in developed countries. Paragraph 30 specifies that at the conclusion of a study, every patient in the study should be assured of access to the best proven treatment, etc. In other words, study participants are entitled to standards of care that are available in the best health care systems, even if they live in countries with poor or no modern health care system. We term this approach universalistic because it does not recognize any distinction between richer developed countries and poorer developing countries. The same standards should be applied to all research regardless of where it is actually conducted. The position embodied here is one that renders the impact of social, economic, and health institutional difference moot. That is, the position insists on applying the identical ethical standards to medical research regardless of the context.

This position generated immediate controversy, much of it based on the "aspirational" implication that research in developing countries should reproduce conditions in developed countries (Macklin, 2001, 2004; Bhutta, 2002). The "relativist" position that embodies the contrasting perspective recognizes the desirability of the aspirations embodied in the *Declaration*, but also argues that the need to do research in developing countries to address matters of direct concern in those countries requires a more flexible and pragmatic approach. That is, social, economic, institutional, and cultural contexts condition the ethical dimensions of intended research but only in so far as they affect the operational definitions of ethical guidelines related to best practice and standards of care. Note however, that the actual effects of context on health are not considered, only the over-all effect on ethical behavior (i.e., the pragmatic consequences of attempting to satisfy universal aspirations).

The CIOMS guidelines, then, can be described as an attempt to align research practice with universal ethical principles while accounting for differing cultural context. The guidelines are largely concerned with assuring research subject autonomy and the protection of dependent or vulnerable populations. While it is recognized that social and economic conditions have sizable effects on health, the document specifically excludes considering these conditions in composing bioethical guidelines, "Sponsors of research or investigators cannot, in general, be held accountable for unjust conditions where the research is conducted…" (CIOMS, 2002, p. 11). But, as we will see shortly, this position leads to problematic solutions to concerns about reasonable availability, standard of care, and placebo-control standards.

The CIOMS document most specifically addresses the two controversial issues related to the 2000 revision of the *Declaration*, research in communities with limited resources (Guideline 10), and the choice of control in clinical trials (Guideline 11). According to these guidelines, research in poor countries must be responsive to the health needs and the priorities of the population or community in which it is carried out, and any intervention or product developed must be made reasonably available for the benefit of that population or community. Further, control groups should receive an established effective intervention rather than a placebo or no treatment (there are also specified exceptions when a placebo or non-treatment control group is deemed appropriate). Definitions of established effective intervention are related to the specification of standards of care.

The CIOMS guidelines while recognizing the importance of respecting the universalistic ethical principles of benefit, autonomy, and justice, suggest that the precise meaning of these principles is contextual and that research design and resource allocation must be assessed in a relativistic manner. These guidelines too, have been subject to much criticism precisely (in our view) because they are written within the limit of not accounting for "unjust conditions." This is both ironic in that the purpose of the guidelines is to address research in the context of unjust conditions and ambiguous because it is very hard to define standards without reference to those same unjust conditions.

According to Fox (1989) bioethics generally has neglected the social context (or institutional contexts of any kind) when constructing bioethical principles. Part of the reason for this is that many of the issues that stimulated the growth of bioethics are very specific to care issues in modern health care systems (including issues of abortion, euthanasia, organ transplants, and the treatment of very low birth weight children). But beyond that is a disciplinary "bias" to view ethical issues as a relationship between a researcher and a test subject (individualistic) and, we would argue, an uncritical use of the biomedical model that also views illness in individual terms. It is precisely this lack of recognition of the role that social and economic context play in causing illness and in treating it that prevents ethicists from formulating sound guidelines to deal with medical research in poor countries where the context plays such a direct and obvious role. Both the *Declaration of Helsinki* and the CIOMS guidelines recognize that the situation is different in poor countries but neither specifically incorporates these conditions into the creation of ethical guidelines. Instead the guidelines encourage researchers to assure certain levels of care and resources that approximate levels in developed countries when testing "protected" or vulnerable populations without dealing with what makes the populations subject to protection or especially vulnerable.

Macklin (2004), however, warns that if the different economic circumstances of developed and developing countries become morally relevant factors in specifying ethical research standards, then one risks creating a double ethical standard that distinguishes developed and developing countries. She argues that this is not acceptable because it does not adhere to *universal* ethical principles of respect for persons, beneficence, and justice. So the dilemma is that universal standards for medical research protocols are highly impractical in developing countries and their use might lead to the termination of all research in developing countries (or at least research sponsored by developed country interests), while a relativist position might create a double-standard that compromises ethical principles to the peril of developing countries and their citizens.

EXPANDING THE DEBATE

The current "debate" among those in the research bioethics community, then, attempts to resolve differences that we summarize as the universal and relativist positions. And as we have already pointed out, despite the origins of the debate in the recognition of the differing social, cultural, and economic contexts of developed and developing countries, there is also an explicit exclusion of these factors from the contrasting ethical positions. These irreconcilable differences have left the discussion sterile for the moment. In our view this has happened precisely because the relevant contextual factors have been excluded from the manner in which the ethical standards were constructed.

Researchers use the shorthand "10/90 divide" to denote the observation that less than 10% of medical research dollars are spent on diseases that account for 90% of the global burden of disease (WHO, 1990). This phrase acknowledges the social, economic, and institutional differences between developed and developing/poor countries that affect both the disease burden and health care resources. But the way that both universalists and relativists incorporate this fact prevents it from contributing more to ethical debates.

There are numerous voices that make it clear that ethical guidelines must account for the social context in more direct ways than either the *Declaration* or CIOMS guidelines now do. These voices are not only sociologists. Benatar and Singer (2000, p. 825) argue that, "considerations of context are required aspects of moral reasoning in the application of universal principals in specific situations and do not entail moral relativism." This approach attempts to resolve the dilemma by insisting that researchers become conscious of the processes and forces that lead to social inequality and then to include this analysis in the creation of specific ethical standards that would apply to a specific research project. Tangwa (2004) agrees with this prescription. He believes that each research situation requires a unique interpretation of ethical guidelines in such a way that the social, economic, and political contexts are specifically considered.

Others have suggested that the ethical issues we have been discussing focus too much on individual rights to the neglect of public health issues (Bhutta, 2002). Bhutta links research in developing countries directly to the public health enterprise. In doing so, he suggests that ethical issues need also to be understood (and specified) relative to the goal of improving the health status of the population. This criterion provides an additional anchor for ethical principles that account for the inequalities of the disease burden and public health status as well as societal economic conditions. Robert and Smith (2004) argue that as we come to recognize that health and illness are determined by social, economic, historical, as well as biological factors, we will need to develop an ethical perspective that focuses on population health. Such a perspective also suggests addressing the previous controversy by expanding its dimensions to include the social, economic, and other contexts. The public health perspective is also emphasized by Tajer (2003) in promoting the Latin American movement for social medicine. This approach emphasizes the political origins of social and health inequalities and ties medicine (and medical research) to the need for social and political reform.

In perhaps the most articulate formulation of these arguments, Farmer and Gastineau Campos (2004, p. 17) call for the "resocializing" of ethics to "contextualise fully ethical dilemmas in settings of poverty." They argue that bioethics "need to be linked to questions of social justice" and to social and health inequality. Bioethics needs to be linked to social analysis because it is clear that the health of individuals and populations are related to social, political, and economic determinants of inequality. If this is so, how shall we "resocialize" ethics and what are the consequences for the content of ethical guidelines?

Each of these arguments provides a basis for incorporating social and economic context into the construction of ethical guidelines based on notions of social justice but none of them are explicitly based on a model of illness causation that weaves these factors into the fabric of the specific subject matter of health and/or research. In our opinion this is precisely the factor that makes the formulation of ethical guidelines so difficult.

THE SOCIOLOGICAL PERSPECTIVE

Consider the typical design of an experimental research study. Let us suppose that we are testing the efficacy of a new drug. At best the study obtains subjects by some random selection process and then assigns these subjects randomly to experimental and control groups. The drug is introduced in one condition and the relevant health outcome is assessed across groups. These comparisons may provide support for the efficacy of the drug.

There are two features of this design that are problematic. First, to the extent that randomization is actually attempted, the selection of character-istics on which to base the randomization (e.g., sex, age, and economic status) may in fact be arbitrary. Second, randomization may have the effect of masking the importance of social and economic conditions for under-standing the outcome of the research. The design model is based on the assumption of biomedical individualism. The design presumes that conditions external to the physical body of the test subject are not relevant for understanding the research outcome and that the external conditions are "controlled" by randomization. This point goes to the heart of our critique. Medical researchers generally use a model of disease/illness causation that focuses on the most proximal aspects of disease/illness which separates the social from the biological. We believe that bioethicists have uncritically accepted this model in formulating ethical guidelines. This is why, for example, the CIOMS guidelines specifically exclude consideration of "unjust conditions" from the responsibility of medical researchers. Consistent with the biomedical perspective social injustice is a matter external to disease and there is no need for bioethicists to consider issues of social justice and beneficence that are related to these external conditions.

Krieger (1994, p. 891) explains that epidemiologists have essentially compiled a list of non-biological factors that can affect health outcomes and they have used this approach to develop multiple factor (multivariate) models of disease. However, these models are not developed theoretically but empirically. As Krieger points out, "As critical as these developments are, it is essential to note what these views of multifactorial etiology omit: discussion of origins..." Krieger also argues that these multifactorial explanations remain embedded in a biomedical model that emphasizes biological determinants of disease and views populations as simply the sum of their individual members.

The emphasis on biomedical individualism represents a limitation on what we can understand about disease and illness (Krieger, 1994; Link & Phelan, 1995). It has also, in our view, limited the scope of how bioethics defines its subject matter. In doing so, it has spawned the current debate regarding ethical guidelines in poor countries and resulted in the current guidelines "stalemate."

In the following we will suggest that the use of a disease causation model that accounts for more distal factors such as social and economic inequality also clarifies the ethical guidelines that must be formulated relative to these factors. Krieger notes that the use of her ecosocial model (or a sociological one) would, "...demand that epidemiologists eschew terms like 'special population'—...—and would instead directly expose what makes these populations 'special': their enforced marginalization (pp. 898–899)." Note that current ethical guidelines refer to residents of poor countries as "special populations."

Unlike either biomedical models or even public health models, the sociological perspective begins with the recognition of the unequal distribution of health/illness in society. It recognizes these inequalities in health/illness as manifestations of more general social and economic inequalities rather than viewing health as a distinctive phenomenon of individuals. Hence, the study of health/illness is the study of inequality and it will stand to reason that ethical principles related to the study of health/illness will be derived from the study of inequality.

In a sociological model of disease causation epidemiological patterns of illness such as those based on race/ethnicity in the United States or extreme poverty in Nepal are explained by arguing that the observed patterns arise because individuals who share common social status are exposed to a certain level of health risk because of their common social status. Low socio-economic status is related to illness not simply because poor people cannot afford health care or because poor people eat the wrong food (and do not get exercise), but also because the consequences of stratification include differences in access to non-stressful occupations, residential segregation, and political alienation (political influence). Relatively poor access to information, instrumental social networks, and power results in higher levels of exposure to health risk factors among individuals in low-status positions.

This is to say that health status follows directly from "unjust conditions" and are a reflection of those unjust conditions. Regardless of whether the unjust conditions exist in the United States or in Nepal, sociologists understand that health is unequally distributed in any society in patterns that reflect general social inequalities. In other words, the sociological explanation for the cause of illness makes unjust conditions a core element of the explanation. This implies that it may not be justifiable to exclude unjust conditions from the specification of ethical guidelines in poor countries.

This is not to say, however, that medical researchers in poor countries must address and correct these unjust conditions in order to fulfill ethical standards. Rather, the sociological model explains that the research design should consider the effects that social and economic inequalities have for the objectives of the researcher. For example, let us reconsider the simple experimental design discussed earlier. A random selection principle would be used to assign research subjects to experimental and control conditions. While randomization of assignment "controls" for the effects of say gender, age, and income, we now realize that those status characteristics also affect the general health of all research subjects and may affect the degree to which efficacious drug effects are observed. Randomization does nothing to account for the significantly poorer health status of all subjects in the research. The general state of health may affect the general biological responsiveness in both the experimental and placebo group. Moreover, other pre-existing medical conditions (i.e., chronic health problems shared in the population) may affect the efficacy of the drug. The side effects and long-term effectiveness of the drug may also differ from what would be observed in developed countries. These highly germane issues should be addressed by researchers for the sake of the success of their experiment and in order to fully understand their findings.

London (2005) refers to this approach as a "human development" perspective. He argues that particularly in developing countries, the meaning of justice in bioethical standards should be "social" justice. This entails considering the ways in which social and economic structures influence health status as well as individual health outcomes including those of medical research subjects. Because it is based on the notion that individual health status is "affected by a matrix of political, social and economic factors," it locates medical research in that same matrix. Thus, it requires that ethical conduct include consideration of how social and economic conditions affect the health status of research subjects. Also, how those same structures affect health-related institutions that address the health needs of research subjects.

What are the ethical responsibilities of researchers in this example? We would argue that this perspective does not mean that medical researchers are now somehow obligated to fix unjust conditions in order to do research. However, it explains why researchers need to incorporate social conditions into their understanding of the initial and resultant conditions in which the research occurs. It does suggest that ethical guidelines need to incorporate these conditions simply because they are part of, not separate from, the subjects who participate in the research study. Rather than resolving the universal-relative dichotomy in order to create ethical guidelines, the issue can be restated in terms of the application of universal guidelines based on concepts of both social and individual justice and benefit.

Considering the ethical issue to include social dimensions expands the ways in which research can be responsive to ethical concerns. The sociological explanation for disease causation also specifies that there are multiple pathways to disease, in general, rather than a single pathology for each specific disease. For example, inequalities in general health status have outlasted the availability of vaccines that in principle should have eliminated such inequalities. The health inequalities have not disappeared because the effects of social and economic structures on health inequality work through multiple pathways. Eliminating one pathway (e.g., providing universal vaccination) does not eliminate other pathways to the same or other diseases. This implies that a given research project does not need to resolve the health-related contextual issues specific to the health condition under study. Rather, a contribution to the welfare of the research population and/or the general population would represent an ethical response.

To illustrate this notion, we now describe a research project in Nepal and the way the project conceived and responded to ethical principles that in our view, meets the sorts of ethical responsibility implied by a sociological perspective. We will use this description finally to make the importance of the sociological perspective for understanding the ethical dimensions of medical research more apparent.

AN EXAMPLE: THE JIRI HELMINTH PROJECT

Jiri is located about 90 km northeast of Kathmandu, Nepal. The local inhabitants of Jiri, known as the Jirels, are the indigenous population of the valley numbering about 4,000–4,500 persons. Jirels speak a Tibeto-Burman language and most make a living by farming and herding animals.

The typical Jirel household consists of an extended family. They occupy a single-story two-room hut constructed of mud and bricks. There is close human–animal interaction. There is a central hearth, which is used for cooking and heat. There are no windows and the hut has no ventilation system. The latrine, which is shared with the general community, is a ravine where the family and neighbors defecate and urinate. The whole area is saturated with feces. This poses a major risk factor to the Jirels because both surface and underground water are jeopardized through such fecal contamination.

The Jiri Helminth project was started in 1994 as part of an international collaboration between investigators at the Southwest Foundation for Biomedical Research, Texas, USA; Miami University, Ohio, USA; and Tribhuvan University, Kathmandu, Nepal. This project, entitled "Genetics of Susceptibility to Helminthic Infection" was funded by a grant from the National Institute of Health, Washington, DC, USA (RO1 AI-37091). The research was designed to evaluate the genetic components of susceptibility to helminthic infection and the resulting disease state. Identification of these genetic components could eventually provide the means for identifying genetically susceptible individuals and suggest new biologic areas to target for intervention. The research involved the following data collection procedures: (1) face-to-face household surveys using structured question-naires to collect data on demographic, sociocultural, behavioral, and environmental conditions; (2) medical history; (3) anthropometric measure-ments; (4) fecal samples, and (5) blood samples. For the study, all Jirels excluding pregnant women and children under three years of age were selected. Potential participants were asked to sign consent forms and voluntarily indicate their willingness to participate in the research. Parents signed/consented for non-adult children. The research also guaranteed confidentiality and protection from physical risks and deception. No monetary compensation was offered for any reason.

Usually, subjects from developing countries gain little benefit from biomedical research. This project was no exception. The only direct benefit to the subjects was one annual dose of Albendazole, a medicine to eliminate worms. Apart from receiving basic health care related to helminthic infections there were no other direct benefits provided by the research protocol. Note that this design is consistent with existing ethical guidelines for conducting research in poor countries.

For collecting information on procedures 2–5 (listed above) the Jiri Helminth Clinic (JHC) was established. The clinic staff consisted of two physicians, two lab technicians, two research assistants, and five individuals who were responsible for collecting fecal samples from subjects' residences. In a typical week 25–35 individuals from a few homes would be selected to come to the clinic.

However, within weeks of the establishment of the clinic, the researchers were confronted by hundreds of patients, not only those sick with intestinal worms, but those coming to the clinic for other sorts of health problems.

The Jirels perceived the clinic to be a substitute for the government-funded hospital which was almost always ill equipped, ill staffed, and most often closed (Subedi et al., 2000).

The researchers were faced with a dilemma: turn away sick individuals or increase the services offered by the JHC to provide basic primary health care services. In the initial phase, the researchers decided to offer basic services, i.e., diagnosis and referrals and to write prescriptions for medicines. It did not take long for researchers to realize that there were no pharmacies in Jiri or nearby, and so most prescriptions were useless. This realization led to an ethical dilemma for researchers – whether to continue to offer diagnosis and make treatment recommendations however meaningless, or begin to offer treatment as well. Some of the ethical questions that the researchers grappled with were: how was the JHC project going to help the subjects in the long term? How could a meaningful impact be made to improve the overall health of the Jirels? How might a balance be struck between carrying out the research effectively, and at the same time benefiting the Jirels through services and initiatives that would affect some of the basic social conditions that led to helminthic infections and a host of other illnesses in the first place? On one hand, it was evident that the research protocol itself would have very little impact on the lives of Jirels as a whole. For Jirels, one tablet of Albendazole given once a year, and a once a year visit to a clinic would not reduce the incidence of helminthic infection. Most Jirels could not afford to buy the medicine on their own. Where was the benefit or social justice for the Jirel community for taking part in the research without any compensation or long-term benefit? On the other hand, the question was, "how extensively must the project respond to the 'unjust social conditions' in which the project takes place?"

This intense ethical discourse led to a turning point for the JHC. Through individual fundraising efforts in Nepal and in the United States, the researchers were able to secure funding for the JHC to offer "free services" for all who came to the clinic. As a result, the JHC began to offer basic primary health care services which included physician consultancy; simple diagnostic tests, e.g., blood, urine, X-ray, etc.; and free medicines. For serious cases, patients were given referrals for hospitals in neighboring districts. There was no transportation available for emergencies or serious cases so additional fundraising efforts led to the purchase of an ambulance for emergencies and transportation to city hospitals.

In addition to these direct health care related activities, a number of other social/community programs were initiated. These included: (1) environmental-teaching Jirels how to dispose of garbage safely, garbage collection and management. In addition, the river in Jiri was polluted with garbage. The "clean river" project was initiated and successfully completed; two local janitors were hired to clean streets and market places; (2) educational-researchers periodically visited schools and local events to give preventive health-related talks; (3) local-community day-to-day items that are necessary for health maintenance such as soap, shampoo, tooth brushes, and tooth paste were distributed regularly to subjects of the research and their families. Also researchers encouraged and taught Jirels to keep homes and the environment clean, and grow flowers and trees for a greener Jiri.

As ambitious and extensive as the JHC program became, it cost approximately $12,000 annually – a small expense by Western standards. The evolution of the JHC reflected an evolution of the ethical response to the participation of Jirels in this research project. While the initial ethical protocol merely obligated the project to provide an effective treatment to worm-infected Jirels (the Albendazole), the expanded program of services represented by the JHC clearly addressed issues of both individual and social justice. Although the clinic arose more from empirical demand than conscious planning, the decision to expand the clinic and its services was made from a social justice perspective.

Praxis and theory

The description of the research ethical component of the Jiri Helminth project illustrates how ethical practice can follow from theory. In this case, several dimensions are germane; the ethical practice is only indirectly linked to the specific disease under study and the ethical practice provides a collective (rather than an individual or aggregate) benefit. From the perspective of the social causation of illness explanation, both of these practice dimensions are consistent with theory. As a result, the example can be viewed as an illustration of the way in which a sociological perspective provides openings to resolve current ethical discussions related to standards of care and benefit.

The notion of benefit (both individual and social) that is currently used in bioethics is consistent with a biomedical explanation of illness in that it isolates a specific medical condition and the research intervention as the target of benefits. That is, benefit is linked to outcomes for individual research subjects or the aggregate of persons experiencing similar health problems. By contrast, the sociological explanation implies that benefit may include a "collective" level of benefit that addresses the distal causes of illness (even those which affect persons not included as subjects of the research or with similar conditions). The sociological explanation emphasizes that there are multiple pathways from social and economic conditions to illness and that the causal pathways are non-disease-specific (Link & Phelan, 1995). The general structure of social and economic relations affects illness in general and not necessarily the specific etiologic pathways that cause particular disorders. This insight suggests that ethical practice does not need to be limited to conceptions of benefit that are linked to specific illness conditions. In the present case, helminthic infection is both a function of specific exposure to the worm, and the general social and economic conditions that sustain this specific exposure and general exposure to health risk. While the clinic treats the consequences of general risk, it indirectly affects specific exposure to intestinal parasitic infection. In short, when we view the specific illness as simply one manifestation of general social and economic structure, we can frame the ethical guidelines related to the investigation of a specific illness in terms that account for the general economic and social context. In doing so, it is not necessary to rectify unjust conditions, but it is possible to incorporate the consequences of those unjust conditions into ethical practice. In addition, it is not necessary to link benefits to the specific illness condition under study. Note that the researcher is not excused from assuring that research subjects have access to the highest standard of care, but additionally the researcher has an obligation to address the unjust conditions that affect the specific health condition under study. The requirement that medical research contain a benefit to research subjects and others remains.

In our view, this perspective on the relationship between theory (illness causation) and practice (ethical practice consistent with guidelines) at least, partially redefines the ethical debate between universalists and relativists. The perspective draws on a universal explanation for illness and requires a relativistic response that represents compliance with universal criteria. Our example suggests that it may be difficult to specify the actual content of the ethically appropriate protocol in advance but that, once a project is in the field, attention to the requirement to address social justice will guide the protocol development.

The intent of this chapter is to make a case for a more dimensioned and nuanced conceptualization of the ethical issues associated with medical research in poor countries. As such we argued that existing guidelines have been constrained by a limited conception of illness that does not include the social context and thus, prevents sensitivity to matters of social justice. In poor countries, the social context of health and therefore, the social context of medical/health research is especially obvious as it affects health and health research outcomes. We have suggested that a sociological perspective on the causes of illness provides the necessary opening for developing more appropriate ethical standards for such research. It is probably also appropriate to consider how this theoretical explanation applies to ethical standards in developed countries as well.

REFERENCES

Andrews, J. (2005). US military sponsored vaccine trials and la resistance in Nepal. *The American Journal of Bioethics, 5,* W1–W3.

Angell, M. (1997). The ethics of clinical research in the third world. *New England Journal of Medicine, 337,* 847–849.

Baral, N., Lamsal, M., Koner, B. C., & Koirala, S. (2002). Thyroid dysfunction in eastern Nepal. *The Southeast Asian Journal of Tropical Medicine and Public Health, 33,* 638–641.

Benatar, S. R., & Singer, P. A. (2000). A new look at international research ethics. *British Medical Journal, 321,* 824–826.

Bhutta, Z. A. (2002). Ethics in international health research: A perspective from the developing world. *Bulletin of the World Health Organization, 80,* 114–120.

Brennan, T. A. (1999). Proposed revisions to the Declaration of Helsinki – Will they weaken the ethical principles underlying human research? *The New England Journal of Medicine, 341,* 527–531.

Council for International Organizations of Medical Sciences – CIOMS. (2002). *International guidelines for ethical review of epidemiological studies.* Geneva: CIOMS.

Del Rio, C. (1998). Is ethical research feasible in developed and developing countries? *Bioethics, 12,* 328–330.

Farmer, P., & Gastineau Campos, N. (2004). Rethinking medical ethics: A view from below. *Developing World Bioethics, 4*(1), 17–41.

Fox, R. (1989). *The sociology of medicine: A participant observer's view.* Englewood Cliffs, NJ: Prentice Hall.

Gorstein, J., Shreshtra, R. K., Pandey, S., Adhikari, R. K., & Pradhan, A. (2003). Current status of vitamin A deficiency and the national vitamin A control program in Nepal: Results of the 1998 National Micronutrient Status Survey. *Asia Pacific Journal of Clinical Nutrition, 12,* 96–103.

Hofman, K. J. (1999). Global forum for bioethics in research: Summary of the first forum, November 7–10, 1999. Fogarty International Center, http://www.fic.nih.gov/programs/bioethics/fl.html

Joshi, D. D., Maharjan, M. M., Johansen, M. V., Willingham, A. L., & Sharma, M. (2003). Improving meat inspection and control in resource-poor communities: The Nepal example. *Acta Tropica, 87,* 119–127.

Khatlwada, N. R., Takizawa, S., Tran, T. V. N., & Inoue, M. (2002). Groundwater contamination for sustainable water supply in Kathmandu valley, Nepal. *Water Science and Technology: A Journal of the International Association on Water Pollution Research, 46,* 147–154.

Krieger, N. (1994). Epidemiology and the web of causation: Has anyone seen the spider? *Social Science and Medicine, 39*, 887–903.

Link, B. G., & Phelan, J. (1995). Social conditions as fundamental causes of disease. *Journal of Health and Social Behavior* (Extra Issue), 80–94.

London, A. J. (2005). Justice and the human development approach to international research. *Hastings Center Report, 35*, 24–37.

Lurie, P., & Wolfe, S. M. (1997). Unethical trials of interventions to reduce perinatal transmission of the human immunodeficiency virus in developing countries. *New England Journal of Medicine, 337*, 853–856.

Macklin, R. (2001). After Helsinki: Unresolved issues in international research. *Kennedy Institute of Ethics Journal, 11*, 17–36.

Macklin, R. (2004). *Double standards in medical research in developing countries.* Cambridge, UK: Cambridge University Press.

Murdoch, D. R., Harding, E. G., & Dunn, J. T. (1999). Persistence of iodine deficiency 25 years after initial correction efforts in the Khumbu region of Nepal. *The New Zealand Medical Journal, 112*, 266–268.

Osrin, D., Tumbahangphe, K. M., Shrestha, D., et al. (2002). Cross sectional, community based study of care of newborn infants in Nepal. *British Medical Journal (Clinical Research Ed), 325*, 1063.

Pharmaceutical Research and Manufacturers Association (PHRMA). (2002). A Q&A on PhRMA's principles of conduct for clinical trials and communication of clinical trial results. http://www.phrma.org/publications/quickfacts/24.06.2002.429.cfm

Rai, S. K., Hirai, K., Ohno, Y., & Matsumura, T. (1997). Village health and sanitary profile from eastern hilly region, Nepal. *The Kobe Journal of Medical Sciences, 43*, 121–133.

Robert, J. S., & Smith, A. (2004). Toxic ethics: Environmental genomics and the health of populations. *Bioethics, 18*(6), 493–514.

Rous, J. J., & Hotchkiss, D. R. (2003). Estimation of the determinants of household health care expenditures in Nepal with controls for endogenous illness and provider choice. *Health Economics, 12*, 431–451.

Shah, S. (2002). Globalizing clinical research. *The Nation.* July 1, 2002.

Shapiro, H. T., & Meslin, E. M. (2001). Ethical issues in the design and conduct of clinical trials in developing countries. *New England Journal of Medicine, 345*, 139–142.

Shrestha, S. (2002). Socio-cultural factors influencing adolescent pregnancy in rural Nepal. *International Journal of Adolescent Medicine and Health, 14*, 101–109.

Shrestha, R. R., Shrestha, M. P., Upadhyay, N. P., Pradhan, R., Khadka, R., Maskey, A., Maharjan, M., Tuladhar, S., Dahal, B. M., & Shrestha, K. (2003). Groundwater arsenic contamination, its health impact and mitigation program in Nepal. *Journal of Environmental Science and Health Part A: Toxic/Hazardous Substances and Environmental Engineering, 38*, 185–200.

Subedi, J., Subedi, S., Sidky, H., Singh, R., Blangero, J., & Williams-Blangero, S. (2000). Health and health care in Jiri. *Contributions to Nepalese Studies, The Jirel Issue*, 97–104.

Tajer, D. (2003). Latin American social medicine: Roots, development during the 1990s, and current challenges. *American Journal of Public Health, 93*, 2023–2027.

Tangwa, G. B. (2004). Between universalism and relativism: A conceptual exploration of problems in formulating and applying international biomedical ethical guidelines. *Journal of Medical Ethics, 30*, 63–67.

Varmuss, H., & Satcher, D. (1997). Ethical complexities of conducting research in developing countries. *New England Journal of Medicine, 337*, 1003–1005.

World Health Organization. (1990). *1990 Report of the Commission on Health Research and Development*. Geneva: WHO.

World Health Organization (WHO). (2001). Selected health indicators. http://www3.who.int/whosis/country/indicators.cfm?country = npl (or usa).

World Medical Association (WMA). (2000). *Declaration of Helsinki: Ethical principals for medical research involving human subjects*. Helsinki: WMA.

CHANGING THE SUBJECT: SCIENCE, SUBJECTIVITY, AND THE STRUCTURING OF ETHICAL IMPLICATIONS

Sara Shostak and Erin Rehel

ABSTRACT

As environmental health scientists increasingly take up genetic/genomic modes of knowledge production and translate their work for applications in biomedicine, risk assessment, and regulation, they "bring the human in" to environmental health issues in novel ways. This paper describes the efforts of environmental health scientists to use molecular technologies to focus their research inside the human body, ascertain human genetic variations in susceptibility to adverse outcomes following environmental exposures, and identify individuals who have sustained DNA damage as a consequence of exposure to chemicals in the environment. In addition to transforming laboratory research, they see in these such practices the opportunity to advance public health, through innovations in biomedical practice and refinement of environmental health risk assessment and regulation. As environmental health scientists produce and translate these new forms of knowledge, they simultaneously assume and instantiate specific notions of the human subject and its agency, possibilities, and responsibilities vis-à-vis health and illness. Because dimensions of human

Bioethical Issues, Sociological Perspectives
Advances in Medical Sociology, Volume 9, 323–347
ISSN: 1057-6290/doi:10.1016/S1057-6290(07)09013-4

*subjectivity remain under-theorized in bioethics, sociological approaches
to understanding and situating the human subject offer an important
means of elucidating the consequences of genetics/genomics in the
environmental health sciences and highlighting the social structures and
processes through which they are produced.*

We are responsible for the world in which we live not because it is an arbitrary
construction of our choosing, but because it is sedimented out of particular practices that
we have a role in shaping.

                                                                    –Barad, 1998

INTRODUCTION

Historically, environmental health scientists worked primarily with animal
models and focused on producing knowledge that would inform the
regulation of chemicals in the ambient environment (e.g., air, water, soil)
(Sellers, 1997). Consequently, neither individual human beings nor
subpopulations generally have been a subject of environmental health
research. However, by the turn of the century, the practices and technologies
of environmental genomics, molecular epidemiology, and toxicogenomics
increasingly enabled environmental health scientists to focus their work on
human biological materials, to ascertain human genetic variations in
susceptibility to adverse outcomes following environmental exposures, and
to identify individuals who have sustained DNA damage as a consequence
of exposure to toxics. Each of these scientific practices and their proposed
applications in biomedical and regulatory settings "bring the human in" to
environmental health research and regulation, instantiating specific notions
of the human subject and its agency, possibilities, and responsibilities vis-à-
vis health and illness.

Many environmental health scientists believe that these new modes of
knowledge production have "ethical, legal, and social implications" (ELSI).
As has been the case with other emergent genetic/genomic projects
(Hedgecoe & Martin, 2003; Reardon, 2005), scientists have turned to
bioethics for help in creating knowledge and guidelines to govern such
"implications." There are many similarities between the human subject who
is the imagined user of applications of genetic/genomic knowledge and that
posited by contemporary American bioethics. This shared understanding of
the human subject facilitates rapprochement between science and bioethics.
However, we contend that the limitations in the bioethical and scientific

notions of the human subject make it difficult to identify or address the broader social factors that shape the potential consequences of molecularization in the environmental health sciences. In contrast, we highlight the contribution of sociological approaches to investigating the relationships between scientific knowledge, forms of subjectivity, and the social structure of the "ethical implications" of science.

The primary data in this analysis come from qualitative and ethnographic research conducted by one of the authors (SS) from August 2001 to September 2002 and from September 2003 to August 2004. These data include in-depth interviews with environmental health scientists, risk assessors, regulators, policy makers, and environmental health and environmental justice activists ($n = 85$). Additionally, we draw on field notes from participant observation at the National Institute for Environmental Health Sciences and National Center for Toxicogenomics, as well as workshops and conferences sponsored by the Society of Toxicology, the National Institutes of Health, the American Association of Cancer Research, and West Harlem Environmental Action. All of the data detailed above were coded and analyzed using the principles of grounded theory (Glaser & Strauss, 1967; Strauss, 1987; Strauss & Corbin, 1990/1998).

CHANGING THE SUBJECT

Molecularizing the Environmental Health Sciences

The molecularization of the life sciences began in the 1930s (Abir-Am, 1985; Kay, 1993; Pauly, 1987); however, it has taken different forms and extended at different rates in specific scientific disciplines (de Chadarevian & Kamminga, 1998). Molecularization consists of not "merely a matter of the framing of explanations at the molecular level. Nor ... simply a matter of the use of artefacts fabricated at the molecular level" but rather a *reorganization* of the life sciences, their "institutions, procedures, instruments, spaces of operation and forms of capitalization" (Rose, 2001, p. 13). Molecularization in the environmental health sciences, in general, and in toxicology, in particular, has lagged behind that in other sciences. In the late 1960s and early 1970s, genetic toxicology brought genetic techniques for assessing the mutagenicity of chemicals firmly within the purview of toxicology (Frickel, 2004). However, while the "regime of truth" in the life sciences – that is, "the body of practices and the types of discourses that a society accepts and makes function as true; the mechanisms and instances that enable one to distinguish true and false statements and the means by which each is sanctioned; the techniques and procedures accorded value in the acquisition of truth; and the status of those who are charged with saying what counts as true" (Lenoir, 1997, p. 48) – is increasingly centered on the molecular level, many of the most important indices of toxicity studied by toxicologists remained at what toxicologists call the "phenomenological" level: body weight, organ weight, level of activity, tumors, death (National Toxicology Program (NTP) Toxicity Reports, abstracts and full reports accessed at URL <http://ehp.niehs.nih.gov/ntp/docs/toxreports.html>). This is due, in large part, to the regulations and mandates governing risk assessment in the federal government. Related, the "gold standard" of toxicological testing, even while it incorporated data from genetic toxicology, continued to center on the 13-week and two-year rodent bioassays and other forms of whole animal studies (NTP, 2002).

Throughout the 1990s, environmental health scientists endeavored to extend their focus from "phenomenology" to mechanisms operating at the molecular genetic/genomic level. These efforts were driven, in part, by a concern on the part of environmental health scientists that "The genomics revolution is washing over us. Either we incorporate it or we'll be left behind" (Field Notes, July 2002).[1] Some toxicologists feared that being "left behind" would not only make their discipline "anachronistic" but also threaten their relevance to environmental health risk assessment, regulation, and policy making (Field Notes, July 2002).[2] For example, one toxicologist stated that he was concerned that if it failed to incorporate genomics, "then the NTP (National Toxicology Program) would be a toxicology program of only historical interest" (Interview 32). In the 1990s, the National Institute of Environmental Health Sciences (NIEHS) began to invest heavily in the molecularization of environmental health research, using both its extramural and intramural grants program to foster the development of molecular epidemiology, environmental genomics, and toxicogenomics.

Molecular epidemiology, environmental genomics, and toxicogenomics emerged from somewhat different disciplinary and institutional contexts and, unsurprisingly, they vary both in the questions they ask about the relationship between the environment and human health and in the technologies they deploy to answer such questions. For example, molecular epidemiologists have focused on the development and validation of molecular biomarkers as a means of improving measurement of exposure, effect, and susceptibility in environmental epidemiology (Christiani, 1996; Hemminki, Grzybowska, Widlak, & Chorazy, 1996; Perera, 1987, 1997, 2000). In contrast, environmental genomics is primarily concerned with identifying genes that confer susceptibility to environmental exposures (NIEHS, 2000b). The goals of toxicogenomics include identifying the mechanisms of action of toxicants, enhancing the sensitivity and interpretability of bioassays, developing biomarkers of exposure, effect, and susceptibility, and elucidating how genetic variation shapes susceptibility to environmental toxicants (Nuwaysir, Bittner, Barrett, & Afshari, 1999). Despite these differences in emphasis and technique, these practices are increasingly isomorphic in their focus inside the human body and in their quest to identify and characterize acquired and/or intrinsic genetic variations that may shape individual and subpopulation susceptibility to diseases following environmental exposures.

In both epidemiology and toxicology, molecular techniques have expanded the scope of environmental research that can be done with human subjects or samples taken from human subjects. Scientists are genuinely excited by this expansion of research practice "inside the black box of the human body." As an environmental epidemiologist recalled:

> What I was interested in is molecular mutagenesis - the basic mechanisms of molecular mutagenesis .... I had been working on bacterial models of mechanisms .... In the 1980s I switched to studying genetic variations in humans. This is when molecular epidemiology was just getting started. The techniques were being developed and I wanted to get into human studies. (Interview 26)

This has implications both for laboratory research and its translations for environmental health risk assessment and regulation. As a toxicologist recounted, he was compelled by the possibility of using molecular techniques as a way of transcending the limitations of extrapolating from animal to human models in assessing the risk of environmental chemicals:

> By the end of the 1980s, I had become very disenchanted with animal experiments .... I was challenged at a committee meeting in the late 80's ... 'what's the alternative?' And I thought that was a good question. So my research went into the direction of biological markers in the late 80's and the beginning of the 90's, with *the idea that we could study people with the latest microbiology and we'd be able to learn a lot more than we could from rats and mice with regard to risk.* What are people actually exposed to? How much are they exposed to? What does the dose response curve look like? Are there susceptible people? All this could be much better answered in people. (Interview 15, emphasis added)

Increasing reliance on molecular techniques and institutional shifts from animal to human studies have changed profoundly the practices of environmental health research:

> It has allowed us to move a lot of our toxicology from animals into humans. In the division that I'm in, the Division of Occupational and Environmental Health, all of our

328   SARA SHOSTAK AND ERIN REHEL

studies are in humans now, whereas ten or fifteen years ago we still used a lot of animal
studies. (Interview 12)

In addition to "moving from animals into humans," molecular techniques
are being used by scientists to identify differences among humans. For
example, environmental genomics is defined by its goal of identifying
"environmental response genes" – those inherited genetic variations that
may affect individuals' responses to environmental exposures (NIEHS,
2000a). In molecular epidemiology, "why similarly exposed people do not
get the same diseases is a target question ... in most disease systems,
susceptibility markers are being identified and evaluated" (Perera, 1997);
molecular epidemiologists also endeavor to use biomarkers of exposure and
effect to identify people who have sustained DNA damage as a consequence
of prior environmental exposures. Likewise, toxicogenomics focuses on both
identifying gene expression profiles that may serve as "fingerprints" or
"signatures" identifying specific chemical exposures and their effects within
human bodies (Hamadeh et al., 2002a, 2002b) and on elucidating "the
relationship between genetic variability and toxicant susceptibility"
(Nuwaysir et al., 1999). In each of its genetics/genomics initiatives, the
NIEHS has prioritized research on genetic variations in susceptibility to
environmental exposures.

Identifying Applications

Molecular epidemiology, environmental genomics, and toxicogenomics also
share the expectation that knowledge about intrinsic or acquired genetic
variation will contribute to public health, either by improving environmental risk assessment regulation and/or by making possible new forms of
biomedical intervention.[3] Specific innovations promised by scientific
entrepreneurs advocating the molecularization of the environmental health
sciences include quicker toxicological assessments, more certain "molecular" identification of chemical classes and chemical exposures (including
mixtures), identification of individuals and subpopulations who are
genetically susceptible to chemicals in the environment, and identification
of individuals and subpopulations who are at increased risk for illness
due to potentially harmful environmental exposures (NCT/NIEHS, 2002;
NIEHS, 2000a, 2000b; Olden, 2002; Paules, Tennant, Barrett, & Lucier,
1999; Perera, 2000; Simmons & Portier, 2002). These "applied aims" shape
contemporary research agendas in the environmental health sciences;
for example, the agenda of the National Center for Toxicogenomics

includes efforts to develop and standardize toxicogenomics for environmental health risk assessment and regulation, bring toxicogenomics to regulators and policy makers, and facilitate public acceptance of regulatory and biomedical applications of toxicogenomic knowledge (NCT/NIEHS, 2002). As such, for these sciences, the goal of producing knowledge that can be translated for applications in risk assessment, regulation, and biomedicine has shaped the conditions and processes of their emergence (Gibbons et al., 1994; Messer-Davidow, Shumway, & Sylvan, 1993; Shostak, 2005).

Certainly, contributing to efforts to protect human health has long been a goal of environmental health science. Traditionally, however, scientists have not placed information about individual and subpopulation genetic variation at the center of such efforts. Rather, in environmental health research, and especially in toxicology, scientists have focused on testing chemicals in animal models (e.g., the two-year rodent cancer bioassay), from which regulatory scientists and risk assessors could extrapolate to a human population of "standard human bodies"(Smith, 1996). Put differently, while environmental health scientists and risk assessors recognized the existence of human genetic variation (Calabrese, 1996), they long regarded it as a source of "noise" in their experiments, rather than a "signal" or parameter of interest (Hattis, 1996). They addressed this noise (as well as that potentially created by extrapolating from animals to humans) with "10-fold factors." For example, in order to protect the "sensitive end of the toxic response continuum," risk assessors will take the value that toxicology testing has determined to be an acceptable exposure limit for a standard human (e.g., the no observed effect level (NOEL)) and multiply it by 10 (Smith, 1996).[4]

Consequently, in their focus on human genetic variation and emphasis on translating knowledge for applications in biomedical and regulatory domains, molecular epidemiology, environmental genomics, and toxicogenomics "bring the human in" to the environmental health sciences in novel ways. Indeed, data about genetic susceptibility to environmental exposures are promoted by scientists, in part, for being able to provide more precise estimations of risk for *specific* humans and subpopulations thereof, replacing a "one size fits all" approach with one that acknowledges variation among human bodies. Testifying in support of the NIEHS's budget for 2002, then Director Olden, told the US Congress that "individuals can vary by more than *two-thousand fold* in their capacity to repair or prevent damage following exposure to toxic agents in the environment" (Olden, Fiscal Year 2002 Budget Statement, emphasis added).

Similarly, writing in *Nature Reviews Genetics*, Olden and the Deputy
Director of the NIEHS, Sam Wilson, assert that

> At present, human genetic variation is not implicitly considered in estimating dose-
> response relationships, nor is it considered when setting exposure limits. Data on the
> prevalence and characteristics of susceptibility genes offers the potential to reduce the
> guesswork in risk assessment and therefore it is likely that the ability to issue fair and
> appropriate regulations concerning human hazards will increase markedly. (Olden &
> Wilson, 2000)

NIEHS scientists express excitement about research on genetic susceptibilities as a means of expanding their disciplines' relevance to public health;
not unrelated, this research also may enhance the standing of their institute:

> .... We started [the genomics initiatives] ... and the National Institute of Environmental
> Health Sciences has become a major player at the National Institutes of Health. It used
> to be, quite frankly, that they didn't see us as important to the mission of the National
> Institutes of Health, to protecting public health. But now we are a major part of the
> Institutes – we are integrated with the National Cancer Institute, the National Human
> Genome Research Institute – and they see how important our work is for public health.
> (Field Notes, 2001)

Or, as another scientist starkly put it, NIEHS had to establish itself as
more than just "a rat toxicology institute" (Field Notes, June 2002).[5]
The molecular biomarkers developed in molecular epidemiology and
toxicogenomics also offer the promise of molecularizing disease phenotypes.
As a molecular epidemiologist commented, "We have used phenotype
forever to diagnosis disease. Now what we're doing is actually looking
at that phenotype at the molecular level" (Interview 20). Specifically,
molecular biomarkers provide the possibility of replacing categorical disease
definitions with definitions based on continuous and quantitative variables.
For example, a "case" (that is, someone who has the outcome of interest)
can now be defined with a continuous variable (e.g., number of deformed
proteins) rather than a categorical one (e.g., normal vs. pathological):

> [The] technologies that are developing are all lending themselves for quantitative
> measures. We're going to start to define cases as 'you've got one hundred thousand
> deformed proteins,' as opposed to ... 'you have emphysema'. (Interview 20)

Related, molecular epidemiological models of disease replace "step
function" models of environmental health and illness with fully normalizing
models based on continuous gradients of quantifiable "markers" of disease.
A step function model, as described by this molecular epidemiologist, would
tell you: "so you're healthy, now you have hypertension, now you have
advanced cardiovascular disease, now you have congestive heart failure,

now you're dead" (Interview 21). In contrast, a continuous model measures accumulation of molecular biomarkers and their associated *risks* over the life course. Therefore, from a molecular epidemiological perspective, one may not be merely "healthy" or "ill"; rather, as this epidemiologist described, "... what we would do is ... use biomarkers as ... measures of disease accumulation ... *you would be dealing with somebody in a variety of gradations of disease*" (Interview 21, emphasis added). This re-conceptualization of disease phenotypes is seen as desirable by environmental health scientists because it may increase the period of time during which the risks of disease can be identified, categorized, prevented, treated and/or managed, thereby potentially expanding options for biomedical intervention.

As we have described elsewhere, scientists face myriad challenges in translating environmental genetic/genomic knowledge for applications in public health, including developing means of communication across disciplines (e.g., toxicology, genomics, epidemiology), articulating emergent technologies and practices with extant ones; managing the tensions generated by grounding genetic/genomic knowledge in traditional standards while working to supplant them, and identifying and stabilizing roles for molecular knowledge in desired markets and service sites (Shostak, 2005). Here, however, we wish to consider the challenges of translating data from the molecular biomarkers, genetically modified mouse models (e.g., mice with genes from humans spliced into their DNA), and cDNA microarrays with which scientists work in their laboratories, to the complexities of the social world in which the human beings who are the intended beneficiaries of such research live, work, and play.

SCIENCE, SUBJECTIVITY AND THE SOCIAL STRUCTURING OF "ETHICAL IMPLICATIONS"

Interrogating the Subject of Bioethics

Environmental health scientists aver that their genetic/genomic research agendas have "implications of an ethical, legal and social nature" (NCT/ NIEHS, 2002). Drawing on the language of the Human Genome Project's ELSI Research Program, the presence of such implications is noted in NIEHS materials describing missions of the Environmental Genome Project (NIEHS, 1997) and the National Center for Toxicogenomics (NCT/NIEHS, 2002). The NCT has sponsored its own ELSI Working Group (Shostak, 2005) and states in its overview that "Bioethicists can and should play an important role in resolving ELSI issues [sic] that arise as toxicogenomics methods are used more widely and begin to impact the general public" (NCT/NIEHS, 2002). The NIEHS has a bioethicist on its faculty, charged with addressing the ethics both of scientific research and of its ELSI (URL: http://dir.niehs.nih.gov/ethics/, accessed8/1/2006). In each of these ways, the social practices of bioethics are an integral part of the emergence of genetics/ genomics in the environmental health sciences.

However, we contend that bioethics is limited, especially by its conceptualization of the human subject, in its ability to fully consider the broader social contexts important to understanding the consequences of genetics/genomics vis-à-vis environmental health and illness. In the following pages, we examine bioethical and scientific notions of the human subject, briefly summarize extant critiques, and then offer an alternative approach to understanding the consequences of genetics/genomics in the environmental health sciences.

There are many similarities between the human subject who is the imagined user of applications of genetic/genomic knowledge and that posited by contemporary American bioethics. Both laboratory research and bioethical reasoning seek generalizable and "universal" truths. Consequently, their methodologies strip away dimensions of social context (Beauchamp & Childress, 2001; cf. Latour, 1987). In both science and bioethics, the human subject is envisioned as an autonomous individual, capable of reasoning, oriented to selecting and carrying out actions that would serve to advance his/ her self-chosen life plan, and participating in the social world via largely autonomous and atomistic modes of engagement (Beauchamp & Childress, 2001; DeGrazia, 2005; Jonsen, 1998; Jonsen, Siegler, & Winslade, 1998; Tauber, 2001). This subject exists largely independent of social context, a "competent, self-sovereign, and unencumbered individual" (Jennings, 1998) inhabiting an imagined social world in which autonomy, equality, and agency are more or less equally available to all.

The autonomous individual subject of bioethics is, of course, a product of the social forces and contexts that shaped the emergence of bioethics in America, including processes of rationalization, the once prominent but then declining influence of religious traditions in bioethics, and bioethicists' engagements with the fields of philosophy, law, and medicine (Bosk, 1999; DuBose, Hamel, & O'Connell, 1994; Evans, 2002; Jennings, 1998; Rothman, 1991). The role of philosophy has been particularly influential, as drawing on the liberal individualism of Mill and the rational autonomy of Kant, philosophers imported Enlightenment notions of the subject to American bioethics. The Enlightenment subject comported well with legal definitions of the human subject as a rational, individual being. It was congruent also with the law's use of rights-based language (e.g., self-determination, self-governance, autonomy) (DuBose et al., 1994).

Broader social trends amplified these inclinations, with 1960's liberal individualism "put[ting] autonomy at the top of the moral mountain" (Callahan, 1999). In principlism (Beauchamp & Childress, 2001), arguably the dominant approach in American bioethics, the autonomous individual is at the center of ethical reasoning and "the proper measure of all things ethical"(Bosk, 1999).[6] Moreover, although four principles are at the center of this approach – autonomy, beneficence, non-maleficence, and justice – autonomy's place in bioethics overshadows and sometimes completely eclipses the other three principles, leading to the observation that "the driving principal in principlism in practice is autonomy" (Callahan, 1999, p. 283).[7]

Critiques of the autonomous Enlightenment subject at the center of bioethics have come from varied positions both within and outside the discipline (Callahan, 1973, 1999; Hoffmaster, 2001; Jonsen & Toulmin, 1988; Toulmin, 1981; Wolpe, 1998). In particular, feminist scholars have highlighted the limitations of this construction of the subject, including its scant attention to the social and cultural dimensions of particular situations and its privileging of individuality over relationships, reason over emotion, autonomy over all else (Anspach, 1993; Anspach & Beeson, 2001; Gilligan, 1982; Sherwin, 1992; Wolf, 1996). Their critiques include a call for bioethicists to pay increased attention to situational details, lived experiences, cultural realities and interconnectedness (Gilligan, 1982).[8] Further, they assert that conceptualizations of subjectivity should incorporate both the rational, autonomous aspects of individuality and the relational reality of acting and participating in the world, including emotionality (Anspach & Beeson, 2001; Gilligan, 1982). Lastly, feminist scholars have alleged that positing the human subject as an autonomous individual reflects the discipline's orientation to privileged members of American society (e.g., White, middle class, males). They argue that it is impossible to discuss health care and medicine without consideration of the many factors that create and perpetuate stark divisions in health-care access and resources. As such, these authors have challenged bioethics to contextualize the human subject and the choices and problems he or she encounters within a social matrix in which intersecting forms of inequality shape the conditions of reflection and action (DeVries & Subedi, 1998; Wolf, 1996).

Related, social scientists (DeVries & Subedi, 1998; Hoffmaster, 2001) have called for a greater role for empirical research in bioethics. They argue

that empirical work is needed both to more fully account for the perspectives of subjects and their family members and to contextualize the
particular situations confronted by bioethicists (Anspach, 1993; Bosk, 1992;
Chambliss, 1996; Haimes, 2002; Hedgecoe, 2004; Rapp, 1998, 1999;
Schneider & Conrad, 1983; Zussman, 1997): "sociologists can show
bioethics how social structures, cultural settings, and social interaction
influence their work" (DeVries & Subedi, 1998). Moreover, because social
scientists are likely to "see legal and ethical issues as primarily social issues,"
they are well positioned to contribute to "understanding of the social
processes through which issues become constituted as ethical concerns"
(Haimes, 2002). Social scientific critiques of bioethics have manifested
recently in calls for a "critical bioethics" (Hedgecoe, 2004). In critical
bioethics, empirical research is used to expand analysis beyond the
individual level, investigate the perspectives of respondents and allow the
categories relevant to their experience to emerge, consider moral and ethical
reasoning outside of clinical settings, and include the social and cultural
dimensions of ethical decision making, which are so often ignored in
traditional bioethics research (Haimes, 2002; Hedgecoe, 2004).

Scholars in science and technology studies (STS) have also made
significant contributions to analyses of bioethical concerns and bioethics
(Casper, 1998; Cussins, 1998; Duster, 2003; Franklin, 2000; Gottweiss, 1995;
Lock, 2002; Novas & Rose, 2000; Reardon, 2005; Rose, 2001). In particular,
in its challenge to the Enlightenment subject of science (and ethics),
scholarship in STS emphasizes that agency and autonomy are not
independent, decontextualized attributes but are located, rather, in "the
ongoing reconfigurings of the world" (Barad, 2003). Moreover, scholars in
STS demonstrate that agency and autonomy are "inextricably tied to the
specific sociomaterial arrangements of which we are part" (Suchman, in
press), which include science, technology, and their applications in multiple
domains of social life (e.g., biomedicine, public policy, law). One goal of
STS is to demonstrate "how capacities for action can be reconceived on
foundations quite different from those of an Enlightenment, humanist
preoccupation with the individual actor living in a world of separate things"
(Suchman, in press). As such, "these scholars align with feminist theorizing
in their emphasis on the always relational character of our capacities for
action; the constructed nature of subjects and objects, resemblances and
differences; and the corporeal grounds of knowing and action" (Suchman,
in press). Scholars in STS have also taken bioethics as their subject, as,
for example, in analyses of how bioethics emerges with and through
new subjects, disciplines, and technologies (Hedgecoe & Martin, 2003;

Rabinow & Rose, 2003; Rapp, 1998, 1999; Reardon, 2005; Shostak, 2005). In the following section of this paper, we demonstrate the importance of these perspectives for fully conceptualizing the processes and consequences of molecularization in the environmental health sciences.

The Social Structure of "Ethical Implications"[9]

To date, the primary regulatory strategy in the domain of environmental health has been the assessment and regulation of chemicals in the ambient environment – the air, water, and soil. Put differently, the classification and regulation of environmental chemicals, rather than the classification and regulation of persons and subpopulations, have constituted the dominant logics of control for protecting human health vis-à-vis the environment. To the extent that scientists and regulators are extending their foci from the ambient environment to individual humans, subpopulations, and their behaviors (e.g., encouraging "susceptible persons" to reduce environmental exposures and/or to access health services to monitor and intervene in the consequences of exposures), they engage with critical questions about the human subject in relation to environmental health and illness. As noted above, environmental health scientists recognize that their molecular research agendas and the intended applications of their knowledge have ELSI and are turning to bioethics as a means of addressing them. Drawing on feminist, sociological, and STS perspectives, we contend that adequately addressing the consequences of genetics/genomic modes of knowledge production in the environmental health sciences requires a broader examination of how scientific knowledge and technologies constitute human subjects, the sociomaterial realities in which these subjects are situated, and the broader social structural conditions that shape subjects' agency and opportunities.

To begin, drawing on contemporary scholarship in STS, we propose that knowledge production in the environmental health sciences, applications of that knowledge (e.g., in biomedicine, risk assessment, and regulation), and associated "ethical implications" must be understood as producing, in part, the entities (e.g., individuals and subpopulations) that they take as their subjects (Casper, 1998; Cussins, 1998; Franklin, 2000; Lock, 2002; Montoya, 2003; Novas & Rose, 2000; Rabinow, 1996; Reardon, 2005; Shostak, 2005). For example, in genetic counseling and testing, individuals are identified as "at risk" and asked to "reshape their form of life – lifestyle, diet leisure activities, alcohol, smoking" as a means of maximizing their life chances, increasing the quality of their lives, and acting ethically in relation to themselves and to others (Novas & Rose, 2000). In this way, knowledge and ethics are linked to "technologies of the self" (Martin, Gutman, & Hutton, 1988) and processes of subject making (Rabinow & Rose, 2003). From this perspective, we see that identifying people who are genetically susceptible to illness as a consequence of environmental exposures is not merely an *implication* of science, but rather an effect that is produced at the intersection of scientific, biomedical, and ethical concerns and practices.

These productive capacities of genetic/genomic practices are especially visible when genetic identifications are used to redefine the possibilities for specific ethical practices and social relations. For example, in the case of environmental genetic/genomic knowledge, advocates of "public health genetics" have suggested that individuals who are genetically susceptible to environmental exposures may be "motivated to take special steps, beyond those taken to protect everyone" (Omenn, 1991) in order to maximize their life chances. Genetic/genomic information creates specific opportunities to act as "responsible genetic subjects" (Novas & Rose, 2000). Thus, scientific knowledge and ethical reasoning together enter into the identities, life practices, and social relations of persons, with the potential to (re)shape their subjectivity (as well as that of their family members and significant others).

Applications of toxicogenomics and their ethical implications are likely also to be productive of new subpopulations of subjects "at risk" due to environmental exposures. As described above, environmental risk assessment, regulation, and policy have been oriented to defining levels of exposure where harms associated with these exposure levels are thought to be minimal (the NOEL). In contrast, molecular epidemiology and toxicogenomics endeavor to identify changes in gene expression, chemical class specific "genomic fingerprints," and other molecular biomarkers of environmental exposure and effect (Bartosiewicz, Penn, & Buckpitt, 2001; Bartosiewicz, Jenkins, Penn, Emery, & Buckpitt, 2001; Christiani, 1996; Hamadeh et al., 2002a, 2002b; Nuwaysir et al., 1999; Perera, 2000). This can be expected to lower NOELs for many environmental agents, increasing the number of individuals who can be identified as having been *exposed* and possibly *affected* by environmental exposures.[10] Changing NOELs would have implications particularly for people seen as having the molecular phenotype of a disease (even if not experiencing any symptoms thereof), who, like people with inherited genetic susceptibilities, will be asked to understand themselves as "at risk" and to modify their life practices (work, leisure, use of health services) accordingly. Again, these proposed applications of scientific knowledge and attendant "ethical stylizations" (Osborne, 1994) thereby co-constitute new subjectivities for individuals and subpopulations "at risk."

While significant for biomedicine and public health more generally, such genetic/genomic relocations of the locus of responsibility for health are likely to be especially consequential in the domain of environmental health and illness. In part, this is due to current approaches to environmental health risk assessment and regulation. Traditionally, environmental protection efforts have focused on categories of risks deemed "involuntary" and beyond individual control (e.g., clean air and water), as opposed to risks that individuals "voluntarily" impose on themselves (e.g., health-related behaviors). As tests for genetic sensitivities to environmental agents become more widely available, however, this new information may significantly expand an individual's so-called voluntary risks by providing estimates of disease likelihood for subjects in specific environments. In other words, the ability to identify genetically sensitive individuals and subpopulations may broaden the class of risks deemed the responsibility of at-risk individuals, rather than matters of public policy. Speaking at a conference on genetics, the environment, and communities of color, sociologist Troy Duster referred to this as the "fracturing of the public health consensus":

> The public health consensus was based on the idea that the environment had to be cleaned up, that we are all vulnerable to disease, so it is in our common interest to clean it up .... Genetics is fracturing this consensus by emphasizing differential vulnerability to diseases. (Field Notes from WE ACT conference, 2002)

At issue in the domain of environmental health is the possibility that scientific capacity to identify individuals and subpopulations with heightened genetic sensitivities to environmental agents may shift the focus of risk-management efforts away from the improvement of unhealthy environmental conditions, in favor of changing the behavior of "high risk" individuals. Indeed, environmental justice activists express great concern that research on genetic susceptibilities to environmental exposures will "shift the perception of who is responsible for environmental health problems from polluters to the individuals living in polluted environments" (Interview P01). Insurers, employers, and landlords might use information about individuals' susceptibility as a means of denying health insurance, workers compensation, or other legal claims (Draper, 1991; Sharp & Barrett, 2000).

Additionally, our present system of environmental laws was not created to protect *individuals*, though under certain circumstances, sensitive groups within the general population, such as children or asthmatics, may be protected (e.g., Clean Air Act 1990; Food Quality Protection Act 1996). Thus, the identification of individuals – and groups of individuals – who are genetically susceptible to environmental exposures raises the possibility of demands for environmental protection *that cannot be delivered under existing laws and regulations.* How genetically susceptible persons and/or groups could be defined and protected under the law remains unclear. Likewise, little is know about how regulators and policy makers will assess the costs of protecting the most vulnerable members of the population.

These issues are made all the more pressing by the extensive body of research on the inequitable distribution of the burden of environmental exposures, with African-Americans and Latinos experiencing the highest rates of exposure and, most likely, disproportionately burdened by their health effects. The groundbreaking research on "environmental racism" was conducted by the Commission on Racial Justice of the United Church of Christ (UCC, 1987). The first UCC study, which was conducted in 1986, found that "those communities with the greatest percentages of minority residents had the most toxic waste facilities ..." and that "percentage of minority population proved to be the strongest predictor of communities with the greatest number of waste facilities and the largest landfills" (Brown, 1995, p. 17). A second UCC study found that "three of five Black and Hispanic individuals resided in a community with a CERCLIS site" and that "three of five of the largest commercial hazardous waste landfills in the US, making up 40% of the nation's total capacity for hazardous waste landfills, were located in predominantly Black or Hispanic communities" (Brown, 1995, p. 17).

In the decades following the UCC reports, studies of multiple regions and geographic units of the United States and of the distribution of a variety of types of environmental hazards have identified multiple ways in which race and class are important determinants of environmental exposure and environmental health effects. First, research on proximity to known environmental hazards and exposure to pollution documents an association between race, class, and exposure. Research has also found that "whether using a general proximity measure or a precise distance measure, race has an independent effect on the locations of waste sites and proves to be a stronger predictor than income" (Brown, 1995, p. 18). Put differently, a person who is Black or Latino is four and a half times more likely than a person who is White to live within a mile of a toxic waste site or facility (Mohai & Bryant, 1992); more than 15 million Blacks and 8 million Latinos live in communities with one or more uncontrolled toxic waste sites (Pinderhughes, 1996). Second, research on race and class differences in exposure to air pollution indicates that "Blacks face higher exposures at all income levels than Whites" (Brown, 1995, p. 20). Third, research on regulation, amelioration, and clean up also finds significant inequalities.[11] Finally, research has found that there are race and class differences in siting proposals for new incinerators, hazardous waste sites, and nuclear storage sites (Brown, 1995, p. 24). This suggests the likelihood of ongoing inequities in environmental exposure and associated risks of disease. This context of social inequality and environmental racism has shaped the response of environmental justice activists to genetics/genomics, who contend that "We cannot get caught in the trap of deepening the discussion about genetics and our illnesses" (Field Notes from WE ACT conference, 2002).[12]

Likewise, it is important to note that many of the ethical issues associated with genetics, which more typically are addressed in the bioethics literature, such as discrimination in employment, health insurance, and life insurance and concerns about the privacy of medical information, are also shaped by broader social contexts. These include the lack of universal health coverage and the absence of federal genetic anti-discrimination legislation in the United States. Inequities in health insurance coverage also render problematic the expectation that people who are identified as "at risk" for illness following environmental exposures will have access to the sophisticated molecular biomedical techniques that would be required to monitor and/or treat "molecular disease phenotypes." Again, we find that broader sociological and political analyses are essential to understanding how ethical dilemmas are produced.

CONCLUSION

Environmental health scientists are developing molecular genetic/genomic research agendas, in part, for their potential to bring the human back into the environmental health sciences. Indeed, molecular epidemiology, environmental genomics, and toxicogenomics offer scientists opportunities for "opening the black box of the human body," ascertaining human genetic variations in susceptibility to adverse outcomes following environmental exposures, and identifying individuals who have sustained DNA damage as a consequence of exposure to toxics. With these new modes of knowledge production also come the possibility of new biomedical and policy interventions to prevent environmentally associated illness.

Translating from the "thin" representations of humans in the laboratory – where molecular biomarkers, transgenic mice, and cDNA microarrays

"stand in" for human beings – to the complex setting where human
subjects live, work, and play poses challenges to scientists and the
practitioners whose work they seek to inform (e.g., policy makers, health-
care providers). Environmental health scientists believe that their molecular
genetic/genomic efforts raise ELSI and have turned to bioethicists for help in
addressing them.

In concert with other critical observers in feminist theory, STS, and the
social sciences, we contend that bioethics' notion of the human subject also
is remarkably thin and decontextualized, especially insofar as it cleaves to
conceptualization of the subject as an autonomous individual, who makes
decision through processes of reason (rather than emotion) with "self" as
the primary referent, and who faces challenges independent of social context
or inequitable distributions of resources. In contrast, we have suggested the
importance of analyses of genetics/genomics in the environmental health
sciences that encompass social process and social structure. As we have
suggested, a more comprehensive sociological analysis of ELSI would
encompass how practices in science, medicine, and bioethics help to
constitute specific human subjects, how extant policy regimes and associated
notions of responsibility for health and illness shape the opportunities and
experiences of those subjects, and how dimensions of structural inequality
(e.g., environmental racism) put people "at risk for risks" and limit their
access to preventive and ameliorative resources (Link & Phelan, 1995).
Put differently, we seek to highlight the social factors shaping the context
in which subjects seek to act on genetic/genomic knowledge and the
sociomaterial relations in which their agency and autonomy becomes
possible and/or is constrained.

The emergence of genetic/genomic practices in the environmental health
sciences does not simply raise ethical implications. Rather, the emergence of
genetic/genomic modes of knowledge production in the environmental
health sciences and their applications across domains of biomedicine, risk
assessment, and policy making *require* the simultaneous production of
ethical norms (Reardon, 2005) and credible systems of environmental health
governance. The social structural dimensions of the production of
environmental health and illness therefore present a challenge to bioethics
that is an opportunity for sociology. To wit, bioethicists already have
commented that the "social implications of the [Environmental Genome]
project have not been adequately discussed in the existing bioethics
literature" and have questioned "the extent to which traditional bioethical
perspectives apply to this new area of research" (Sharp & Barrett, 2000).[13]
More recently, bioethicists have begun to consider ethical issues in the

environmental health sciences more broadly, including "the choice of research topics to study, the methods employed to examine these topics, the communication of research findings to the public, and the involvement of scientific experts in the shaping of environmental policy and governmental regulation" (Sharp, 2003). For decades, social scientists, feminist theorists, and scholars in STS have been developing theoretical frameworks and methodological approaches that allow us to understand "the effects of particular assemblages, and assess the distributions, for better and worse, that they engender"(Suchman, in press). These approaches have the potential to deepen the understandings of what gets frames as "ethical issues," to challenge the "assumption that the right thinking with the right values will suffice to silence ... conflict" (Bosk, 1999), and to broaden the discourse of ELSI into a wider discussion about social structure, public policy, inequality, and the social production of environmental health and illness.

NOTES

1. Per the requirements of the IRB protocol under which this research was conducted, we do not reveal the names of any of individual respondents. Institutional affiliation has been revealed only for those subjects who consented to be interviewed "on the record," as well as for those whose comments were recorded in my field notes during ethnographic observation. In order to better contextualize quotations from interviews, we provide the respondents' scientific background (for example, "epidemiologist," "toxicologist") whenever possible. We also have provided codes for interview respondents (for example, "Interview 45"), so that they may be understood as unique "voices," while remaining anonymous.

2. Risk assessment refers to "the systematic scientific characterization of potential adverse health effects resulting from human exposures to hazardous agents or situations" (National Research Council, 1983, p. 1). Along with political and economic considerations, the results of risk assessment are part of decision making about regulatory standards or policy actions to deal with hazards identified in the risk assessment.

3. In many ways, this is the latest expression of environmental health scientists' belief that toxicology is "not science for the sake of science, as are many other areas of research," but rather is "largely driven by issues that relate to safety of consumer products, occupational exposures, human exposure from substances in the environment, as well as the effects of chemicals on environmental species"(Schwetz, 2001).

4. Most regulatory scientists believe that this is a conservative practice and express confidence that it is successful in protecting susceptible individuals. However, such 10-fold factors are seen as arbitrary and burdensome by regulated industries (Interview P03), while environmental health advocates question whether they are truly protective (Interview P06).

5. Ironically and unfortunately, while "rat toxicology" has made significant contributions to protecting public health and safety, many scientists regard it as of lower status than "basic" research. As one scientist noted, "Toxicology needs to go beyond kill 'em and count 'em. But the other side of that is that this way has served the public well." (Interview 29).

6. For example, the Belmont Report, published in 1978 by the National Commission for the Protection of Human Subjects of Biomedical and Behavioral Research, states clearly that individuals should be treated as autonomous agents. Many of the criticisms leveled against principlism more broadly similarly are directed at the Belmont Report (Hedgecoe, 2004).

7. Now in its 5th edition, Beauchamp and Childress have "thoroughly revised" their classic text, taking into consideration the criticisms of their earlier work and the many developments in the field. Intent on presenting "a conception of autonomy that is not excessively individualistic ... not excessively focused on reason ..., and not unduly legalistic" (2001: p. 57), Beauchamp and Childress do offer a slightly more relational understanding of autonomy in the 2001 version. The chapter on autonomy in the 3rd edition contains a sub-section on "Autonomy and Authority"; in the 5th edition, this sub-section is revised and entitled "Autonomy, Authority, and Community." Despite the recent revision, the impact of the earlier editions of their work and the vast bioethical literature supporting their initial conception of autonomy can hardly be overlooked. While they may be repositioning their own work, their widespread influence on the field has left bioethics with a definition of subjectivity emphasizing reason and autonomy.

8. Gilligan (1982) proposes that there are two different approaches to ethics in our society: the ethic of justice and what she refers to as the ethic of care. An ethic of care prioritizes actual people, their context and situation specific details. Gilligan's study found that women are more likely to employ an ethic of care and men more likely to employ an ethic of justice. However, she also asserts that all moral agents should look to both types of ethics, as each can be appropriate in different situations.

9. Portions of this analysis began in conversations that one of the authors (SS) had with Dr. Richard R. Sharp, who was the director of the Program in Environmental Health Policy and Ethics (PEHPE) at the NIEHS during her PEHPE internship in 2002.

10. To be sure, this will require that scientists and biomedical practitioners find means of differentiating between adaptive, stochastic, and adverse effects; this is currently a priority of many scientists working on the application of genomic technologies to environmental health research.

11. For example, a study which gathered information from a computer-assisted analysis of census data, the civil court case docket of the EPA, and the agency's own record of performance at 1,177 Superfund sites came to the following conclusions: (1) Penalties under hazardous waste laws at sites having the greatest white population were about 500 percent higher than penalties at sites with the greatest minority population. Hazardous waste ... is the type of pollution most concentrated in minority communities; (2) For all the federal environmental laws aimed at protecting citizens from air, water, and waste pollution, penalties in white communities were 46 percent higher than in minority communities; (3) Under the Superfund clean-up program, abandoned hazardous waste sites in minority areas take 20 percent longer to be placed on the national priority action list than those in white areas; (4) In more than one half of the 10 autonomous regions that administer

EPA programs around the country, action on Superfund sites begins from 12 to 42 percent later at minority sites than at white sites; (5) At the minority sites, the EPA chooses "containment," the capping- or walling-off of a hazardous dump site, 7 percent more frequently than the clean-up method preferred under the law, that is, permanent "treatment," which eliminates the waste or rids it of its toxins. At white sites, the EPA orders treatment 22 percent more often than containment (Lavelle & Coyle, 1992, p. 137).

12. Already there are examples of studies of genetic susceptibility that report their findings in terms of genetic differences across sex/gender or "racial" groups. Environmental justice activists are particularly concerned about this research and the ways in which it is reported, interpreted, and utilized, as it seems to contain the potential for a re-emergence of scientized racism (Shostak, 2004).

13. Sharp and Barrett's (2000) discussion of the ELSI of environmental genomics does address broader issues of notions of responsibility for health and illness.

ACKNOWLEDGMENTS

We are grateful to the scientists, activists, and policy makers who chose to share their experiences, perspectives, and insights and without whose generosity this analysis would not have been possible. We thank Elizabeth Armstrong, Charles Bosk, Peter Conrad, and others for the incisive and constructive comments we received during the Sociology of Bioethics panel at the 2006 meeting of the American Sociological Association. Dr. Shostak gratefully acknowledges the support of the National Science Foundation (Award # 035381), the University of California Toxic Substances Research and Teaching Program, and the Robert Wood Johnson Health & Society Scholars Program at Columbia University.

REFERENCES

Abir-Am, P. (1985). Themes, genres, and orders of legitimation in the consolidation of new scientific disciplines. *History of Science, 23*, 73–117.

Anspach, R. (1993). *Deciding who lives: Fateful choices in the intensive care nursery*. Berkeley: University of California Press.

Anspach, R., & Beeson, D. (2001). Emotions in medical and moral life. In: B. Hoffmaster (Ed.), *Bioethics in a social context* (pp. 112–136). Philadelphia: Temple University Press.

Barad, K. (1998). Getting real: Technoscientific practices and the materialization of reality. *Differences: A Journal of Feminist Cultural Studies, 10*, 88–128.

Barad, K. (2003). Posthumanist performativity: Toward and understanding of how matter comes to matter. *Signs: Journal of Women in Culture and Society, 28*, 801–831.

Bartosiewicz, M., Penn, S., & Buckpitt, A. (2001a). Applications of gene arrays in environmental toxicology: Fingerprints of gene regulation associated with cadmium chloride, benzo(a)-pyrene, and trichloroethylene. *Environmental Health Perspectives, 109*, 71–74.

Bartosiewicz, M. J., Jenkins, D., Penn, S., Emery, J., & Buckpitt, A. (2001b). Unique gene expression patterns in liver and kidney associated with exposure to chemical toxicants. *Journal of Pharmacology and Experimental Therapeutics, 297*, 895–905.

Beauchamp, T., & Childress, J. (2001). *Principles in biomedical ethics.* Oxford: Oxford University Press.

Bosk, C. (1992). *All god's mistakes: Genetic counseling in a pediatric hospital.* Chicago: University of Chicago Press.

Bosk, C. (1999). Professional ethicist available: Logical, secular, friendly. *Daedalus, 128,* 47–68.

Brown, P. (1995). Race, class, and environmental health: A review and systematization of the literature. *Environmental Research, 69,* 15–30.

Calabrese, E. J. (1996). Biochemical individuality: The next generation. *Regulatory Toxicology and Pharmacology, 24,* S58–S67.

Callahan, D. (1973). Bioethics as a discipline. *Hastings Center Studies, 1,* 66–73.

Callahan, D. (1999). The social sciences and the task of bioethics. *Daedalus, 128,* 275–294.

Casper, M. (1998). *The making of the unborn patient: A social anatomy of fetal surgery.* New Brunswick, NJ: Rutgers University Press.

Chambliss, D. (1996). *Beyond caring: Hospitals, nurses, and the social organization of ethics.* Chicago: University of Chicago Press.

Christiani, D. (1996). Utilization of biomarker data for clinical and environmental intervention. *Environmental Health Perspectives,* 921–925.

Cussins, C. (1998). Ontological choreography: Agency for women patients in an infertility clinic. In: M. Berg & A. Mol (Eds), *Differences in medicine* (pp. 166–201). Durham, NC: Duke University Press.

de Chadarevian, S., & Kamminga, H. (1998). *Molecularizing biology and medicine: New practices and alliances, 1910s-1970s.* Amsterdam: Harwood Academic Publishers.

DeGrazia, D. (2005). *Human identity and bioethics.* Cambridge: Cambridge University Press.

DeVries, R., & Subedi, J. (Eds). (1998). *Bioethics and society: Constructing the ethical enterprise.* Upper Saddle River: Prentice Hall.

Draper, E. (1991). *Risky business: Genetic testing and exclusionary practices in the hazardous workplace.* Cambridge: Cambridge University Press.

DuBose, E. R., Hamel, R. P., & O'Connell, L. J. (Eds). (1994). *A matter of principles? Ferment in US bioethics.* Valley Forge: Trinity Press International.

Duster, T. (2003). *Backdoor to eugenics.* New York: Routledge.

Evans, J. E. (2002). *Playing god?: Human genetic engineering and the rationalization of public bioethical debate.* Chicago, IL: University of Chicago.

Franklin, S. (2000). Life itself: Global nature and the genetic imaginary. In: C. Lury, S. Franklin & J. Stacey (Eds), *Global nature, global culture* (pp. 188–277). London: Sage.

Frickel, S. (2004). *Chemical consequences: Environmental mutagens, scientist activism, and the rise of genetic toxicology.* New Brunswick, NJ: Rutgers University Press.

Gibbons, M., Limoges, C., Nowotny, H., et al. (1994). *The new production of knowledge: The dynamics of science and research in contemporary societies.* Thousand Oaks, CA: Sage.

Gilligan, C. (1982). *In a different voice: Psychological theory and women's moral development.* Cambridge: Harvard University Press.

Glaser, B. G., & Strauss, A. L. (1967). *The discovery of grounded theory.* Chicago, IL: Aldine.

Gottweiss, H. M. (1995). *Governing molecules: The discursive politics of genetic engineering in Europe and the United States Cambridge.* Massachusetts: MIT Press.

Haimes, E. (2002). What can the social sciences contribute to the study of ethics? Theoretical, empirical, and substantive considerations. *Bioethics, 16,* 89–113.

Hamadeh, H. K., Bushel, P. R., Jayadev, S., Martin, K., DiSorbo, O., et al. (2002a). Gene expression analysis reveals chemical specific profiles. *Toxicological Sciences, 67.*

Hamadeh, H. K., Bushel, P. R., Jayadev, S., DiSorbo, O., Bennet, L., et al. (2002b). Prediction of compound signature using high density gene expression profiling. *Toxicological Sciences, 67,* 232–240.

Hattis, D. (1996). Variability in susceptibility - how big, how often, for what responses to what agents? *Environmental Toxicology and Pharmacology, 2,* 135–145.

Hedgecoe, A. (2004). Critical bioethics: Beyond the social science critique of applied ethics. *Bioethics, 18,* 120–143.

Hedgecoe, A., & Martin, P. (2003). The drugs don't work: Expectations and the shaping of pharmacogenomics. *Social Studies of Science, 33,* 327–364.

Hemminki, K., Grzybowska, E., Widlak, P., & Chorazy, M. (1996). DNA Adducts in environmental, occupational, and life-style studies in human biomonitoring. *Acta Biochimica Polonica, 43,* 305–312.

Hoffmaster, B. (Ed.) (2001). *Bioethics in a social context.* Philadelphia: Temple University Press.

Jennings, B. (1998). Autonomy and difference: The travails of liberalism in bioethics. In: R. DeVries & J. Subedi (Eds), *Bioethics and society: Constructing the ethical enterprise* (pp. 258–269). Upper Saddle River, NJ: Prentice Hall.

Jonsen, A. (1998). *Birth of bioethics.* Oxford: Oxford University Press.

Jonsen, A., Siegler, M., & Winslade, W. (1998). *Clinical ethics: A practical approach to ethical decisions in clinical medicine.* New York: McGraw-Hill.

Jonsen, A., & Toulmin, S. (1988). *The abuse of casuistry: A history of moral reasoning.* Berkeley: University of California Press.

Kay, L. (1993). *The molecular vision of life: Caltech, the Rockefeller foundation and the new biology.* New York: Oxford University Press.

Latour, B. (1987). *Science in action: How to follow scientists and engineers through society.* Cambridge, MA: Harvard University Press.

Lavelle, M., & Coyle, M. (1992). Unequal protection: The racial divide in environmental law. *National Law Journal, 15,* S1–S12.

Lenoir, T. (1997). *Instituting science: The cultural production of scientific disciplines.* Stanford, CA: Stanford University Press.

Link, B., & Phelan, J. (1995). Social conditions as fundamental causes of disease. *Journal of Health and Social Behavior, 35.*

Lock, M. (2002). *Twice dead: Organ transplants and the reinvention of death.* Berkley, CA: University of California Press.

Martin, L. H., Gutman, H., & Hutton, P. H. (1988). *Technologies of the self: A seminar with Michel Foucault.* Amherst, MA: University of Massachusetts Press.

Messer-Davidow, E., Shumway, D. R., & Sylvan, D. J. (1993). *Knowledges: Historical and critical studies in disciplinarity.* Charlottesville, VA: University of Virginia.

Mohai, P., & Bryant, B. (1992). *Race and the incidence of environmental hazards.* Boulder, CO: Westview Press.

Montoya, M. (2003). *Genetics of inequality: Configurations of race and Mexican ethnicity in diabetes genetic epidemiology.* Ph.D dissertation, Department of Anthropology, Palo Alto: Stanford University.

National Institute of Environmental Health Sciences (NIEHS) (1997). A summary of the environmental genome project symposium. Presented at environmental genome project symposium, National Institutes of Health. Bethesda, MD.

National Research Council (NRC). (1983). *Risk assessment in the Federal Government: Managing the process.* Washington, DC: National Academy Press.

NCT/NIEHS. (2002). *Using global genomic expression technology to create a knowledge base for protecting human health*. Research Triangle Park, NC: National Institute of Environmental Health Sciences.

NIEHS. (2000a). Environmental Genome Project Overview.

NIEHS. (2000b). Toxicogenomics Research and Environmental Health Introduction.

Novas, C., & Rose, N. (2000). Genetic risk and the birth of the somatic individual. *Economy and Society, 29*, 485–513.

NTP. (2002). *Current directions and evolving strategies*. Washington, DC: Department of Health and Human Services.

Nuwaysir, E. F., Bittner, M., Barrett, J. C., & Afshari, C. A. (1999). Microarrays and toxicology: The advent of toxicogenomics. *Molecular Carcinogenesis, 241*, 153–159.

Olden, K. (2002). New opportunities in toxicology in the post-genomic era. *Drug Discovery Today, 7*, 273–276.

Olden, K., & Wilson, S. (2000). Environmental health and genomics: Visions and implications. *Nature Reviews Genetics, 1*, 149–153.

Omenn, G. S. (1991). Future research directions in cancer ecogenetics. *Mutation Research, 247*, 283–291.

Osborne, T. (1994). Sociology, liberalism and the historicity of conduct. *Economy and Society, 23*, 484–501.

Paules, R. S., Tennant, R. W., Barrett, J. C., & Lucier, G. W. (1999). Bringing genomics into risk analysis: The promises and problems. *Risk Policy Report, 17*, 30–33.

Pauly, P. J. (1987). *Controlling life: Jacques Loeb and the engineering ideal in biology*. New York, NY: Oxford University Press.

Perera, F. P. (1987). Cancer epidemiology: A new tool in cancer prevention. *Journal of the National Cancer Institute, 78*, 887–898.

Perera, F. P. (1997). Environment and cancer: Who are susceptible? *Science, 278*, 1068–1073.

Perera, F. P. (2000). Molecular epidemiology: On the path to prevention. *Journal of the National Cancer Institute, 92*, 602–612.

Pinderhughes, R. R. (1996). The impact of race on environmental quality: An empirical and theoretical discussion. *Sociological Perspectives, 39*, 231–248.

Rabinow, P., & Rose, N. (2003). Thoughts on the concept of biopower today. Presented at vital politics: Health, medicine and bioeconomics into the twenty first century. London School of Economics, 5-7 September 2003.

Rabinow, P. (1996). Artificiality and enlightenment: From sociobiology to biosociality. In: P. Rabinow (Ed.), *Essays on the anthropology of reason*. Princeton, NY: Princeton University Press.

Rapp, R. (1998). Refusing prenatal diagnosis: The meanings of bioscience in a multicultural world. *Science, Technology, and Human Values, 23*, 45–70.

Rapp, R. (1999). *Testing women, testing the fetus: The social impact of amniocentesis in America*. New York: Routledge.

Reardon, J. (2005). *Race to the finish: Identity and governance in an age of genomics*. Princeton, NJ: Princeton University Press.

Rose, N. (2001). The politics of life itself. *Theory, Culture, and Society, 18*, 1–30.

Rothman, D. (1991). *Strangers at the bedside: How law and bioethics transformed medical decision making*. New York: Basic Books.

Schneider, J. W., & Conrad, P. (1983). *Having epilepsy: The experience and control of illness.* Philadelphia, PA: Temple University Press.

Schwetz, B. A. (2001). Toxicology at the food and drug administration: New century, new challenges. *International Journal of Toxicology, 20,* 3–8.

Sellers, C. (1997). *Hazards of the job: From industrial disease to environmental health science.* Chapel Hill, NC: University of North Carolina Press.

Sharp, R. R. (2003). Ethical issues in environmental health research. *Environmental Health Perspectives, 111*(14), 1786–1788.

Sharp, R. R., & Barrett, C. J. (2000). The environmental genome project: Ethical, legal, and social implications. *Environmental Health Perspectives, 108,* 279–281.

Sherwin, S. (1992). *No longer patient: Feminist ethics and health care.* Philadelphia: Temple University Press.

Shostak, S. (2004). Environmental justice and genomics: Acting on the futures of environmental health. *Science as Culture, 13,* 539–562.

Shostak, S. (2005). The emergence of toxicogenomics: A case study of molecularization. *Social Studies of Science, 35,* 367–403.

Simmons, P. T., & Portier, C. J. (2002). Toxicogenomics: The new frontier in risk analysis. *Carcinogenesis, 23,* 903–905.

Smith, E. (1996). Variability in toxic response - relevance to chemical safety and risk assessment at the global level. *Environmental Toxicology and Pharmacology, 2,* 85–88.

Strauss, A. L. (1987). *Qualitative analysis for social scientists.* New York: Cambridge University Press.

Strauss, A. L., & Corbin, J. (1990/1998). *Basics of qualitative research.* Newbury Park, CA: Sage.

Suchman, L. (in press). Agencies for technology design: Feminist reconfigurations. In Londa Schiebinger (Ed.), *Gendered Innovations in Science and Engineering.* Palo Alto, CA: Stanford University Press.

Tauber, A. I. (2001). Historical and philosophical reflections on patient autonomy. *Health Care Analysis, 9,* 299–319.

Toulmin, S. (1981). Tyranny of principles. *Hastings Center Report, 11,* 31–39.

UCC. (1987). Toxic wastes and race in the United States: A national report on the racial and socio-economic characteristics of communities with hazardous waste sites. Commission for Racial Justice, United Church of Christ.

Wolf, S. (1996). *Feminism and bioethics: Beyond reproduction.* Oxford: Oxford University Press.

Wolpe, P. R. (1998). The triumph of autonomy in bioethics: A sociological view. In: R. DeVries & J. Subedi (Eds), *Bioethics and society: Constructing the ethical enterprise.* Upper Saddle River, NJ: Prentice Hall.

Zussman, R. (1997). Sociological perspectives on medical ethics and decision-making. *Annual Review of Sociology, 23,* 171–189.

SET UP A CONTINUATION ORDER TODAY!

Did you know that you can set up a continuation order on all Elsevier-JAI series and have each new volume sent directly to you upon publication? For details on how to set up a **continuation order**, contact your nearest regional sales office listed below.

To view related series in Sociology, please visit:

www.elsevier.com/sociology

The Americas
Customer Service Department
11830 Westline Industrial Drive
St. Louis, MO 63146
USA
US customers:
Tel: +1 800 545 2522 (Toll-free number)
Fax: +1 800 535 9935
For Customers outside US:
Tel: +1 800 460 3110 (Toll-free number).
Fax: +1 314 453 7095
usbkinfo@elsevier.com

Europe, Middle East & Africa
Customer Service Department
Linacre House
Jordan Hill
Oxford OX2 8DP
UK
Tel: +44 (0) 1865 474140
Fax: +44 (0) 1865 474141
eurobkinfo@elsevier.com

Japan
Customer Service Department
2F Higashi Azabu, 1 Chome Bldg
1-9-15 Higashi Azabu, Minato-ku
Tokyo 106-0044
Japan
Tel: +81 3 3589 6370
Fax: +81 3 3589 6371
books@elsevierjapan.com

APAC
Customer Service Department
3 Killiney Road #08-01
Winsland House I
Singapore 239519
Tel: +65 6349 0222
Fax: +65 6733 1510
asiainfo@elsevier.com

Australia & New Zealand
Customer Service Department
30-52 Smidmore Street
Marrickville, New South Wales 2204
Australia
Tel: +61 (02) 9517 8999
Fax: +61 (02) 9517 2249
service@elsevier.com.au

30% Discount for Authors on All Books!

A 30% discount is available to Elsevier book and journal contributors on all books *(except multi-volume reference works)*.

To claim your discount, full payment is required with your order, which must be sent directly to the publisher at the nearest regional sales office above.